CONTENTS

PREFACE

Some years ago I was invited to give a lecture at a conference organized by a food allergy support group in Ontario, Canada. As I made my way to the lecture theatre, I was confronted by a distressingly macabre scene: emergency health professionals in full uniform with ambulance stretchers and hospital gurneys and displays of resuscitation equipment complete with face masks, IV tubing, oxygen cylinders, and syringes ready for injections. Of course, such a scenario is not unusual when a patient is at risk of anaphylactic shock. However, as an exhibit, the message was too stark and frightening for a conference on food allergy in children.

Unfortunately, the exhibit set the tone for the whole meeting. Hair-raising stories of fatal and near-fatal anaphylactic reactions, frantic emergency calls, and terrifying races to the hospital by car and ambulance were recounted with relish. The attendees were, for the most part, parents whose children had been diagnosed with food allergy. Those new to the allergy scene were clearly distressed and upset. It is always important for anyone associated with food allergy, especially parents and care-givers of atopic infants and children, to be aware of all the potential dangers. But, to present the rare threat of anaphylaxis in such frightening and uncompromising terms amounts to quite unnecessary fear-mongering. Anaphylactic resuscitation is rarely required in the day-to-day management of food allergy. To generate such fear and anxiety at the outset of a conference designed to equip parents to handle food allergy in their children has the potential to jeopardize the well-being of not only the atopic child but also the whole family and the family's support network. A story from my years as head of the Allergy Nutrition Program at Vancouver Hospital and Health Sciences Centre in British Columbia illustrates this well.

Jason[a] was a 14-year-old boy. He was referred to the Allergy Nutrition Clinic by his family doctor who was becoming concerned about his growth

[a] Name has been changed

and development. Jason was an only child and came into the Clinic with his mother and father. His mother was a nurse and his father worked in retail sales. Jason appeared much smaller than would be expected for his age even though both parents were of normal height and stature. He was pale and fragile-looking and wore a baseball cap that hid his thin, sparse hair. His mother told his story.

Jason had been a colicky baby and had developed eczema at about two months of age. At six months his mother had consulted an allergist who performed skin tests for food allergy. The parents were informed that the skin tests were "positive to everything." A list of foods that Jason must avoid was provided by the allergist. Faithfully, the mother had eliminated all of the "allergy foods," and Jason had never eaten any of them. His diet consisted of about eight foods that were not on the allergist's "avoid list." Jason had consumed only these foods since the age of six months. He had been given no nutritional supplements because his mother did not think they were "safe." Jason added his own story. He felt very unhappy in school. He was teased by the other children because of his sparse hair and his small size, which was more typical of a 9-year-old than a boy in his early teens. Jason's father said little throughout the interview but made it clear that he felt his wife was "overprotective" of the child. Nevertheless, he thought that because his wife was a nurse she was entitled by her training to be in charge of Jason's health. The father was obviously unhappy about his child's situation but felt powerless to intervene in any way.

It was clear to me that Jason needed to start eating a much wider range of foods than he was presently consuming. His small size, fragile appearance, and obvious lack of development were unmistakable indicators that multiple nutritional deficiencies were very real risk factors for his health and well-being.

We arranged for Jason to undergo challenge tests, starting with small amounts of individual foods and monitoring his reactions in a safe environment. I waited to hear the outcome, hoping for some encouraging news about his progress. Two weeks later, Jason and his mother came into the office; both were noticeably ill-at-ease. Apparently, the challenge test had been cancelled. No new foods had been introduced. Gradually, the sad story unfolded. Prior to the day scheduled for the first trial, Jason became extremely anxious and upset. He had become nauseated, vomited continuously, and was unable to sleep. Apparently, he was convinced that he was going to die as a result of eating the "bad foods" and was so frightened that it would have been impossible for him to proceed with the food challenge test plan.

The father refused to take any further part in the process. He disagreed with his wife's handling of Jason's diet and felt she was over-protective of the boy to the point of obsession. The father had felt optimistic about the original plan for introducing new foods into the boy's diet but was defeated when he was again faced with the fears of his wife and son. The father was distressed by the outcome of the proposed management strategy. He later left the family and the parents subsequently divorced.

These two scenarios represent extreme examples of the fears and stresses that a diagnosis of food allergy can impose on individuals and families. But the stories are representative of the anxiety and uncertainties that people experience when faced with the challenge of managing food allergies, especially in the infants and children who are so utterly dependent on them for their well-being and survival. Sometimes the responsibility seems overwhelming. When presented in such graphic terms as the first example, food allergy appears to be a loaded gun, primed and ready to end the life of an innocent child. However, a loaded gun has to be aimed and fired in order to pose a threat and even the family car can be an instrument of destruction. So, let us be realistic as well as responsible. *Be careful—not fearful*—and all will be well.

My message to those caring for an allergic child is simple. A diagnosis of food allergy is not a sentence of death; it is merely a signal that special caution and knowledge is required in the feeding of the precious life that has been entrusted to your care. This book has been written to provide the knowledge you need to care for you child with food allergies.

INTRODUCTION

A baby with food allergies is clearly suffering and the baby's distress frequently persists despite the best efforts of parents and care-givers to provide relief. This so often leads to enormous stress for everyone involved, especially for first-time parents who are not only faced with the challenges associated with adjusting to this seemingly fragile and needy little person who is completely dependent on their care but who also have to cope with demands over and above the expected nourish, clean, and cuddle that satisfies most babies (or so they are led to believe!).

Sleepless nights and the inability to console a new baby cause a great deal of stress for everyone. Studies on infants with colic, which may often accompany food allergy, show that their mothers tend to be more concerned about their infants' temperament, and even to feel rejection, compared with mothers with infants without colic.[1] Even more distressing is the finding that mothers seem to be less responsive to and interact less with infants they feel are "difficult" at 3 months old. Strong negative emotions are still evident when these infants are 8 months old. Further, the associated feelings of guilt and inadequacy may last long after the child's infancy.

If the baby with food allergy can be recognized early, there is a great deal that parents and care-givers can do to relieve the baby's distress. These steps often completely avoid the negative consequences of failing to console a suffering infant. I have lost count of the number of mothers who have passed through my practice who have expressed their immeasurable happiness when, after recognizing and avoiding the offending foods, they are rewarded with a calm and contented baby. These mothers battled with a "screaming tyrant" (their words) for far too long. Observing their obvious joy in bonding with their happy baby is a gift that I cherish every time I see it happen.

Food allergy in older children can cause even greater distress both for the child and their family. The child who is ostracized by his or her peers as a result of the unsightly skin of eczema is at risk of emotional scars that can persist long after the discomfort of the condition has been outgrown. A child who is unable to sleep as a result of the pain and distress of the symptoms of food allergy is often unable to function well during the day; they may suffer the consequences of poor school performance and related behavioral problems. An inability to join in childhood activities may cause distancing from peers, with the result that the allergic child's social interactions are impaired for many years. The well-meaning family members who are doing their best to protect a potentially anaphylactic child from exposure to their food allergens can unwittingly compound the problems of social isolation, adding unnecessary fear and uncertainty on top of the burden of coping with the stressful symptoms of food allergy.

Some interesting studies, using health-related quality of life (HRQL) evaluation questionnaires, have revealed surprising information. Contrary to the prevailing assumptions, it is the fear of allergic reactions and the measures taken to avoid them, rather than the symptoms of allergy, that cause the greatest distress among food-allergic children and their families. In one study, more than half (55 percent) of the children had not experienced any food reactions in the past 12 months. Still, all the children were reported to have lower psychosocial HRQL than the general population.[2]

It is very important for you to realize that most of these negative consequences can be reduced—or completely avoided—with knowledge, understanding, and the careful management of your child's food intake.

FOOD ALLERGY IN CHILDHOOD

Childhood is the period of life when allergies to food are most prevalent. Food allergy is much more common in babies and young children than in adults. Most food allergies are outgrown by the age of five years. Food allergy in adults is relatively uncommon. Estimates of food allergy in adults indicate an incidence of less than 2 percent. However, intolerance of food components, naturally occurring chemicals, and food additives is a frequent experience, and some practitioners estimate the incidence of these conditions as high as 50 percent of the adult population. Food allergy is a response of the immune system; a food intolerance can be broadly defined as a sensitivity mechanism that does not involve the immune system. Food intolerance is usually due to a physiological reaction such as an enzyme deficiency. We shall talk about the differences between food allergy and food intolerance later in this book.

Incidence of Food Allergy in Childhood

It is difficult to determine exactly how many babies and children are sensitive to foods and suffer symptoms as a result of eating or drinking. There is no single reliable laboratory test that can prove that a child is allergic or intolerant to a specific food or food additive. This makes estimating how frequently such reactions occur very difficult. Because there are so many different immunological and nonimmunological reactions involved in food sensitivity symptoms, it would be unrealistic to expect that a laboratory test alone could identify them all. In the end, the only accurate way to determine a child's reactivity to a food, drink, or food additive is elimination and challenge, and this process is too expensive and time-consuming to be a routine procedure.

However, based on the statistics that are available, it is usually estimated that food allergy occurs in up to 8 percent of children under the age of five years, and that 2 percent of children in this age group have an allergic reaction to cow's milk proteins. Based on specific studies, 4 to 6 percent of children had documented food allergy.[3] The overall incidence of cow's milk allergy ranged from 1.9 to 7.5 percent in different populations.[4] Other reports suggest the incidence of food allergy in childhood to be up to 8 percent and "food-related complaints" to afflict as many as 28 percent of children.[5]

An Australian study[6] indicated that at the age of two years, egg was the most frequent food allergen (3.2 percent), while cow's milk (2.0 percent) and peanut (1.9 percent) were fairly equal in frequency. Allergy to wheat, soy, sesame seed, cashew nuts, hazelnuts, and walnuts was less frequent and about equal in prevalence. Allergies to fish, Brazil nuts, and shell fish were quite uncommon. In Asian countries the reported frequency was remarkably similar to that in Australia, except allergy to seafood was more common than for nuts, peanuts, and wheat, if seafoods were a regular part of the infant's diet. Rice hypersensitivity was rare in Australia and in Asian countries.

Progress of Food Allergy in Children

Early infancy is a particularly critical time because the baby might be at maximum risk of being sensitized to allergens. From birth to about two years of age, the baby's immune system is relatively immature and the layer of cells lining the digestive tract (known as the gastrointestinal epithelium) may be more permeable than in the mature human. From the age of two years onward, children appear to outgrow their early food allergies. Based on research in animals, it is thought that tolerance to foods develops as the immune system matures and the lining of the digestive tract changes so that food molecules of the size required for an allergic reaction to occur cannot pass through the digestive tract tissues (the epithelium becomes less permeable).

Many experts believe that if a baby can be protected from becoming sensitized to the most highly allergenic foods when the immune system and the digestive tract are in the most vulnerable stage for allergy to develop, the incidence of lifelong food allergy and potentially life-threatening anaphylactic reactions to foods will be reduced and hopefully entirely prevented. When a baby has been identified to be at risk for developing allergy, measures to reduce allergic sensitization might be implemented at birth and the problems associated with future food allergy may be significantly reduced. However, as we shall see in later discussions, experts disagree on the best way to avoid this early allergic sensitization.

Nutrition for the Allergic Child

The most important aspect of managing food allergy in babies and children is to be sure that the developing child has each and every nutrient that is essential for its optimum growth and development. Deficiency in a critical nutrient in the early days can have enormous negative consequences that can, in some instances, last a lifetime. The words of a British group of practitioners eloquently express this most important aspect of infant feeding:

> "Few other aspects of food supply and metabolism are of greater biological importance than the feeding of mothers during pregnancy and lactation, and of their infants and young children. Nutritional factors during early development not only have short-term effects on growth, body composition and body functions but also exert long-term effects on health, disease and mortality risks in adulthood, as well as development of neural functions and behavior, a phenomenon called "metabolic programming.""[7]

In the diligent search for and avoidance of the foods that cause the distressing symptoms of allergy, no one must forget that every nutrient that is eliminated as a result of its being part of allergenic food must be replaced by an equal amount of the nutrient from an alternative source. Information about the nutrients that may be deficient when some important foods are eliminated and the sources of these nutrients in alternative foods is provided in Appendix E.

The management of an allergic child's diet is not achieved without some effort. It takes time, knowledge, and skill. However, all these things can be learned; it is truly not a demanding process. Once you have understood the underlying concepts of food allergy management, you will be surprised how easy and gratifying it can be to provide a safe, healthy, and enjoyable eating plan for your child and the whole family.

Foods That Cause Food Sensitivity Reactions

In theory, any food is able to trigger an allergic reaction. All foods contain molecules capable of triggering a response of the immune system. However, for many reasons—including both the structure of the food molecules and a child's immunological responses—the foods that cause the majority of allergic reactions tend to be few in number.

Although people often look for the ideal "hypoallergenic diet," and often hear about the latest "allergy diet" from popular publications and zealous friends, such a thing does not exist. What is "hypoallergenic" for one child could be life-threatening for another. Each person is an individual. Inherited tendencies, medical history, family lifestyle, and response to both food and nonfood factors (such as airborne and environmental allergens) will all contribute to the way in which one child's body reacts to the "foreign" foods and chemicals that enter it.

There is no reason that any baby, child, or family should suffer as a consequence of food allergy. However, the management of the condition does require understanding and patience. This book provides information and guidelines that can help you meet the challenge of providing relief for both you and your allergic child.

References

1   Rogovik AL, Goldman RD. Treating infants' colic. *Canadian Family Physician* 2005; 51(9):1209–1211.

2   Marklund B, Ahlstedt S, Nordstrom G. Health-related quality of life in food hypersensitive schoolchildren and their families: parents' perceptions. *Health and Quality of Life Outcomes* 2006; 4:48.

3   Zeigler RS. Food allergen avoidance in the prevention of food allergy in infants and children. *Pediatrics* 2003; 111:1662–1671.

4   Jarvinen KM, Suomalainen H. Development of cow's milk allergy in breast-fed infants. *Clinical and Experimental Allergy* 2001; 31:978–987.

5   Bock SA. Prospective appraisal of complaints of adverse reactions to foods in children during the first 3 years of life. *Pediatrics* 1987; 79:683.

6   Hill DJ, Hosking CS, Ahie CY, Leung R, Baratwidjaja K, Iikura Y, Iyngkaran N, Gonzalez-Andaya A, Wah LB, Hsieh KH. The frequency of food allergy in Australia and Asia. *Environmental Toxicology and Pharmacology* 1997; 4(1–2):101–110.

7   Koletko B, Agget PJ, Bindels JG, Bung P, Ferre P, Gil A, Lentz MJ, Robefroid M, Strobel S. Growth, development and differentiation: a functional science approach. *British Journal of Nutrition* 1998; 80(Suppl 1):S6–S45.

*Dedicated to my own children, Sunil and Nalini,
with whom I learned so much about food allergies,
and who continue to inspire me to look further
and search deeper for answers.*

*I also dedicate this book to all parents
and care-givers of allergic babies and children.*

DISCLAIMER

The information provided here is as up-to-date, accurate, and as practical as possible in a field that is moving very quickly and is full of controversy. However, we cannot guarantee or warrant the quality, accuracy, completeness, timeliness, appropriateness or suitability of the information provided. This book is not intended to provide specific medical advice, but rather is intended to provide users with information to better understand their health. You should not use the content of this book for diagnosing or treating a medical or health condition, and reliance on the content of this book is solely at your own risk.

Any information and advice in this book is not meant to take the place of that provided by a medical practitioner. If you have or suspect that you may have a medical problem, you should contact your professional healthcare provider. Any strategies suggested in this book should be discussed with and managed by a suitably qualified physician, and implementation should be supervised by a registered dietitian/nutritionist for maximum benefit. Never disregard medical advice or avoid seeking it because of something that you have read in this book.

The author and publisher disclaim any responsibility for any adverse consequences resulting from the use of drugs, foods, diets, or procedures mentioned in this book.

Food lists are never exhaustive. There will always be omissions and modifications. Manufactured products and their ingredients are constantly changing. Those listed in this book. although current at the time of publication, may not be up-to-date when accessed by the consumer. The reader should apply to the manufacturer to confirm all such listings.

Trade names of foods, drugs, medical devices, and other products are used only as examples. The trade names given are not meant as a complete list of those available or as recommendations of any particular product(s).

CHAPTER 1

What Is Food Allergy?

THE SIMPLE EXPLANATION

A simple explanation of food allergy is that it is an inappropriate response by the immune system that results in symptoms. Our immune systems keep us free from disease by recognizing a "foreign invader" when it enters the body and by releasing in response a battery of defensive chemicals (called "inflammatory mediators") into local tissues and into the circulatory system. All the food we eat comes from foreign sources—plants and animals—that we consume as nourishment. Normally our immune systems see this material as "foreign but safe" due to a complex process of tolerance that occurs when food is processed through the digestive system. When something goes wrong during this processing, a person becomes "sensitized" to the food, and thereafter the immune system perceives it as foreign and a threat. Whenever that food enters the body again, the immune system treats it as if it could cause disease. The symptoms that we experience as a result of this defensive action are called allergy.

Unlike allergy, *food intolerance* does not involve a response of the immune system. The chemicals released in the immune response are not involved in an intolerance reaction. Most intolerance reactions that we understand (and there are many that we do not!) involve a defect in the processing of the food, either during digestion, or later, after the food parts, or components, have been absorbed into the body. The symptoms of food intolerance are often caused by an excess of a component that has not been digested completely (for example, lactose intolerance) or a component that, for some reason, cannot be processed efficiently after it has entered the body.

Whatever the mechanism that causes the symptoms, in the final analysis the only way to avoid distress is to avoid the foods that trigger the response. The first stage in avoidance, of course, is the correct identification of the foods and food components that are the triggers for the adverse reactions.

These are the simple "bare bones" explanations for the ways in which our bodies react to foods when we experience food allergies or intolerances. However, these processes are complex and diverse. If you want a more detailed, scientific explanation of the mechanisms leading to food allergy and food intolerance, please read on.

This chapter explains food allergy; the rest of the book discusses how this knowledge applies to your child. Understanding these processes will take some time and effort for the "nonscientist," but it will ultimately be worthwhile. You will not only understand and appreciate how your child's body functions when he or she is experiencing the distressing symptoms of an allergic reaction, but you will also understand what you can do, with the help of your pediatrician, dietitian, and other health care providers, to prevent or alleviate these symptoms at various stages in your child's development. Furthermore, this chapter will help you to understand and evaluate information on allergy that you find in other sources.

THE BASICS OF ALLERGY

The symptoms of an allergic reaction are caused by biologically active chemicals produced by the immune system in its attempt to protect the body from a foreign invader. Our immune systems are designed to protect us from anything that might cause disease. Usually this is a microorganism such as a virus, bacterium, or other pathogen. However, the immune system of an allergic (atopic) person attempts to protect the body not only from potential pathogens but also from harmless substances such as pollens, animal dander, dust mites, mold spores, and food.

What is it that causes the immune system of one individual to fight a harmless substance, while another's system recognizes the same materials as innocuous? Although we do not know the entire answer to this question, research is starting to reveal parts of the puzzle. The difference lies right at the beginning of the process of recognition of what is safe and what may be harmful to the body.

First, it is important for you to understand that food itself is incapable of causing any disease in the way that viruses, bacteria, and cancer cells can. There are no "bad foods"! It is the body's response to components of the food that results in the miserable symptoms we call *food allergy, food intolerance, food sensitivity*, or *adverse reactions to foods*. The reason that one child's body responds to food by developing distressing symptoms, and that another's uses the same food for comfort and nurture, may be found in several factors:

- The child's inherited genetic makeup

- The circumstances under which the child first encountered the food

- The microorganisms that live within a child's digestive tract

- The medications the child may have taken by mouth or been exposed to, for example, in mother's breast milk

- Other factors that we are only just beginning to (often incompletely) understand

Food sensitivity is unlike any other disease entity. It has many different causes, since *any* food is capable of triggering an allergic reaction in a child who has been sensitized to it, or who lacks the systems required to process it adequately when it enters the body. The same food may be absolutely safe for other children. Furthermore, food allergy can result in many different symptoms in diverse organ systems. For example, one child may develop symptoms in the skin, such as eczema or hives; another may have symptoms in the digestive tract, such as stomachache, diarrhea, nausea, or vomiting; yet another develops symptoms in the lungs, such as asthma; or the upper respiratory tract, with a stuffy, runny nose; or earache; or all body systems at the same time (anaphylaxis). All this may occur as a result of eating the *same* food, such as peanuts or shellfish for example. Each allergic child differs in the way his or her immune system responds to food and which foods it responds to.

The usual medical model of disease that your doctor traditionally follows has several distinct steps that lead from symptoms to therapy:

- The symptoms ("presentation") suggest several possibilities as to their cause.

- Tests are carried out that will lead to a diagnosis.

- The diagnosis arrived at as a result of the tests determines the treatment.

- Treatment usually consists of medications and/or surgery.

- As a result of treatment (therapy) the symptoms are alleviated.

This protocol works extremely well for conditions that are caused by a single entity such as a bacterium, virus, cancer, injury, or other agents that cause harm to the body. It does not work well for food allergy, where there are many different agents responsible for triggering a response of the immune system, which results in a diverse array of symptoms that differ from person to person, and even within the same person at different times.

What this means in practice is that, because there are a number of different processes that can occur when body systems deal with the diverse chemicals that make up a food, it would be unrealistic to expect that the specific food responsible for triggering the body's adverse reaction could be identified by any single laboratory test. Consequently, even a clear definition of the term "food allergy" using symptoms, causative factors, physiological processes, or diagnostic tests (which are the usual ways we define a disease) has always eluded clinicians and scientists.

In the popular literature it has become convenient for all adverse reactions that result from eating to be labeled "food allergy," but in medical and scientific fields, there are several defined conditions within this broad category that indicate the probable mechanism of the reaction that is taking place within the body. These defined conditions help in determining the possible cause of the symptoms, predicting the probable severity and duration of the reaction, and suggesting the most appropriate treatment.

Definition of Food Allergy Terms

It will be helpful for you to have some understanding of the terms that are currently being used by practitioners in the field of allergy so that you can understand the medical literature as you search for information on your child's allergy. Understanding the terms will also pave the way for our discussion of why your child has allergies and what is happening in his or her body when an allergic reaction is occurring.

The most recent attempt at a definition of adverse reactions to foods from the European Academy of Allergy and Clinical Immunology in 2001[1] includes the following:

- *Allergy* is a hypersensitivity reaction initiated by immunologic mechanisms.

- An adverse reaction to food should be called *food hypersensitivity*.
  - When immunologic mechanisms have been demonstrated, the appropriate term is *food allergy*.
  - If the role of IgE is highlighted, the correct term is *IgE-mediated food allergy*. [We shall discuss IgE and other antibodies later in this chapter.]
  - All other reactions, previously sometimes referred to as "food intolerance," should be referred to as nonallergic food hypersensitivity.

- Severe, generalized allergic reactions to food can be classified as *anaphylaxis*.

- Anaphylaxis is a severe, life-threatening, generalized or systemic hypersensitivity reaction.

- *Atopy* is a personal or familial tendency to produce IgE antibodies in response to low doses of allergens, usually proteins, and to develop typical symptoms such as asthma, hay fever (rhiniconjunctivitis) or eczema/dermatitis.

Previously, the American Academy of Allergy and Clinical Immunology (AAACI) and the National Institute of Allergy and Infectious Disease (National Institutes of Health (NIH))[2] defined the diverse terms in use thus:

- An *adverse food reaction* is a generic term referring to any untoward reaction after the ingestion of a food.

- Adverse food reactions can be
  - Food allergy.
  - Food intolerance.

- A *food allergy* is the result of an abnormal immunologic response after ingestion of a food.

- A *food intolerance* is the result of nonimmunological mechanisms.

In spite of (or more likely, because of) these seemingly precise, but some-times conflicting academic definitions, authors of research papers and articles on food allergy now frequently define their own use of the terms in any pub-lished work so that the reader is quite clear about their meaning in that spe-cific context. In accordance with this sensible practice, I will do likewise (see Table 1-1). I have used the 1984 definition of the AAACI/NIH in all my pre-vious publications and still find this the least confusing; I will continue that practice here. The terms *anaphylaxis* and *atopy* I use in the way they are defined by the EAACI.

Table 1-1
DEFINITION OF TERMS AS USED IN THIS BOOK

- An *adverse food reaction* and *food sensitivity* are generic terms referring to any troublesome reaction after the ingestion of a food.

- Adverse food reactions can be
  - Food allergy.
  - Food intolerance.

- A *food allergy* is the result of an abnormal immunologic response after ingestion of a food.

- Immunological *hypersensitivity* is the same as allergy.

- A *food intolerance* is the result of nonimmunological mechanisms.

- *Anaphylaxis* is a severe, life-threatening, generalized (systemic) allergy or hypersensitivity reaction.

- *Atopy* is a term used to indicate IgE-mediated allergy.

Now that you understand what each of the terms means, we can go on to discuss the subject much more easily. If you want to refresh your memory until the terminology becomes quite familiar to you, please look at the Glossary (page 511). We can start with a discussion of what happens in the body when an allergic reaction takes place.

The Immunological Process in an Allergic Reaction

When an allergen enters the body of a person at risk for allergy, an extremely complex series of events is set in motion that will finally result in the release of chemicals (called inflammatory mediators) that act on body tissues to cause the symptoms of allergy. All immunological processes involve the various white blood cells (leukocytes), and the different types of chemicals they produce. For a more detailed description of the immunological process of allergy, you may wish to read Chapter 3 in the companion book in this series.[3]

The first stage of the immunological response involves recognition of the invading *antigen*. An antigen is a protein within the cells of any living (or previously living) material that enters the body causing the immune system to react to it. All foods contain numerous antigens. When the antigen causes an immune response that results in allergy, we call it an *allergen*. Not all foreign proteins (antigens) cause allergy, and therefore not all antigens are allergens. On the other hand, all allergens are antigens.

When an antigen enters the body, the white blood cells called *lymphocytes* are activated. Lymphocytes are the first cells of the immune system that recognize and respond to anything foreign entering the body. We can visualize them as the sentinels of the immune system. There are two different types of lymphocytes in blood: T cells and B cells. T-cell lymphocytes are the ultimate "gatekeepers" and controllers of the immune system. We will discuss B cells later in this chapter.

T-cell Lymphocytes Detect a Foreign Invader

Certain types of T cells, called *helper T cells* (Th cells), are responsible for identifying foreign materials that enter the body through any route, such as the mouth, nose, and skin. Th cells initiate and direct the subsequent activities of the immune system if the foreign material is deemed a threat to the health of the body. T cells exert their control of the whole immune response by means of a number of different types of "messenger chemicals" called *cytokines*. The responses of helper T cells in allergic and nonallergic individuals are different. The two types of responses have been designated Th2 and Th1 response, respectively (see Figure 1-1). Different cytokines are released in each response, and they control the way in which the body reacts to the foreign material.

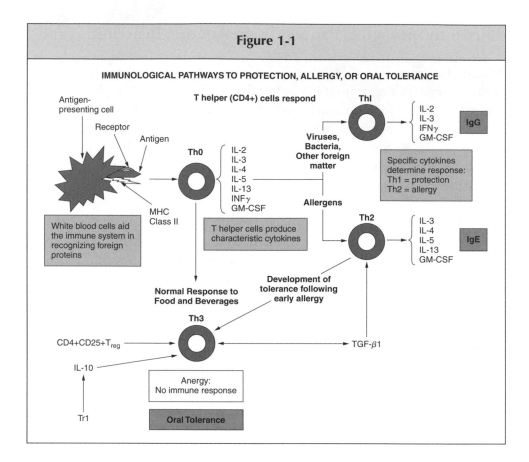

Figure 1-1

IMMUNOLOGICAL PATHWAYS TO PROTECTION, ALLERGY, OR ORAL TOLERANCE

Cytokines Direct the Immune Response

When a pathogen (disease-causing microorganism) enters, the immune system protects the body by a Th1 response. Cytokines such as interleukin 1 (IL-1), interleukin 2 (IL-2), interferon-gamma (INF-γ), and others are produced. They stimulate the formation of antibodies of the IgG class, which eventually destroy the invading microorganism by means of a complex series of events known as the complement cascade.[a] Symptoms such as fever, aching

---

[a] *Complement* is a group of over 20 enzymatic proteins in the blood that act together, in response to antigen and antibody, to destroy foreign cells by splitting them apart (*lysis*). This process is known as the *complement cascade*, which releases various chemical byproducts that act as opsonins, chemotaxins, and anaphylatoxins to help destroy a threat to the body and results in inflammation in various tissues.

muscles, fatigue, and general malaise (typical of an infection such as flu) are the result of the body's response to cytokines and other inflammatory mediators produced during this battle between the immune system and the foreign invader.

In an allergic reaction, a similar battle is engaged, but this time it is between the immune system and a nonthreatening invader such as a food. In this case, the Th2 cytokines control the immune response. Instead of the IL-2, INF-γ, and similar cytokines of the Th1 response, an entirely different set of cytokines is produced. Interleukins 4, 5, 6, and 13 (IL-4, IL-5, IL-6, and IL-13) are typical of the Th2 response, and result in production of antibodies of the IgE type. (We discuss the different types of antibodies and their functions later on in this chapter.) Unlike IgG, IgE antibodies do not trigger the complement cascade. Instead, they initiate a series of reactions that result in the release of inflammatory mediators (such as histamine) and other reactive chemicals from specialized cells called *mast cells*. The inflammatory mediators act on body tissues and produce the itching, swelling, reddening (flushing), and smooth muscle contraction (such as the bronchospasm of asthma) that are typical of allergy.[4]

Simply stated,

- The Th1 response protects the body from disease, and the IgG antibodies are responsible for the ultimate destruction of the invader.

- The Th2 response results in allergy, and IgE antibodies are responsible for the release of inflammatory mediators that cause the symptoms of allergy.

The next question of course, is why does one individual experience a Th2 response while another does not?

Allergy Is an Inherited Characteristic

There is strong evidence that the potential to develop allergy is an inherited characteristic. The incidence of allergy in children of allergic parents is significantly greater than in children of nonallergic parents (nonatopics). Family history is the most important indicator that a child is likely to develop allergy and is the factor that is most frequently taken into consideration when preventive measures are being considered. It is probable that the characteristic that is inherited is the potential to respond with a Th2 response when harmless foreign materials enter the body. Some researchers have suggested that the Th2 is a more primitive response than the Th1 and that, as a baby matures, the potential for the immune system to respond with a Th2 response is gradually diminished. This decline, together with maturation of the digestive tract (which provides a barrier between food molecules and the immune cells that could respond to them) would explain why children usually outgrow their early food allergies.

Sensitization to Allergens

Early infancy is a particularly critical time when the baby might be at maximum risk of being sensitized to allergens. From birth to about two years of age, the baby's immune system is relatively immature. During this period the baby with an inherited potential to develop allergy is likely to respond to a foreign protein with the Th2 response that results in allergy. As the immune system matures, the chance of a Th2 response is significantly reduced. In addition, the lining of the digestive tract changes and becomes less permeable to food molecules of the size required for an allergic reaction to occur. From the age of two years onward, most children start to outgrow their early food allergies. Many experts believe that, if the baby can be protected from exposure to the most highly allergenic foods during the period in which the immune system and the digestive tract are in the most vulnerable state for allergy to develop, the incidence of lifelong food allergy and potentially life-threatening anaphylactic reactions to foods will be reduced and, hopefully, prevented.

The last trimester of pregnancy, the newborn (neonatal) period, and the first few months of life have been cited as critical periods for allergic sensitization. Many authorities suggest that if exposure to the most highly allergenic foods can be avoided during these periods, the likelihood of the baby's becoming allergic to these foods may be considerably reduced, or entirely prevented. This is further discussed in Chapter 3, Prevention of Food Allergy.

On the other hand, recent research suggests that this same time period in a baby's life might be a critical stage during which *tolerance* to foods occurs. The idea of immunological tolerance is a fairly new concept in food allergy, although in reality it is the most important event in digestive tract immunology. *Oral tolerance* is the term that we use to indicate that, although the immune system of the digestive tract can recognize that all of the material that we consume as food is completely foreign to our bodies, a tolerizing event has occurred that has taught the T cells that this particular foreign material is harmless and can be safely allowed to enter the body.

Oral Tolerance and Antigenic Proteins in Food

All of the food we eat is derived from plants and animals that—without exception—are foreign to the human body. The immune system's sole function is to protect the body from invasion by foreign materials that might cause harm. Thus, the question that has always intrigued scientists is, "Why does the immune system not fight and reject the foreign materials that we consume as food?" Of course, if it did so, we could not survive! So, what is it that allows food to apparently evade the barrier of immune cells and be taken up into our bodies to become an integral part of our tissues and organs, or to be used as fuel for essential body processes? Over the past decade, research has begun to uncover part of the answer to this important question: the complex series of events known as oral tolerance.

The Immune System of the Digestive Tract

The immune system associated with the digestive tract is different from that in other parts of the body. It is composed of specialized cells that make up the gut-associated lymphoid tissue (GALT). The processing of food through this system allows the uptake of nutrients through the walls of the digestive tract (the intestinal epithelium) without triggering the protective response that would otherwise form a barrier to the foreign materials in food. At the same time, any potentially disease-causing microorganisms taken in through the same route are effectively excluded by the GALT. So we have a system that can—at the same time and in the same place—recognize and differeniate foreign material that is safe (food) and foreign material that is a threat (microorganisms, toxins, and other noxious agents).

Microorganisms in the Large Intestine: The Resident Microflora

But even that process is not the whole story. In addition to distinguishing between food and potential pathogens, the GALT must also distinguish between invading microorganisms and others that are permanent residents of the large intestine, called the gut microflora, or microbiota. It is estimated that there are about 10^{12}–10^{14} fairly innocuous microorganisms per mL in the gastrointestinal tract of the healthy human,[b] mostly in the large bowel. They break down the undigested food that moves into the bowel from the small intestine (where most of our digestion of food and absorption of nutrients takes place). Micronutrients such as vitamin K, biotin, thiamin, vitamin B12, and folate are produced as a result of their metabolic activities. We absorb these vitamins, and they form an essential part of our nutritional resources.

In addition, microorganisms in the large bowel defend the bowel from invasion by nonessential, or frankly harmful, microorganisms by competing with them for space and nutrients. They also perform a vital role in keeping the surrounding tissues healthy by stimulating the GALT in a positive manner. We shall talk more about these resident microorganisms in Chapter 25, where we discuss probiotics and their role in digestive tract health.

The Process of Immunological Tolerance to Food in the Digestive Tract

As in all immunological responses, the process of oral tolerance involves T cells and their "messenger chemicals," cytokines. As far as we know at present, in the normal healthy (nonallergic) human, T cells that first encounter the "foreign food" when it enters the body for the very first time (perhaps in mother's breast milk, or as a solid food after weaning) are of the Th1 type[c]. The food molecules are picked up by special cells (usually dendritic cells) in

---

[b] To understand these numbers, write down 1 and add the number of 0s in the superscript (10^{12} = 1,000,000,000,000 or one trillion). One milliliter (mL) is approximately one fifth of a teaspoon.

[c] Sometimes these cells are called Th3 cells to distinguish them from the Th1 response that results in immunological protection.

the infant's digestive tract. The antigenic parts of the food[d] are then "presented" to the T cells where they couple with special receptor molecules on the T cell surface. The T cells with the attached food molecules are then transported in the lymphatic system to the thymus gland. In the thymus gland, the regulatory T cells (sometimes written as T_{reg} cells) stop any further action on the part of the Th1 cells when it is discovered that the "foreign molecules" pose no threat to the body. This process of inhibiting T-cell action is carried out by cytokines, especially TGF-β (transforming growth factor–beta) and possibly IL-10 (Interleukin-10).

The "educated" T cells are then transported, in the blood circulatory system, back into the digestive tract GALT as "memory cells." Whenever the same food is eaten again, the memory T cells remember that this material is safe and remain quiescent, without any further attempt to protect the body from this particular foreign material. As far as we know, this process occurs every time a new food enters the body for the first time.[5]

Immunological Sensitization to Food Allergens

The process of oral tolerance allows a healthy (nonallergic) human to eat any food, absorb its essential nutrients, and excrete the residue that is unnecessary to the body in the form of feces, while maintaining healthy tissue along the whole length of the digestive tract.

However, not all food is tolerated by all people. The immune system of individuals who have food allergies is in effect rejecting the foreign proteins in food. But the process is not the same as when the immune system fights the foreign protein in a virus or bacterium, even though both the food and the invading microorganism enter the body through the same route (the mouth and digestive tract). We have already discussed the difference between the way in which the immune system defends the body against disease-causing microorganisms (the Th1 pathway) and how it functions during an allergic reaction (the Th2 pathway), as well as the way in which most babies' immune

---

[d]The antigenic parts of the food are proteins that have the potential to trigger a response of the immune system. See above, and the Glossary for a discussion and description of "antigen."

systems are educated to allow food to pass into the body without any adverse effect whatsoever. (You might want to look back at Figure 1-1 to understand the ways in which T cells interact with food molecules and lead to nurture or harm.)

Now we are going to look a little more closely at exactly what happens when the Th2 response causes the symptoms of food allergy. The link between the response of the T helper cells and the release of the inflammatory mediators that cause allergy consists of B-cell lymphocytes. These are the cells that produce the extremely important *antibodies.*

Antibodies and the Immune Response

B cells

The main function of B cells is to produce antibodies. Antibodies are complex molecules produced by the immune system in response to antigens. As mentioned previously, antigens are foreign proteins or glycoproteins (a sugar linked to a protein) that trigger the immune response. Every living cell produces several different proteins, each unique to its own cell type and species. The antibody produced against the antigen is entirely specific to that antigen. The two fit together like a lock and key, forming an antigen-antibody complex. When the body is invaded by a microorganism such as a bacterium or virus, B cells will make an antibody precisely designed to couple with molecules of that specific microorganism and no other. The molecules of the microorganism that trigger that response are antigens. Similarly, if a pollen or a food causes B cells to make an antibody in the allergic response, the molecules of the pollen or food causing antibody production are antigens. When we talk about allergy, we call the antigens *allergens.* In the process of making antibodies, B cells first convert into plasma cells. The antibody is then generated from plasma cells.

The antibodies produced by B cells are of five different types, or classes, called IgA, IgG, IgM, IgE, and IgD. The Ig stands for immunoglobulin. Each antibody molecule is made up of a special protein called a globulin. Because the globulin is associated with the immune system, the prefix immuno- is attached to it. Each of the five antibodies has a very specific role in immune protection and in the reactions that are responsible for adverse reactions to foods.

IgM

IgM is the largest of the antibodies and is found circulating in blood. It acts by seeking out antigens and attaching them to an end of one or more of its five "arms." It has ten attachment sites (two per arm) and can mop up many antigens at a time. IgM is the first line of defense against a foreign molecule when it reaches the blood stream. As we shall see later, IgM is the first *protective* antibody to be produced by the fetus in the womb (in utero).

IgA

IgA is found mainly in mucous secretions (secretions from surfaces exposed to the outside world through orifices such as the mouth, respiratory tract, vagina, etc.), where it is called *secretory IgA* (sIgA) to distinguish it from the IgA found in blood (usually called *serum IgA*). sIgA acts as the first line of defense against foreign molecules entering through external orifices, before they can enter the bloodstream. sIgA is extremely important in defending the digestive tract of the newborn baby against anything entering through its mouth. However, as we shall discuss later, the newborn baby (neonate) has no sIgA of its own, and its early digestive tract protection comes entirely from its mother's colostrum—the first fluid that passes through the breast before mature milk is produced—which contains an abundant supply of sIgA.

IgG

IgG is the most important antibody in the immune system's defense against invading disease-causing microorganisms. It is found in the bloodstream after the first-line IgM has started to mop up the invader. In effect, B cells first produce IgM and then switch over to IgG once it has been established that the invader is a real threat to the body. Even after the disease has been successfully suppressed, IgG remains to ensure that the same microorganism is "neutralized" when it enters the body on a subsequent occasion. IgG is the resident guardian that looks for a known dangerous invader that can cause the same infection again. This same process occurs when you receive an immunization shot that contains killed or "attenuated" microorganisms and defends the body against the real live virus or bacterium.

We shall be looking at the role of IgG in reactions to foods in some detail, so a little more information about IgG is important. There are four different types of IgG antibodies; each type functions in different situations. These four types are called IgG1, IgG2, IgG3, and IgG4. In general, IgG4 antibodies are important in certain types of immunological (or hypersensitivity) reactions against foods. IgG1, IgG2, and IgG3 are important in the defense against invading pathogens and other agents that can cause disease in the body.

IgE

IgE is the most important antibody in allergy of all types, including the "classic allergy" of hay fever, asthma, skin reactions such as hives and angioedema (tissue swelling), and the potentially life-threatening anaphylactic reactions. The only other role for IgE, apart from the allergic reaction, is in fighting parasites and intestinal worms (helminths and nematodes).

IgD

The role of IgD is less well defined and is usually associated with aiding other immune functions such as "switching" from one antibody type to another. It is mentioned here simply for completeness. Its role in allergy is probably minimal.

The Production of Antibodies in the Fetus, Baby, and Child

Each of the different types of antibody is produced at different times during development of the fetus and child, and each has a specific role to play in defense against pathogens and other agents that could cause harm to the developing baby.

Figure 1-2 is a visual depiction of the way in which antibodies develop from fetal life through to 9 years of age. This is a comparative graph in which levels of antibodies are shown as a percentage of the adult level (designated

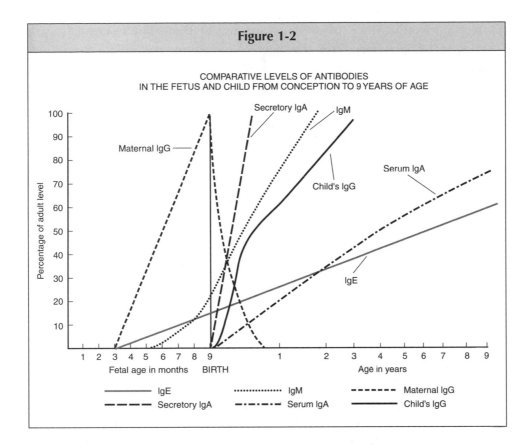

Figure 1-2

COMPARATIVE LEVELS OF ANTIBODIES
IN THE FETUS AND CHILD FROM CONCEPTION TO 9 YEARS OF AGE

100%) of each antibody. Antibody values may be expressed in milligrams per deciliter (mg/dL) or other units of measurement, such as international units (IU), units (U), or kilounits (kU) per liter. As an example, the adult level of IgM is about 100 mg/dL, whereas the adult level of IgG is about 1300 mg/dL.

IgG

IgG is the only antibody that is able to cross the placenta from mother to fetus. All of the other antibodies that can be detected in the fetus or newborn baby are actually made by the immune system of the fetus while in the womb.

When the mother has been exposed to a specific microorganism, such as a bacterium or virus, her immune system makes antibodies of the IgG class to protect her from further infection or invasion by that same microorganism. The IgG antibodies then cross the placenta to become part of the blood circulation of her unborn child. They will protect the fetus from the same microorganism while it is in the womb and during the first few months of life. In most cases this system is extremely efficient in protecting the fetus from infections to which the mother is exposed.

The IgG in the fetus and newborn baby is solely of maternal origin. After birth, maternal IgG declines quite rapidly and by 9 months has disappeared altogether. Production of IgG by the baby begins at birth and increases quite rapidly. By the age of 12 months, the baby is producing a level of IgG that is about 60 percent of that of an adult.

IgE

The earliest of the antibodies of nonmaternal origin detectable in the fetus is IgE. Antibodies of this class are made by the immune system of the fetus itself as early as 11 weeks gestation. IgE is the antibody whose *protective* role (in contrast to its role in allergy) is defending the body from parasites such as intestinal helminths and nematodes. Babies with high levels of IgE at birth are the most effectively protected from these parasites. Under the "natural conditions" of what we now consider to be developing countries, parasite infestations are endemic. In these areas, babies with high levels of IgE are the survivors. However, a baby with a high IgE level in our sanitized Western world is unlikely to encounter intestinal parasites at birth and is consequently the one most likely to develop allergies.

The levels of IgE in the baby and child are extremely variable between different individuals. The level is often dependent on the allergic status of the child; the more allergens to which he or she is sensitized, the higher the level of IgE. Conversely, the higher the IgE level, the more likely the infant is to become sensitized to allergens in its food and its environment. The specific relationship between IgE level and clinical symptoms, however, is currently unknown. Some children with low levels of IgE may develop symptoms of allergy, while others with high levels of IgE may not show signs of allergy. Factors in addition to IgE, as yet not understood, are important in the process.

IgM

IgM levels in the fetus and newborn baby are entirely of fetal origin. Production of IgM may start as early as 22 weeks gestation and reach 15 to 20 percent of the adult level at birth. Thereafter, the level of IgM rises rapidly and typically reaches 75 percent of the adult level at 12 months of age. However, if the fetus becomes infected by a virus in the womb (in utero), the fetal immune system is capable of producing a higher level of IgM in an attempt to protect the unborn baby. There are a few viruses that do infect the fetus directly, for example, the HIV virus that is responsible for AIDS and the rubella virus that causes German measles. When such viruses gain access to the fetus, the level of IgM in the fetus and newborn becomes much higher than shown in the graph.

IgA

The newborn baby is born without any IgA. However, starting at birth, IgA is produced rapidly by the baby's immune system. Secretory IgA (sIgA) may reach the adult level as early as six months of age. The lack of sIgA at birth, however, means that the baby is vulnerable to invasion by infective microorganisms, or other foreign material, through orifices that are normally protected by a coating of mucus. The digestive tract is especially vulnerable, because at every feeding, foreign material enters through the mouth. Fortunately, sIgA is adequately supplied to the newborn baby in the form of maternal sIgA in mother's colostrum, and continues in her mature milk. Ninety percent of the antibodies in mother's colostrum and breast milk is sIgA. This sIgA will protect all of the baby's mucous membrane-lined cavities[e] until he or she is making sufficient sIgA. Thus, every effort should be made to provide the newborn baby with colostrum as soon after birth as possible, and certainly before any other material, such as an infant formula, is given to the baby by mouth. Ideally, breast-feeding should commence within half an hour of birth, and exclusive breast-feeding should continue until solid foods are introduced at 4 to 6 months of age; for the allergic infant, 6 months is preferable and recommended.

---

e Mucous membranes line all of the organs that have external orifices. These include the digestive tract from the mouth to the anus; the respiratory tract including the mouth, nasal passages, inner ear canals, upper respiratory tract and lungs; and the urogenital tract.

IgE-Mediated Allergy

After the Th2 reaction produces IgE in response to an allergenic food, a series of events takes place that finally results in the symptoms of allergy. Biologically active chemicals, called inflammatory mediators, are released from mast cells. Mast cells are specialized white blood cells that are present in all tissues but are particularly abundant in the digestive tract, the lungs and respiratory tract, and the skin. Mast cells produce and store the inflammatory mediators that are then ready to defend our cells and tissues whenever an event that threatens the body's health takes place. In the case of food allergy, this event is eating the allergenic food that has triggered the Th2 response and sensitized the child to the allergen.

The reaction can be considered as occurring in two phases, the early response and the late response:

- The early phase results in the release of inflammatory mediators from mast cells in tissues and circulating basophils in blood.

- The late phase results in the recruitment of additional granulocytes,[f] which are drawn to the reaction site by chemotactic factors (agents that move cells by a process of chemical attraction) released in the early phase. The newly recruited granulocytes are stimulated to release their own inflammatory mediators, which augment the allergic reaction by increasing the levels of those already present.

Early Phase: Release of Inflammatory Mediators

As soon as IgE antibodies are produced by the activated B-cell lymphocytes, they migrate to the surface of specific white blood cells that have receptors on their surface with which to couple with the antibody. These receptors are designated FcεR1 receptors; the ε indicates that they are compatible with the IgE

---

[f] A granulocyte is a white blood cell with a lobed nucleus, characterized by numerous granules within its cytoplasm. The granules contain a variety of biologically active chemicals called inflammatory mediators that are important in immunological protection. Mast cells, basophils, neutrophils, and eosinophils, are examples of granulocytes.

type of antibody. Mast cells in tissues and basophils, which circulate in blood, possess these IgE-compatible receptors. The mast cell is the essential granulocyte in the allergic response. It has been estimated that there may be as many as 500,000 receptors for antibody molecules on the surface of each mast cell.

Mast cells, basophils, and other granulocytes manufacture and store inflammatory mediators in internal granules (hence the name "granulocyte"). The process of releasing inflammatory mediators is called *degranulation*. It is the action of these biologically active chemicals on body tissues that causes the symptoms of allergy.

The process of degranulation is initiated when an allergen cross-links two IgE molecules on adjacent receptors on the surface of a mast cell, forming a bridge between them. The allergen needs to be a certain size (estimated at 10 to 70 kilodaltons[g]) to effect this bridging. At the same time there must be a sufficient number of IgE molecules on the surface of the cell to ensure that two are close enough for the allergen to bridge them.

Often the first exposure to an allergen does not result in a sufficient number of IgE molecules to allow the allergen-antibody bridges to form. Therefore, a single exposure to an allergen rarely results in the release of inflammatory mediators and is usually symptom-free. The process in which a person is exposed to an allergen but does not exhibit symptoms is generally referred to as the *sensitizing event*. On subsequent exposure, when sufficient IgE molecules are present on the surface of the mast cells, degranulation will occur and overt symptoms are experienced.

Late Phase: Amplification of the Allergic Response

During the late phase of the allergic response, neutrophils, eosinophils, monocytes, and basophils are attracted to the reaction site by the chemotaxins produced in the early phase. A measurable increase in eosinophils can be taken as an indication that the symptoms are due to a hypersensitivity reaction. When the granulocytes release their intracellular inflammatory mediators, the allergic reaction is powerfully augmented. This can be experienced in the late-phase reaction of asthma or anaphylaxis when an initial reaction seems to be

---

[g] Daltons and kilodaltons are the units used to measure the size of molecules.

resolving but suddenly becomes extremely acute; without warning the patient is in serious danger. The second phase of an anaphylactic reaction that has been assumed to have resolved often proves fatal. The second phase may occur several hours after the initial response but is usually exhibited within a maximum of 4–6 hours after the first phase.

Clinical Expression of Allergy (Atopy)

Even when the potential to produce antigen-specific IgE has been inherited, further genetic elements appear to be required for atopic disease to be expressed clinically and for symptoms to appear. For example, the ability of granulocytes such as basophils to release inflammatory mediators appears to be determined by genetic factors, but exposure to the allergens that trigger the response is dependent on life-style events.

Other Antibodies in Food Sensitivity

It is common to find anti-food IgG antibodies circulating in blood, even in people who have no signs or history of adverse reactions to foods. In fact, some authorities think that an increase in anti-food IgG in some cases might be indicative of successful resolution of an IgE-mediated allergy. The subject of IgG-mediated food allergy is extremely complicated because of the nature of the antibody and the immunological reactions associated with it. The present knowledge about food allergy-associated IgG may be summarized as follows:

- Four distinct subclasses of IgG have been identified, designated IgG1, IgG2, IgG3, and IgG4.

- IgG4 seems to be the subclass that has a high affinity for food antigens.

- IgG4 represents a very small proportion of total IgG in normal sera; reports of the normal level of IgG4 differ from laboratory to laboratory, the range being 0.7 percent to 4.9 percent of total IgG.[6]

- In the newborn baby, levels of IgG1 and IgG3 rise rapidly. IgG1 may reach concentrations close to the adult level at 8 months: In contrast,

IgG4 is still only a fraction of the adult level at 2 years of age and may not reach adult levels until 12 years.

- Anti-food IgG4 may be associated with allergy, in particular to the milk protein β-lactoglobulin in atopic dermatitis (eczema) in children.[7]

- There is some evidence that *total* anti-food IgG (all classes of IgG measured together) might represent some protection from IgE-mediated food allergy: In one study, symptom-free children had higher levels of IgG antibodies to milk and egg proteins than those who developed allergic symptoms, and a high IgG/IgE ratio in cord blood was suggested to be a sign of a decreased risk for food allergy.[8]

- Food allergy in infants is frequently associated with an increase in gut permeability ("leaky gut"). It is likely that antigenic food molecules passing into circulation trigger production of anti-food IgG. Thus, in cases of IgE-mediated food allergy that result in inflammatory reactions within the gastrointestinal tract causing a non-intact digestive epithelium, it is logical to expect to find higher than normal levels of anti-food IgG. Some authorities think that these anti-food IgG antibodies represent a protective mechanism, rather than a source of allergic pathology.[9]

It remains for future research to determine the role of IgG, and especially IgG4 anti-food antibodies, in allergy. We shall be discussing the role of IgG in allergic sensitization and tolerance in the fetus and newborn in Chapter 3.

In Chapter 4 we shall look at the consequences of all this immunological activity in our discussion of the symptoms of allergy in the baby and child.

But first we should start right at the beginning, and ask the most important question: Is there anything that we can do to recognize the baby who is likely to develop allergy and thereby prevent the development of allergy in the first place? That is the subject of Chapter 2.

References

1. Johansson SGO, Hourihane JOB, Bousquet J, Bruijnzeel-Koomen C, Dreborg S, Haahtela T, Kowalski ML, Mygind N, Ring J, van Cauwenberge P, van Hage-Hamsten M, Wüthrich B. A revised nomenclature for allergy. An EAACI position statement from the EAACI nomenclature task force. *Allergy* 2001;56:813–824.

2. American Academy of Allergy and Clinical Immunology/NIAID. *Adverse Reactions to Foods.* NIH Publication 84-2442: 1–6, 1984.

3. Joneja JMV. *Dealing with Food Allergies.* Boulder CO: Bull Publishing Company, 2003. 27–50.

4. Joneja JMV. *Dealing with Food Allergies.* 42–44.

5. Strobel S, Mowat A. Oral tolerance and allergic responses to food proteins. *Current Opinion in Allergy and Clinical Immunology* 2006;6(3):207–213. Online ref: http://www.medscape.com/viewarticle/532236

6. Oxelius VA. IgG subclass levels in infancy and childhood. Acta Paediatrica Scandinavica 1979 68(1):23-27

7. Jenmalm MC and Bjorksten B. Exposure to cow's milk during the first 3 months of life is associated with increased levels of IgG subclass antibodies to beta-lactoglobulin to 8 years. *Journal of Allergy and Clinical Immunology* 1998;102(4 Pt 1):671–678.

8. Dannaeus A, Inganas M. A follow-up study of children with food allergy. Clinical course in relation to serum IgE- and IgG-antibody levels to milk, egg and fish. *Clinical Allergy* 1981;11:533–539

9. Sampson HA. Food allergy. Part 1: Immunopathogenesis and clinical disorders. Current reviews of allergy and clinical immunology. *Journal of Allergy and Clinical Immunology* 1999;103(5 Pt 1):717–728.

CHAPTER 2

Dealing with Food Allergy in Babies and Children

During the years that I have been involved in the management of adverse reactions to foods I have seen several very important changes in our approach to food allergy. In the early 1970s when I was desperately trying to cope with allergy in my own two children, I was told quite bluntly by the doctor who was treating my son's asthma, "There is no such thing as food allergy." This in spite of the fact that our son was anaphylactic to peanuts and on several occasions needed emergency treatment for his reactions. In those days anaphylaxis was considered a "medical emergency," but the underlying cause—food allergy—was not part of the medical lexicon.

Our son's pediatrician was convinced that his asthma and other reactions, including severe and often infected eczema, were the result of stress in the home caused by a dysfunctional marital relationship. She prescribed a "parentectomy"—the removal of our son from the family home. (I took him to a children's asthma and allergy clinic in Denver, Colorado, for a year when he was 7 in response to this advice.)

At age 13 our son's frequent severe migraine headaches were investigated during a week's hospitalization, when he underwent every test available (his father being a neurologist). The migraine headaches cleared amazingly when—reasoning that meat and milk made him "feel sick"—our son made the independent decision to follow a strict vegan diet. We finally discovered that he was very allergic to pork, and to a lesser extent to beef. Both pork and beef triggered migraine headaches with vomiting and nausea.

Still, his doctors denied the existence of food allergy! According to then-prevailing medical opinion, food allergy was the product of the parents' overprotective and neurotic focus on the child—especially the mother's!

Although I was a university professor involved for many years in immunology research and teaching—including the immunology of allergy, on which subject I wrote a book, published in 1990[1]—it was not until I earned the designation of registered dietitian in 1990 that I began the long and sometimes difficult road to managing food allergy in the clinical setting. At the time very few dietitians were dealing with food allergy because so little was known about how to do it effectively. Scientific research papers on food allergy were few and far between, with perhaps no more than ten good papers a year being published. The field seemed to be the province of naturopaths, homeopaths, and other practitioners of alternative medicine. In a tradition as old as the ages, when this novel thinking appeared to originate on the fringes of medical science, mainstream doctors tended to shun it and ignored the whole thing, hoping it would go away like so many other medical fads. However, with increased public awareness that eating certain foods made adults and children sick, doctors found ever more patients in their offices and clinics claiming to suffer food allergies. They finally had to acknowledge that food allergy, contrary to their hopes, was an established scientific fact that had to be dealt with.

Beginning in the mid-1990s an increasing number of doctors embraced the facts of food allergy. I was amused to see that the respirologist who in 1975 had told me that food allergy did not exist now made a practice of skin-testing every patient who entered his office, and included many foods in his arsenal of allergens. Many general practitioners ordered a supply of skin test kits, and I was called on more than once to tutor an aspiring allergist who was moving into the field from another specialty and who needed help passing the immunology part of the qualifying exam.

Far from the few sparse research papers in the early years, today we see the publication of a new paper on some aspect of food allergy almost daily. Position papers, consensus documents, and evidence-based practice guidelines by learned allergy societies appear frequently (some contradicting others, unfortunately). The result of all this activity is that we now have some solid science on which to base our understanding of and approach to food allergy. In practical terms, this means that we have moved from the early strategies based mainly on anecdote and "doing what we've always done" to some quite different ways of looking at the subject.

One of the most drastic changes in recent years is in the prevention of food allergy in early infancy. Previously the idea prevailed that withholding foods from the infant until the immune and digestive systems are more mature would serve to prevent allergic sensitization. The common advice regarding introduction of the most highly allergenic foods was frequently "the later the better." It was hoped this would in turn prevent not only allergy to food, but inhalant and contact allergies in later life. We now know that in many cases this is not the best advice. In fact, new research seems to indicate the very opposite: it is exposure to allergens in early life that may tolerize the immune system, and may prevent allergic sensitization to food (a complete reversal of our previous thinking). One example is allergy to fish. Previously it was thought that fish, a highly allergenic food, should be avoided until the child is at least 1 year old. Some authorities suggested delaying the introduction of fish until even later for children considered to be at high risk for allergy.[2] However, recent research has provided evidence that children of both allergic and nonallergic mothers are less likely to develop allergy to fish if the mother consumes fish two or three times a week during pregnancy[3] (provided, of course, that the mother herself is not allergic to fish). Another paper provides evidence that regular fish consumption during the first year of life is associated with reduced risk of allergic disease by age 4.[4]

Even more revolutionary is evidence published in the past two years that indicates it is possible that adverse reactions to certain foods might be prevented by introducing these foods to the baby during a window of opportunity limited to the few months when the baby's immune system is most likely to become tolerant.[5] This likely applies to not only food allergy but also to other conditions triggered by food, such as celiac disease.[6] These studies seem to suggest, for example, that wheat should be introduced after 3 months but before 7 months. It is possible that there exist specific optimal introduction stages for different foods. However, more research must be done before we can confidently advise parents when to introduce specific foods to their allergic babies. The best we can do at the moment is rely on consensus documents and practice guidelines, based on extensive reviews of studies published in peer-reviewed, reputable medical and scientific journals—and wait for more good studies.

FOUR-STAGE APPROACH TO FOOD ALLERGY IN BABIES AND CHILDREN

The process of dealing with your child's allergies will be more easily understood if examined in four distinct stages: prediction; prevention; identification; and management:

- **Prediction.** If the baby at risk for allergy can be identified before exposure to allergens—especially food allergens—it is thought that the development of allergy can be prevented or be greatly diminished in incidence and severity.

- **Prevention**. When the potentially atopic baby is identified, measures to prevent initial allergic sensitization may be taken to attempt to reduce the development of allergic disease. This is usually referred to as primary prevention of allergy.

- **Identification**. If primary prevention has been unsuccessful, accurate identification of the culprit allergen(s) must be made to decrease the chances of allergic reaction and to reduce the severity of allergic symptoms. This is especially important when there is risk of anaphylactic reaction.

- **Management**. When the culprit allergen(s) have been identified it is vitally important that they be avoided. Most children will outgrow their early food allergies, so reevaluation of the child's reaction to foods is necessary at regular intervals. A dietary regimen must be followed to ensure that the infant receives all the nutrients essential to growth and maturation during this critical stage in its development.

I have designed the remainder of this book to follow these four stages.

Prediction: This chapter discusses the factors that might predict which babies are likely to become allergic.

Prevention: Chapter 3 looks at the ways it may be possible to prevent the onset of food allergy, based on our current knowledge of the processes of immunological sensitization and tolerance.

Identification: Chapters 4, 5, and 6 deal with the accurate identification of the foods responsible for your child's food allergy symptoms.

Management: Chapters 7 through 17 describe ways to manage your child's diet to address specific food allergies once they are already established. Chapters 18 through 24 discuss several conditions in which food allergy is an important contributing factor but not the primary or sole cause of the condition. In these cases, removing the contributing foods will improve or even entirely alleviate the symptoms, while the underlying cause persists. Chapter 25 looks at probiotics and the possibility of managing food allergies with bioactive foods.

Additional dietary information is provided in the appendices.

EARLY ALLERGY PREDICTORS

Allergic diseases result from a strong relationship between genetic and environmental factors. Sensitization to food allergens occurs mainly in the first year of life. Cow's milk allergy is often the first food allergy to appear in susceptible infants. The incidence of allergy in children of allergic parents is significantly greater than in children of nonatopics. It is estimated that genetic factors account for 50 to 70 percent of cases of asthma and allergy.[7] However, many children who develop atopic diseases during the first years of life come from families with no history of allergy.

It is important to remember that inheritance of the potential to develop allergy is actually the inheritance of the Th2 response to allergens, not the inheritance of a specific allergy. In other words, a baby's immune system is primed at birth to respond to certain harmless proteins as if they posed a threat to the body, but the system is not programmed to respond to any allergen in particular. For example, even if both parents are allergic to peanuts, their baby does not inherit peanut allergy—he or she inherits an increased likelihood of responding to an allergen. The development of peanut allergy in the baby would require sensitization to the peanut allergen under conditions appropriate to that sensitization. The baby is just as likely to develop allergy to milk, soy, or some obscure tropical fruit—or to nothing at all. (Some foods are more likely than others to lead to allergy; see Table F-1 [Food Allergen Scale] in Appendix F.) Whether or not a baby develops allergy depends on the infant's exposure to the allergen and the response of his or her immune system at the time of exposure.

Many authorities have tried to provide parameters to identify those babies who are most likely to develop early allergies based on their inherited allergic potential. As these babies are identified, it is hoped that strategies can be implemented to reduce their sensitization to allergens during the period in which they are most likely to become allergic. Various definitions of the "high-risk infant" have been used. The prevailing definition, published as a joint statement of the European Society of Paediatric Allergology and Clinical Immunology (ESPACI) and the European Society for Paediatric Gastroenterology, Hepatology and Nutrition (ESPGHAN), describes high-risk infants as those with at least one first-degree relative (parent or sibling) with documented allergic disease,[8] and most authorities rely on this definition in their assessment of the pediatric population at risk for allergy.

Scientific Tests to Predict Atopy

Several different types of scientific tests have been considered over the years in attempting to find an objective measure to predict which babies will develop allergies. For a time, measuring the IgE levels in cord blood at birth seemed promising. This idea was based on the theory that IgE produced in utero may be responsible for early IgE-mediated allergy. However, large-scale studies indicated no difference in cord blood IgE levels in infants with and without allergy. In the final analysis the general consensus is that "a family history of atopy is far more sensitive in detecting infants at risk for atopy and little is added by knowledge of cord IgE."[9]

IgE as a predictive measure has also been considered by researchers looking for inheritance factors in predicting atopy. Maternal and paternal levels of IgE were measured at various stages throughout pregnancy. The results have not been conclusive, but the authors of one such study found evidence that the maternal, but not paternal, total IgE level correlated with higher levels of IgE in the newborn infant, and with an increased incidence of infant atopy. The authors suggest that "maternal factors, placental factors, or both have an impact on perinatal allergic sensitization."[10] The significance of maternal allergy in fetal and neonatal potential for allergy is discussed in Chapter 3.

Another attempt to develop a scientific test to predict atopy examined the levels of other indicators of allergy in cord blood at birth. As discussed in Chapter 1, T-cell lymphocytes and the cytokines they produce are extremely important in the process of the allergic reaction, and can be measured as indicators that a reaction is taking place. Specific populations of T cells and their cytokines have been measured in the cord blood of a large number of babies at birth, but no difference was found to distinguish infants born to atopic parents from infants born to nonatopic parents.[11]

The bottom line here is that we have no objective scientific tests by which to determine exactly which babies will develop allergy. The best we can do is make an informed guess, based on the number of an infant's close relatives with a positive history of allergy.

References

1. Joneja JMV and Bielory L. *Understanding Allergy, Sensitivity and Immunity: A Comprehensive Guide.* New Brunswick, NJ: Rutgers University Press, 1990.

2. Fiocchi A, Assa'ad A, Bahna S. Food allergy and the introduction of solid foods to infants: A consensus document. *Annals of Allergy, Asthma and Immunology* 2006;97(1):10–21.

3. Calvani M, Alessandri C, Sopo SM, Panetta V, Pingitore G, Tripodi S, Zappalà D, Zicari AM. Consumption of fish, butter and margarine during pregnancy and development of allergic sensitizations in the offspring: Role of maternal atopy. *Pediatric Allergy and Immunology* 2006;17(2):94–102.

4. Kull I, Bergstrom A, Lilja G, Pershagen G, Wickman M. Fish consumption during the first year of life and development of allergic diseases during childhood. *Allergy* 2006;61(8):1009–1015.

5. Poole JA, Barriga K, Leung DY, Hoffman M, Eisenbarth GS, Rewers M, Norris JM. Timing of initial exposure to cereal grains and the risk of wheat allergy. *Pediatrics* 2006;117(6):2175–2182.

6. Norris JM, Barriga K, Hoffenberg EJ, Taki I, Miao D, Haas JE, Emery LM, Sokol RJ, Erlich HE, Eisenbarth GS, Rewers M. Risk of celiac disease autoimmunity and timing of gluten introduction in the diet of infants at increased risk of disease. *Journal of the American Medical Association* 2005;293:2343–2351.

7. Moat MF and Cookson WOCM. Gene identification in asthma and allergy. *International Archives of Allergy and Immunology* 1998;116:247–252.

8. Host A, Koletzko B, Dreborg S, Muraro A, Wahn U, Aggett P, Bresson JL, Hernell O, Lafeber H, Michaelsen KF, Micheli JL, Rigo J, Weaver L, Heymans H, Strobel S, Vandenplas Y. Dietary products used in infants for treatment and prevention of food allergy. Joint statement of the Committee on Hypoallergenic Formulas of the European Society of Paediatric Allergology and Clinical Immunology (ESPACI) and the Committee on Nutrition of the European Society for Paediatric Gastroenterology, Hepatology, and Nutrition (ESPGHAN). *Archives of Disease in Childhood* 1999;(8):80–84.

9. Hide DW, Arshad SH, Twiselton R, Stevens M. Cord serum IgE: An insensitive method for prediction of atopy. *Clinical and Experimental Allergy* 1991;21(6):739.

10. Liu CA, Wang CL, Chuang H, Ou CY, Hsu TY, Yang KD. Prenatal prediction of infant atopy by maternal but not paternal total IgE levels. *Journal of Allergy and Clinical Immunol* 2003;112(5):899–904.

11. Hagendorens MM, Van Bever HP, Schuerwegh AJ, DeClerck LS, Bridts CH, Stevens WJ. Determination of T-cell subpopulations and intracellular cytokine production (interleukin-2, interleukin-4, and interferon-gamma) by cord blood T-lymphocytes of neonates from atopic and nonatopic parents. *Pediatric Allergy and Immunology* 2000;11(1):12–19.

CHAPTER 3

Prevention of Food Allergy

As you will understand after reading Chapter 1, babies are born with a fairly immature immune system, and allergy seems to be a consequence of sensitization to allergens after exposure to food molecules under conditions that promote a Th2 response. Every parent with this knowledge will inevitably ask the question, "If we could somehow avoid that exposure, or ensure that it take place under conditions that do not elicit an allergic response, could we prevent the distress of allergy symptoms in our babies, and our own stress in dealing with it?" This is a question that all of us who research or manage food allergy constantly ask ourselves.

For many years it was assumed that if we could prevent the early onset of allergy, we could avoid what allergists used to call the "allergic march"—the progression from food allergy to inhalant-triggered respiratory allergy and asthma, which have their onset at a later age. It was assumed that the early expression of allergy in the form of allergic reaction to foods primed the immune system to take the Th2 route, and that once started—like a train rolling down the track—the Th2 response would progress to respiratory allergy and asthma. However, more recent research has demonstrated that this is not the case. Prevention of food allergy in early infancy prevents or reduces *food allergy*. It has little or no effect on the development of allergy to airborne and environmental allergens. Nevertheless, it is extremely important to prevent, reduce, or relieve food allergy as early as possible because of its central role in many allergic diseases (particularly eczema) and its contribution to asthma and allergic rhinitis, and because of the real danger of life-threatening anaphylactic reactions.

This brings us to an important concept in understanding food allergy: allergy to food is not a stand-alone disease. The mediators released in an allergic reaction affect many different tissues and organ systems, resulting in a variety of different symptoms. Therefore, a reaction to a food may cause a flare-up of eczema; may trigger an asthma attack or make existing asthma worse; may increase the severity of hay fever, especially in the pollen season; may cause digestive tract upset—or all of the above simultaneously. Of course, each of these conditions may have a primary allergy trigger apart from food, such as airborne pollens, dust mites, mold spores, animal dander, and so on. This means that in most cases mediators released in a food allergy can impact any vulnerable area of the body, depending on the individual's sensitivity. Figure 3-1 shows the central role that food allergy plays in all types of allergy. Successfully managing a child's food allergy will not only prevent the direct effects of food sensitivity, but will also relieve or reduce the impact of other allergies at the same time.

Our next questions ask how we can make a difference in a baby's risk of developing allergy and how early in life we can implement strategies to avoid the baby's sensitization to allergens. Our first question considers when atopic disease begins.

DOES ATOPIC DISEASE START IN FETAL LIFE?

During pregnancy immune responses in the uterus are skewed to the Th2 type, not the Th1 type, because the fetus must be protected from rejection by the mother's system. (Obviously, having inheritance from both father and mother, the fetus has a cellular composition different from its mother's.) The developing baby would be at risk of rejection by the mother's immune system, which is designed to reject anything foreign inside her body. This rejection would be a Th1 response. (Please read Chapter 1 for a detailed discussion of Th1 and Th2 immune responses.) To avoid this rejection, the fetal environment develops a predominantly Th2 milieu, which suppresses the mother's natural defense system. This effectively bathes the fetus in Th2-type cytokines that keep it safe in its environment.

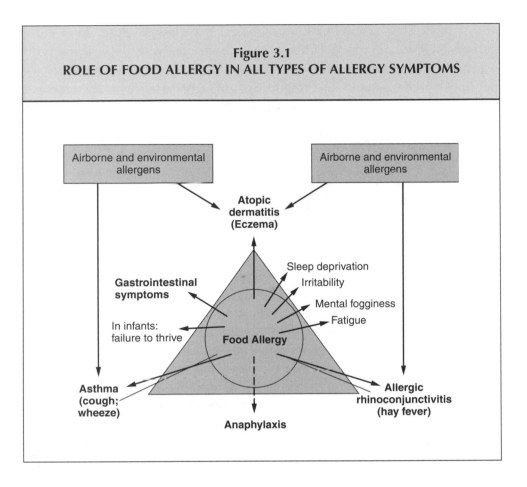

Figure 3.1
ROLE OF FOOD ALLERGY IN ALL TYPES OF ALLERGY SYMPTOMS

Because the fetus is enveloped by Th2-type cytokines in the womb, it is logical to question whether allergic sensitization to foods in the mother's diet might gain access to the developing baby's system, and thereby start allergic sensitization even before birth. In fact, allergens have been detected in amniotic fluid, indicating that allergens to which the mother has been exposed can cross the placenta.[1] However, there is no real evidence to suggest that the fetal immune system is primed to respond to these allergens.[2] In fact some authorities suggest that exposure to food antigens in utero may promote fetal *tolerance*.[3] That is, the immune system may be educated to recognize the food as foreign but safe, and is deterred from mounting a defensive action against it when the food is encountered in the future. So, in utero exposure to food molecules may mark the beginning of the baby's ability to consume food with impunity.

At birth all newborn babies (neonates) have low levels of interferon-gamma (IFN-γ) and produce the cytokines associated with the Th2 response, especially interleukin (IL)-4. Newborns of both atopic and nonatopic parentage have a predominantly Th2 response to antigens. As babies mature, there is a switch from the Th2 response to the so-called protective Th1 response. An exception is atopic babies, in whom the Th2 response continues to predominate and set the stage for allergen sensitization and allergy.[4] Here the important question becomes, why don't all neonates have allergy? New research indicates that the answer lies with the immune system of the mother, which plays a significant role in the *expression* of allergy in her baby.[5]

The only antibody that crosses the placenta from mother to fetus is immunoglobulin (Ig)G. As mentioned in our discussion of antibodies (Chapter 1), there are four subtypes of IgG, designated IgG1, IgG2, IgG3, and IgG4. IgG4 is frequently associated with IgE in allergy. The nonatopic mother produces abundant IgG1 and IgG3, which cross the placenta to protect her fetus in utero. Because food proteins can cross the placenta, it is thought that fetal exposure to these antigens in the environment of the uterus protected by mother's IgG1 and IgG3 may promote fetal tolerance to these foods, and that the tolerance continues in the neonatal period. In contrast, the allergic mother tends to produce IgE and IgG4; IgG4 is very inefficient at crossing the placenta. It is thought that the mother's IgE:IgG ratio has the greatest consequences for the offspring.[6] In allergic mothers, there is likely to be insufficient IgG1 and IgG3 to reduce the level of (down-regulate) fetal IgE. At birth, these mothers' babies may thus be primed to become sensitized to allergens and to develop allergic symptoms very early.

Although there is no evidence that the fetus of the allergic mother can mount an IgE-mediated response to specific allergens in utero, the potential to produce allergen-specific IgE predominates at birth. The only defense against susceptibility to allergens at present is to reduce the allergic mother's exposure to her own allergens throughout pregnancy in the attempt to decrease her production of IgE and IgG4 and enhance production of the protective IgG1 and IgG3. The mother should avoid foods to which she is allergic at all times, and obtain complete balanced nutrition from alternative sources. There is no evidence to suggest that avoidance of any foods other than the mother's own allergens will improve the allergic status of her baby. A 1988 report[7] indicated that excluding highly allergenic foods from the mother's diet from week 28 through the end of pregnancy had no effect on the atopic status of the infant.

Several studies suggest that women tend to have a weaker immune response to allergens with each successive pregnancy, which might explain why children born later tend to suffer less from eczema, hay fever, and asthma than do their older siblings. In addition, first-born children generally have a higher level of IgE in their blood (measured in cord blood at birth) than children born subsequently. The authors of these studies suggest that the mother's immune response influences the baby's immune system, which subsequently affects the child's later sensitivity to allergens.[8]

THE NEWBORN BABY: CONDITIONS THAT PREDISPOSE TO ALLERGY

There are three topics that are often discussed when exploring conditions that may predispose a newborn baby to allergy: the immaturity of the infant's immune system, the permeability or "leakiness" of the baby's digestive tract, and breast-feeding. Each of these items is discussed below.

Immaturity of the Infant's Immune System

The major elements of the immune system are in place at birth, but do not function at a level that provides adequate protection against all infections. The level of antibodies (except maternal IgG) is a fraction of that of the adult, and secretory IgA (sIgA), the "first-line defense" of all mucous membranes, is absent at birth. Babies at risk of developing atopic disease are commonly described as having impaired function or delayed maturation of various immunologic processes, including cytokine production.[9]

Permeability, or "Leakiness," of the Digestive Tract

The infant's intestine is highly permeable. During the first 3 years of life—in particular, between the first 6 and 12 months—the intestine can absorb large molecules of food. Larger food molecules (i.e., between 10,000 and 70,000 daltons in molecular size) trigger the Th2 response and production of food-specific IgE. During the period when the digestive tract is most permeable, therefore, sensitization to food allergens can occur, and food allergy is most likely to develop.

The newborn baby is consequently at risk for the development of food allergies caused by the predominance of the Th2 response, the lack of protective secretory IgA (sIgA) at mucosal surfaces, and the hyperpermeable digestive epithelium. The offspring of the allergic mother has the additional risk factors associated with the increased potential to mount an IgE-mediated response and the lack of the maternal IgG1 and IgG3 that would normally down-regulate the production of Th2 cytokines.

Breast-feeding and Allergy

Breast milk provides the ideal nutritional, immunologic, and physiologic nourishment for all newborns. Components of human milk enhance the baby's natural defenses and promote maturation of the immune system.[11] Ninety percent of antibodies in human colostrum and milk are secretory IgA (sIgA), and provide the baby with protection at mucosal surfaces until he or she is able to independently produce adequate quantities of sIgA, at about 6 months of age.[12] However, the effect of breast-feeding on the development of allergic diseases in the breast-fed infant remains controversial.

Some studies report that breast-feeding is protective against allergy with a definite improvement in infant eczema and associated gastrointestinal complaints, and reduced risk for asthma in the first 24 months, when the baby is exclusively breast-fed and the mother eliminates highly allergenic foods from her diet.[13] However, other studies seem to indicate that breast-feeding has no effect on the infant's symptoms of allergy, or may even be associated with increased prevalence of atopic eczema.[14] One of the reasons for this apparent contradiction may be explained by data that indicate that the breast milk of atopic mothers differs immunologically from that of nonallergic mothers.[15]

Atopic mothers tend to have a higher level of the cytokines and chemokines associated with allergy in their breast milk. In addition, they tend to have a lower level of the cytokine known as transforming growth factor-beta 1 (TGF-β1) that promotes tolerance of food components in the intestinal immune response. A normal level of TGF-β1 in mother's colostrum and breast milk is likely to facilitate tolerance of food molecules encountered by the infant in the mother's breast milk and later to formula and solids.[16] Evidence is accumulating to indicate that breast-feeding is protective against allergies when the mother is nonatopic,[17] but that babies of allergic mothers may be at greater risk of developing allergies, especially to foods, during breast-feeding.

In view of substantial evidence regarding the role of breast milk in promoting the well-being of all babies and based on careful analysis of all research on the topic, the European Society of Paediatric Allergology and Clinical Immunology (ESPACI) and the European Society for Paediatric Gastroenterology, Hepatology, and Nutrition (ESPGHAN) strongly recommend 4 to 6 months' exclusive breast-feeding. The American Academy of Pediatrics (AAP)[18] recommends 6 months' exclusive breast-feeding as the hallmark of allergy prevention.[19]

PREVENTION OF FOOD ALLERGEN SENSITIZATION DURING THE FIRST 6 MONTHS

From the results of epidemiological studies, it is thought that initial sensitization to food allergens in the exclusively breast-fed baby occurs predominantly from external sources, as from a single feeding of infant formula, or perhaps by accident. It is thought that thereafter, the baby's immune system responds to the same allergen in the mother's milk.

In an important study of 1749 newborns in Odense, Denmark, 39 (2.2%) were identified as being sensitized to cow's milk proteins soon after birth. Of these, 9 developed symptoms of cow's milk allergy before 3 months of age, in spite of being exclusively breast-fed. Records from the newborns' nursery revealed that all 9 infants had been exposed to cow's milk formula in amounts corresponding to approximately 0.4–3.0 g of beta-lactoglobulin (BLG) during the first 3 days of life. Similar proteins were detected in their mothers' breast milk, to which the infants reacted with allergic symptoms. The authors concluded that early occasional, inadvertent exposure to cow's milk proteins may initiate sensitization in predisposed neonates. Subsequent exposure to minute amounts of bovine milk proteins in human breast milk may act as a booster dose, eliciting allergic reactions.[10]

Whether allergens in breast milk from the mother's diet can act as the initial sensitizing dose for development of food allergy in the breast-fed baby has been widely investigated, but the answer is not clear.[20] Consequently, recommendations on the lactating mother's diet are still being debated. The AAP recommends the elimination of peanuts and tree nuts, and possibly eggs, cow's milk , fish, and other foods.[21] The European groups do not recommend elimination of any specific foods from the maternal diet during breast-feeding unless the baby has been diagnosed with allergy to one or more foods, in which case the mother should avoid the baby's allergenic food as long as she continues to breast-feed.

A compromise endorsed by most authorities[22] is that the breast-feeding mother be instructed to avoid the most highly allergenic foods, following evaluation of each family's atopic risk. The exception is peanuts. Because of the seriousness and persistence of peanut allergy, the increasing prevalence of sensitization, and the decreasing age of onset of peanut allergy in childhood,[23] the British Medical Council recommends avoidance of peanut products for all pregnant and lactating mothers of offspring at high risk for allergy.

At present, the most important diet advice to the breast-feeding mother is to maintain a detailed food record and strictly avoid her own allergens. Should the infant exhibit signs of food allergy while being exclusively breast-fed, foods in the mother's diet that are implicated as possible allergens on the basis of observation and the food record can be tested by elimination and challenge. When the culprit foods have been identified, these should be excluded from the maternal diet as long as breast-feeding continues.

Formula Feeding

It is not always possible for a baby to be breast-fed. When the infant is at risk for, or has already developed allergies, making the best choice of formula is extremely important.

Most authorities suggest that if a baby has no signs or symptoms of cow's milk allergy, a conventional cow's milk–based formula is safe and appropriate for infant feeding, even when there is a strong family history of allergy. However, some allergists suggest an extensively hydrolyzed casein formula (ehf) as a safer choice for babies at high risk for allergy, as determined by having one or two close relatives (e.g., a parent or sibling) with allergy.[24]

Hydrolyzed casein formulas include Similac Alimentum (Abbott Nutrition), Nutramigen (Mead-Johnson), and Enfamil Pregestimil (Mead-Johnson). These formulas may be prohibitively expensive for some families. Therefore they are usually used for babies who already have a milk allergy, rather than as a preventive measure. (Please refer to Chapter 7 for details about infant formulas for the milk-allergic baby.)

An alternative formula shown by research to possibly help prevent milk allergy and eczema is a partially hydrolyzed formula (phf) based on whey, called GoodStart and manufactured by Nestlé Foods. Goodstart has the advantage of being the same price as a conventional cow's milk–based formula. GoodStart is *not* an appropriate formula for the baby who has already developed an allergy to cow's milk because it contains whey (see Chapter 7, Milk Allergy). A 2003 German study compared conventional cow's milk–based formulas (CMFs), an ehf formula (Nutramigen), and a phf formula (GoodStart) in their performance in preventing allergic disease in the first year of life. The results showed the incidence of allergy to be significantly reduced in babies fed the ehf formula Nutramigen compared to the incidence of allergy in infants fed CMF. The incidence of eczema was significantly reduced in babies fed ehf or phf, compared to eczema in those fed CMA.[25]

INTRODUCING SOLID FOODS

Answers to the questions of when to introduce foods into the diet of the allergic or potentially allergic infant and of which foods to introduce have been largely matters of previous practice, not evidence-based or consensus-based guidelines. In fact, there exists no standard schedule for weaning infants, be they healthy or be they at risk for allergy. The first consensus document on the introduction of solid foods to the food-allergic infant was published in July 2006 by the Adverse Reactions to Foods Committee of the American College of Allergy, Asthma, and Immunology.[26] The committee recommends not introducing to the allergic infant the multiple allergens in solid foods until after 6 months of age. Before this age, the authors suggest, the immaturity of the infant's digestive tract and immune system may increase his or her risk for sensitization and development of allergy.

Most pediatric allergists recommend delaying introduction of the most highly allergenic foods until 1 year of age or later.[27] The AAP recommends specific timing for the addition of specific allergenic foods—cow's milk at 12 months; egg at 24 months; peanut, tree nut, and fish at 3 years.[28]   The European committees suggest adding only foods with low allergenicity and limited in variety when starting infants on solids. The European allergists do not specify any particular order for the introduction of any specific food. Table 3-1 summarizes diet recommendations to help prevent development of allergies in the infant.[29]

Table 3-1
INFANT DIET RECOMMENDATIONS TO HELP PREVENT ALLERGY[29]

- Breast-feed exclusively for the first 6 months. The benefit of protection against allergic symptoms will continue long after baby has been weaned from the breast.

- Avoid cow's milk–based formulas (CMFs) and other supplemental foods during the first 6 months. Avoiding CMFs has proven effective in preventing cow's milk allergy.

- Introduce complementary foods (formulas and solid foods) at the start of the sixth month.

- In the developed world, the main foods posing allergy risk are
    - Cow's milk
    - Egg
    - Peanut
    - Tree nuts
    - Fish
    - Shellfish

  Avoid these until the baby is 12 months old.

- Introduce foods individually and gradually.

- Give mixed foods that contain several potentially allergenic foods only after each component has been individually evaluated and shown to be tolerated.

- Because cooking reduces the allergenicity of many foods—especially fruits and vegetables—give baby the cooked, homogenized (puréed) form of a food before giving the food in raw form.

There is no general agreement about the relative allergenicity of foods, but the majority of practitioners rate milk (of any species except human), egg, peanut, tree nuts, soy, shellfish, and fish as potentially highly allergenic. Some practitioners also include corn, wheat, citrus fruit, beef, and chicken on the list of potentially highly allergenic foods.

Appendix F provides a chart as a suggested sequence of introducing solid foods to the allergic baby, starting with the foods least likely to cause allergic sensitization.

The Sequential Incremental Dose Method of Introducing Solid Foods

The guidelines of all pediatric societies and consensus committees agree that solid foods should be introduced individually and gradually, starting at about 6 months of age. The most highly allergenic foods should not be given until after 12 months.

For many years I have introduced solid foods to allergic babies using the sequential incremental dose method. This protocol introduces graded quantities of individual foods, starting with very small amounts, and requires the baby's response to be monitored as each food is tested. These are the steps that compose the incremental dose method employed in my practice with great success:

- Before introducing a new food to an infant who has previously demonstrated any type of allergic reaction, apply the food to the baby's cheek. Wait 20 minutes to see whether a reddened area appears at the site of application. A reddened area would be an "early warning sign" indicating the release of histamine and a probable allergic response to the food.

- If no reddened area appears, apply a little of the food to the outer border of the baby's lower lip (not inside the mouth). If there is no response to this—no reddening, swelling, or irritation (as indicated by baby rubbing the area)—feed the infant a small amount (half a teaspoon or less) of the food. Carefully observe the baby for any reactions for the next 4 hours.

- If no adverse signs appear, the infant can be fed more (from one-half to one teaspoon) of the food.

- If no adverse reactions occur during the next 4 hours, one to two teaspoons of the food can be given.

- The next 24 hours are a time to monitor for delayed reactions, which may include disturbed sleep patterns, irritability, and overt allergic symptoms.

- If no adverse reactions are observed, introduce more of the same food on the third day, providing slightly greater quantities than on the first day. End with feeding the baby as much of the food as he or she wants.

- The fourth day is a second monitoring day on which none of the test food is eaten. Observe the baby for any signs of delayed reaction.

- If the baby is free from any signs of allergy after the 4-day introduction period, assume the food is safe and include it in the regular diet.

- Now proceed to a new food, repeating the steps of this method of introduction.

Sequence of Introducing Solids

There is no preferred order in which to introduce the different categories of foods. However, if the baby has been exclusively breast-fed, it is a good idea to introduce meats early because it is important to take in a food source of iron by age 6 months, and thereafter.

Many dietitians and nutritionists advocate the use of iron-enriched baby cereals for early infant feeding. Babies from 6 to 11 months old require 7 milligrams of iron a day. Once babies start ingesting solid food, the iron they consume in breast milk is not as easily absorbed.

People have somehow forgotten that the best source of iron is heme iron, a form of the mineral that is present in animals and is abundant in red meat. The mistaken belief that babies cannot digest red meats has for some reason become entrenched in popular thought—but without the support of any scientific evidence. It is ironic to recall that before the advent of "hypoallergenic" formulas based on extensively hydrolyzed casein, babies who were allergic to milk were fed a meat-based infant formula from birth.[30] In the majority of cases, these milk-allergic babies did extremely well, and they continue to.[31] Every hospital developed its own meat-based formula for newborns unable to breast-feed and unable to tolerate cow's milk–based formula.

The idea that red meat should be one of babies' first solid foods seems rarely considered, in spite of the fact that humans have more digestive enzymes to break down foods from animal sources than foods from plant sources. Humans lack the digestive enzymes that break down much of the plant material we ingest. We are unable to digest the structural parts of plants—those we designate as fiber—and sometimes have difficulty with certain starches (those known as "resistant starch"). These plant materials move unchanged into the colon, where they are "digested" by microbial, not human, enzymes. In contrast, the healthy human can digest almost every part of an animal-derived food, a fact that is as true for babies as it is for adults.

Meats are readily prepared for early introduction to the baby: cook ground meat well in water; then purée into a soft paste, diluting with water as required.

Despite this ease in preparation, it has become traditional in Western countries to introduce grains as babies' first solid food, probably owing to the presumption that cereals are easier to cook into purée for infant feeding. Grains should be introduced in their pure grain form, not in manufactured baby cereals that contain the grain, among other things. Some baby cereals contain added ingredients other than the grain. If such a cereal is a baby's first exposure to the grain and an allergic reaction occurs, it will not be possible to tell whether the baby is reacting to the grain or to the additional ingredients (unless the grain and the other ingredients were introduced separately). Above all, it is important that your baby's introduction to a specific food be to the individual food alone, in cooked and puréed form.

Homemade Baby Foods

The best foods for your baby are those made from pure ingredients in your own kitchen. Many Web sites post free recipes for all ages, starting at 6 months. The best sites include everything you need to know about puréed foods for early feeding, and about finger foods to serve as your baby gets older. Run an Internet search of "homemade baby foods" and you'll find countless numbers of good recipes.

Making your own food for your baby puts you in charge, meaning you can avoid all the highly allergenic foods, and all the foods your baby may have become sensitized to if he or she already has food allergies. Making your own food ensures that your baby eats only the purest ingredients. For an allergic or potentially allergic baby, this is crucial. You wouldn't feed yourself and the rest of your family a diet of prepackaged and jarred foods; why would you consider such a diet for your family's most vulnerable member? The breast is best—and homemade is the next best!

The next sections provide guidelines for preparing a few of baby's first foods.

Cereals

It's easy to make your own baby cereal (sometimes called "pablum"). Grind dry grain in a blender or coffee grinder. Use whole grains such as brown rice (more nutritious than white rice), oatmeal, wheat flakes, barley grain or flakes, and millet grain. Grind the grain or flakes into a powder.

This powder becomes your baby cereal. Add the powder to water in a saucepan and bring it to a boil. Turn the heat down and cover with a lid. Simmer until the mixture reaches a smooth, soupy consistency. This usually takes about 15 minutes. Add breast milk or formula (if your baby is already consuming and tolerating formula) to achieve the texture your baby prefers.

Meats

Cook ground meat of any type in water. Whir in a blender until the meat becomes a smooth purée or paste. Add water as necessary to achieve the consistency of a thickened soup.

Fruits and Vegetables

Remove the peel of vegetables; remove the peel and the core, pit, stone, or seed(s) of fruit. Boil in water in a saucepan, cooking until soft. Whir the softened fruit or vegetable in a blender to achieve a smooth purée. Add water as needed.

Babies' First Vegetables

Babies' first vegetables should not include those that are stringy or contain small seeds. These will not break up in the blender and may cause choking in very young babies. Exclude these vegetables from babies' first foods:

- Celery (too stringy)

- Tomatoes with seeds (remove the seeds)

- Sweet peppers with seeds (remove the seeds)

- Cucumber with seeds

Start with vegetables that easily form a smooth purée, such as root vegetables (potato, sweet potato, yams, squashes, carrots, parsnips), and others that soften readily, such as green peas and beans and broccoli and cauliflower.

Babies' First Fruits

In offering babies' first fruits, avoid those with tiny seeds, such as:

- Berries

- Figs

Babies' first fruits should not include those with fibrous layers, such as:

- Oranges

- Grapefruit

- Similar fruits

Start with fruits that soften when cooked and readily form a smooth purée, such as peaches, pears, and apples. Always cook bananas. Use either a conventional or microwave oven. Although raw bananas can easily be mashed to the right consistency, banana contains a great deal of resistant starch,[32] which some babies in the first months are unable to digest. Undigested banana starch moves into the colon where it is fermented by microorganisms. This can cause great distress in the form of gas, bloating, pain, and sometimes diarrhea. Cooking banana converts its starch into a form that is readily digested. Cooking baby's banana will prevent the distress of gas and bloating.

Remember that your baby has no preconceived notion about taste, making it unnecessary to add anything to his or her pure foods. Fruits are naturally quite sweet and need no sugar added; nor does the pure taste of vegetables require the addition of salt or other seasoning.

A Cautionary Note

When making baby foods in a blender or coffee grinder, reserve an appliance that is used for no purpose other than making baby foods. An anecdote from my practice will illustrate the reason for this rule.

When one of my small clients—a baby who was extremely allergic to milk—reached the age of 6 months, it was time to introduce him to solid foods. He had been breast-fed from birth, and continued to be. His parents were very receptive to making their own baby foods because the baby had endured such difficulty with symptoms of allergy in early infancy. The little boy had been symptom-free since we removed his allergens from mother's diet. Naturally, the parents wanted to keep him that way. They decided to start with rice as the first solid food. As I recommended, they cooked the pure grains and made a purée in the blender. Following my instructions, they applied a small amount of the cereal to the baby's cheek. To their dismay, a very noticeable red patch developed, so of course they did not give the baby that cereal. We then decided to try a different type of rice. Later that same day I took a call from the baby's mother. They had discovered the source of the baby's reaction: Father had made a milk shake in the blender, and in spite of careful washing, traces of milk remained, which were transferred to the baby's rice. The baby had reacted to the traces of milk in the blender. Subsequent batches of rice cereal prepared in the baby's own blender caused no problems. He is now successfully eating a range of homemade foods, including meats, and is progressing beautifully.

Manufactured Baby Foods

Only when a baby tolerates a food in its pure form should the same food be given in its commercially prepared or prepackaged form.

Make sure that any manufactured food you give your baby contains only the food you intend to feed. So many store-bought baby foods contain additional ingredients, almost hidden from the consumer, that it is essential to read labels carefully. Typical of the obscure ingredients added to commercial foods are:

- Milk solids or formula, added to baby cereals

- Soy derivatives such as soy lecithin, added to baby cereals and other foods

- Citrus, added to lamb for babies

- Preservatives, thickeners, and stabilizers, added to prolong the shelf life of many products

Many of the foods marketed as "organic" or "natural" are free from additional ingredients, but it would be wrong to assume this is the case. Always read a product's label, including the small print.

ORAL TOLERANCE AND ALLERGY PREVENTION

The recommendations discussed in this chapter are based on current directives from leading allergy and pediatric specialists in the United States and other Western nations. The work of a number of clinicians and researchers suggests there may be alternative, perhaps more effective, ways to reduce allergy. The most plausible contra arguments suggest that delaying exposure to foods until after the first year or later may bypass the stage at which oral tolerance may be most effectively achieved. Furthermore, advising avoidance of any foods by the breast-feeding mother (apart from her own and her baby's known allergens) may preclude the infant's development of tolerance to those foods. It is well known that continuous exposure to small quantities of antigen is an effective means of "informing" the immune system that the material is safe. As discussed earlier, this may be how the immune system of the fetus is first primed in utero to become tolerant of the molecules of food in the amniotic fluid in the womb. The next step toward achieving tolerance to food may be exposure to the small quantities of food molecules that find their way into breast-milk from the mother's diet. By excluding these foods, the mother may in fact be denying her baby the opportunity to develop tolerance of the foods he or she will eat later.

On the other hand, we know that an excess of allergen can cause an immunological response as a result of "allergen overload." Anecdotal evidence supports the theory that consumption of a large quantity of a single food (especially a highly allergenic food like peanut butter) will cause sensitization of the breast-feeding baby, and even the fetus in utero. For this reason, mothers are advised to avoid bingeing on any food during pregnancy and lactation, and to eat all foods (except their own and their baby's allergens) in moderation.

A great deal more research must be conducted before we can provide universally acceptable guidelines for the optimal ages at which exposure to specific foods will promote immunologic and clinical tolerance to them. The best advice we can offer at present is summarized in Table 3-2, which lists dietary recommendations for allergy prevention.

HYGIENE THEORY IN ALLERGY PREVENTION

Before concluding the discussion of allergy prevention, we should consider what has been called the "Hygiene Hypothesis." Research indicates that when the Th1 pathway of immunological protection is triggered against potentially disease-causing bacteria and viruses, a corresponding reduction (a down-regulation) occurs in the Th2 pathway that would lead to allergy. It is therefore logical to assume that if babies and children were exposed early on to a wide range of microorganisms, the Th1 pathway would predominate, and the incidence of allergy would be reduced. This theory appeared to be validated by observations that children in the developing world, those living in lower socioeconomic conditions, and those living on farms, had a lower incidence of allergy than babies and children in highly sanitized homes in urban centers of the developed world.

Further evidence supporting the idea that early exposure to microorganisms may reduce allergenic sensitization comes from a study on allergic children and their pets. A team of researchers compared 184 children who were exposed to two or more dogs or cats in their first year of life with 220 children who didn't have pets. To their surprise, the scientists found that children raised with pets were 45 percent less likely to test positive for allergies than those without pets.[33]

Another recent study showed that children who drank unpasteurized milk (which would contain many more microorganisms than pasteurized milk)

Table 3-2
DIETARY RECOMMENDATIONS FOR ALLERGY PREVENTION

- It is essential that mother obtain complete balanced nutrition appropriate for pregnancy,[a] and that she eat as wide a range of foods as possible.

- No special diets are recommended for mother during pregnancy but the allergic mother must strictly avoid her own allergens.[b] This means that even before she becomes pregnant, mother should undergo investigations, including elimination and challenge, to determine her own food allergies.

- The allergic mother must take care to consume equivalent nutrients in the alternative foods she eats as substitutes for her allergens.

- During lactation, avoidance diets may be determined on an individual basis.[b] The allergic mother should continue to avoid her own allergens.

- If the baby develops symptoms, and if allergy to a specific food or foods is definitively diagnosed, mother must eliminate the baby's allergenic foods from her own diet as long as she continues to breast-feed.

- Mother should breast-feed baby exclusively for at least 4 months, while making every effort to continue exclusive breast-feeding for 6 months.

- Supplement breast-feeding with conventional cow's milk–based formula, as advised by European pediatric allergists. If baby develops signs of milk protein allergy, choose an extensively hydrolyzed casein formula. Alternatively, as advised by U.S. pediatric allergists, supplement with a hydrolyzed formula until milk is introduced at age 12 months.

- Avoid offering solid foods until baby is at least 4 months old, but try to delay offering solid foods until after 6 months.

- Introduce solid foods one at a time starting at 6 months.

- Give baby mixed foods only after each food in the mixture has been introduced separately and been proven safe.

---

[a] See Appendix I: Pregnancy Diet

[b] Many authorities in Western countries recommend that mother avoid peanuts during pregnancy and lactation. However, current evidence suggests that unless either mother or baby is allergic to peanuts, a moderate quantity of peanut in the mother's diet should promote tolerance in the fetus and breast-feeding infant.

had fewer eczema symptoms and a generally lower incidence of overall allergies than children who had never drunk unpasteurized milk.[34] Consumption of unpasteurized milk was associated with a 59 percent reduction in total IgE levels and higher production of whole blood IFN-γ compared with levels in children who only drank pasteurized milk, indicating that the former had less allergy than the latter group. Of course this is not to advise all children to drink unpasteurized milk because the risk of exposure to a disease-causing pathogen is too great. However, these types of studies do suggest that the hygiene hypothesis is probably valid in its basic assumption that exposure to microorganisms early in life may reduce or prevent allergen sensitization and development of allergy by promoting Th1-type immune development.

These observations suggest that exposing babies and children to appropriate "safe" microorganisms early in life may reduce the incidence of allergy. This is currently being attempted by feeding probiotic foods, a topic discussed in some detail in Chapter 25.

References

1. Szepfalusi Z, Loibichler C, Pichler J, Reisenberger K, Ebner C, Urbanek R. Direct evidence for transplacental allergen transfer. *Pediatric Research* 2000; 48(3):404–407.

2. Prescott S. Early origins of allergic disease: A review of processes and influences during early immune development. *Current Opinion in Allergy and Clinical Immunology* 2003; 3(2):125–132.

3. Prescott S. Early origins of allergic disease: A review of processes and influences during early immune development. *Current Opinion in Allergy and Clinical Immunology* 2003; 3(2):125–132.

4. Prescott S, Macaubas C, Smallcombe T, Holt B, Sly P, Holt P. Development of allergen-specific T-cell memory in atopic and normal children. *Lancet* 1999; 353:196–200.

5. Jones CA, Holloway JA, Warner JO. Does atopic disease start in foetal life? *Allergy* 2000 55:2–10.

6. Jones CA, Holloway JA, Warner JO. Does atopic disease start in foetal life? *Allergy* 2000 55:2–10.

7. Kjellman N-IM. Allergy prevention: Does maternal food intake during pregnancy or lactation influence the development of atopic disease during infancy? In: Hanson, LA (ed) *Biology of Human Milk.* Nestle Nutrition Workshop Series 15, New York: Vevey/Raven Press, 1988.

8. Karmaus W, Archad SH, Sadeghnejad A, Twiselton R. Does maternal immunoglobulin E decrease with increasing order of live offspring? Investigation into maternal immune tolerance. *Clinical and Experimental Allergy* 2004;34(6):853–859.

9. Jones CA, Holloway JA, Warner JO. Does atopic disease start in foetal life? *Allergy* 2000 55:2–10.

10. Host A, Husby S, Osterballe O. A prospective study of cow's milk allergy in exclusively breast-fed infants. Incidence, pathogenetic role of early inadvertent exposure to cow's milk formula, and characterization of bovine milk protein in human milk. *Acta Paediatrica Scandinavica* 1988;77(5):663–670.

11. Goldman AS. The immune system of human milk: Antimicrobial, anti-inflammatory and immunomodulating properties. *Pediatric Infectious Disease Journal* 1993; 12:664–671.

12. Joneja JMV. Breast milk: A vital defense against infection. *Canadian Family Physician* 1992;38:1849–1855.

13. Arshad SH. Primary prevention of asthma and allergy. *Journal of Allergy and Clinical Immunology.* 2005 July;116(1):3–14.

14. Miyake Y, Yura A, Iki M. Breast-feeding and the prevalence of symptoms of allergic disorders in Japanese adolescents. *Clinical and Experimental Allergy* 2003 33:312–316.

15. Wright AL, Sherrill D, Holberg CJ, Halonen M, Martinez FD. Breast-feeding, maternal IgE, and total serum IgE in childhood. *Journal of Allergy and Clinical Immunology* 1999 104:584–589; Bottcher MF, Jenmalm MC, Garofalo RP, Bjorksten B. Cytokines in breast milk from allergic and nonallergic mothers. *Pediatric Research* 2000 47:157–162; Bottcher MF, Jenmalm MC, Bjorksten B,

Garofalo RP. Chemoattractant factors in breast milk from allergic and nonallergic mothers. *Pediatric Research* 2000 47:592–597.

16. Saarinen KM, Vaarala O, Klemetti P, Savilahti E. Transforming growth factor-β1 in mothers' colostrums and immune responses to cow's milk proteins in infants with cow's milk allergy. *Journal of Allergy and Clinical Immunology* 1999 104(5):1093–1098.

17. Jarvinen KM, Suomalainen H. Development of cow's milk allergy in breast-fed infants. *Clinical and Experimental Allergy* 2001 31:978–987.

18. American Academy of Pediatrics, Committee on Nutrition. Hypoallergenic infant formulas. *Pediatrics* 2000 106:346–349.

19. Zeiger RS. Food allergen avoidance in the prevention of food allergy in infants and children. *Pediatrics* 2003 111:1662–1671.

20. Saarinen KM, Juntunen-Backman K, Jarvenpaa AL, Kuitunen P, Renlund M, Siivola M, Savilahti E. Supplementary feeding in maternity hospitals and the risk of cow's milk allergy: a prospective study of 6209 infants. *Journal of Allergy and Clinical Immunology* 1999 104:457–461.

21. Jarvinen et al. Development of cow's milk allergy in breast-fed infants.

22. Jarvinen et al. Development of cow's milk allergy in breast-fed infants.

23. Hourihane JOB. Peanut allergy: current status and future challenges. *Clinical and Experimental Allergy* 1997; 27:1240–1246.

24. American Academy of Pediatrics, Committee on Nutrition. Hypoallergenic infant formulas.

25. Von Berg A, Koletzkop S, Grubl A, Filipiak-Pittroff B, Wichmann HE, Bauer CP, Reinhardt D, Berdel D. The effect of hydolyzed cow's milk formula for allergy prevention in the first year of life: The German Infant Nutritional Intervention Study, a randomized double-blind trial. *Journal of Allergy and Clinical Immunology.* 2003;111(3):533–540.

26. Fiocchi A, Assa'ad A, Bahna S. Food allergy and the introduction of solid foods to infants: A consensus document. *Annals of Allergy, Asthma, and Immunology.* 2006;97(1):10–21.

27. Host A, Koletzko B, Dreborg S, Muraro A, Wahn U, Aggett P, Bresson JL, Hernell O, Lafeber H, Michaelsen KF, Micheli JL, Rigo J, Weaver L, Heymans H, Strobel S, Vandenplas Y. Dietary products used in infants for treatment and prevention of food allergy. Joint statement of the Committee on Hypoallergenic Formulas of the European Society of Paediatric Allergology and Clinical Immunology (ESPACI) and the Committee on Nutrition of the European Society for Paediatric Gastroenetrology, Hepatology, and Nutrition (ESPGHAN). *Archives of Disease in Childhood* 1999;8:80–84.

28. American Academy of Pediatrics, Committee on Nutrition. Hypoallergenic infant formulas.

29. Saarinen et al. Supplementary feeding in maternity hospitals and the risk of cow's milk disease; Hourihane. Peanut allergy: Current status and future challenges.

30. Weisselberg B, Dayal Y, Thompson JF, Doyle MS, Senior B, Grand RJ. A lamb meat–based formula for infants allergic to casein hydrolysate formulas. *Clinical Pediatrics* 1996;35(10):491–495.

31. Cantani A. A homemade meat-based formula for feeding atopic babies: A study in 51 children. *European Review for Medical and Pharmacological Sciences* 2006;10(2):61–68.

32. Joneja JMV. Effect of cooking and processing on the digestibility of starch. In: *Digestion, Diet, and Disease.* New Brunswick, NJ: Rutgers University Press, 2004: 96–97.

33. Ownby DR, Johnson CC, Peterson EL. Exposure to dogs and cats in the first year of life and risk of allergic sensitization at 6 to 7 years of age. *Journal of the American Medical Association* 2002;288:963–972.

34. Perkin MR, Strachan DP. Which aspects of the farming lifestyle explain the inverse association with childhood allergy? *Journal of Allergy and Clinical Immunology* 2006;117(6):1374–1381.

CHAPTER 4

Symptoms of Food Sensitivity in Babies and Children

The most important question that parents ask is: "How do I know if my child has food allergies?" With older children who are eating solid foods this can sometimes be apparent when symptoms develop in minutes, and usually within 2 hours, after he or she eats a specific food or foods. With exclusively breast-fed infants it is more difficult to spot a food allergy because the culprit food may come from mother's diet and her baby may show symptoms several hours (typically 2 to 8 hours) after she has eaten the meal that contains the allergen. Most importantly, though, any other causes for the baby's or child's symptoms must be ruled out before food allergy is considered. Your family doctor and pediatrician will always carry out a thorough physical examination, take into account your child's medical history, and order appropriate tests to determine if your child's problems are due to conditions other than allergy.

AGE RELATIONSHIP BETWEEN FOOD ALLERGY AND ALLERGY SYMPTOMS IN THE MAJOR ORGAN SYSTEMS

In the majority of cases, the first sign of allergy (atopy) in a baby is an allergic reaction to foods. In the exclusively breast-fed baby, this is a response to components of the mother's diet. In these cases, the food components are absorbed by the mother from her food and pass into her breast milk. Symptoms frequently start in the digestive tract and skin of the baby. These may be followed by symptoms in the upper respiratory tract and lungs. Respiratory tract symptoms in the first year are frequently triggered by food allergy. As early food allergies are outgrown, allergy to airborne allergens may prolong the symptoms, often into adulthood.

Digestive Tract

The first signs of a food allergy problem may appear in the digestive tract soon after birth. The common signs include persistent colicky pain, frequent spitting up or even projectile vomiting after a feeding, and abnormally liquid or frothy stool. These signs continue for several weeks. Of course, not all food-allergic babies start with these symptoms, but these early signs should alert the parents to the possibility that an adverse reaction to foods might be the problem if no other cause for the symptoms is found.

In older children, food allergy might appear as nausea and vomiting, frequent stomachaches, bloating, and/or diarrhea. Although not usually considered to be a common symptom of food allergy, chronic constipation that does not respond to laxatives is being increasingly recognized as a possible symptom of food allergy in children.[1] Further studies need to be carried out to obtain firmer evidence for the role of allergy in constipation and to clarify the pathogenic mechanisms involved.

Irritable Bowel Syndrome (IBS)

Other causes of digestive tract problems in children include irritable bowel syndrome (IBS). It is not unusual for symptoms such as abdominal pain ("stomachache"), bloating, diarrhea, and gas to persist after an infection in the gastrointestinal tract. This condition is not due to a food allergy. The symptoms are a result of an "irritated" digestive tract lining, which can be made worse when the child eats certain "irritant" foods. The foods most frequently associated with distress include free starches and sugars. These pass quickly and only partially digested into the large bowel. There the starches and sugars are fermented by the resident microorganisms. The fermentation products include excessive gas, which results in bloating, pressure, and pain. The sugars and other products of fermentation cause an imbalance in the contents of the bowel, an imbalance that causes the diarrhea.

Raw fruits and vegetables are often not tolerated when the digestive tract is irritated. This condition can be successfully managed with an IBS diet that takes into account all of the ways in which foods aggravate the irritated area. In most cases the "damaged" cells heal, and the child can gradually return to a normal diet when the irritant foods are removed for a period of time. For details of the IBS diet, please see reference.[2]

Lactose Intolerance

Lactose intolerance is not uncommon in babies and young children, when infection in the digestive tract results in damage to the epithelial cells lining the small intestine. These epithelial cells produce lactase, an enzyme that is essential for the digestion of the sugar (lactose) in milk. As long as the cells are not producing lactase, the child will be unable to tolerate lactose. Symptoms of diarrhea, colicky abdominal pain, bloating, and gassiness usually follow consumption of milk. These symptoms mimic milk allergy, but differ in the fact that the symptoms are confined to the digestive tract. In milk allergy typically there are additional symptoms, especially in the skin. Lactose intolerance is usually a temporary condition in early childhood, and the ability to tolerate lactose returns once the brush-border cells that produce the enzyme return to normal functioning. (See Chapter 8 for more details about lactose intolerance.)

Skin

Allergic skin reactions may also start early. Eczema (sometimes called atopic dermatitis) can appear soon after birth or, in some unusual cases, a baby may have signs of eczema at birth. In the early stages, eczema may be present on the baby's cheeks, upper surfaces of the feet, legs, hands, and arms. Later, the eczematous patches are more commonly found in the creases in the elbow and behind the knees, behind the ears and where the ear meets the face, and sometimes in the ear itself. A baby with eczema often has dry, flaky skin which is easily irritated. It has been my experience that when the mother has allergies, eczema frequently starts within the first few weeks of life. When the mother has no allergies and the father is the allergic parent, eczema seems to appear later, typically after about 2 months. However, this is by no means invariably the case, and I have not yet seen this observation reported in controlled scientific studies.

Hives (urticaria) and facial reddening and swelling (angioedema) may also be indicators of an allergic reaction to foods in a baby or young child. These signs may appear and disappear with very little apparent association with specific foods. However, careful observation often provides some indication of frequent triggers in the diet of either the baby or the mother. Persistent rashes that have no other cause (such as infection) may also be associated with early food allergy.

Respiratory Tract

Symptoms of nasal stuffiness, congestion, runny nose, itchy, irritated eyes, cough, and the wheeze associated with asthma are unusual as symptoms of food allergy in babies. These types of symptoms are more commonly associated with airborne allergens (such as pollens from trees, grasses and weeds, dust mites, mold spores; and animal danders) than they are with foods. Respiratory allergies to airborne allergens usually start to appear about the age of 18 months to 2 years. Respiratory allergies are uncommon in infants.

Respiratory symptoms in babies under the age of about 18 months may be associated with foods, but symptoms in the respiratory tract in this age group rarely occur alone. There is usually some sign of reactions in other organ systems, such as the digestive tract (often as prolonged or unusually severe colic) or skin reactions such as eczema.

Anaphylaxis in the Young Infant

The whole body involvement of an anaphylactic reaction is rare in babies and very young children. Most life-threatening anaphylactic reactions tend to occur in the teens and early twenties. Occasional reports of anaphylactic reactions to foods in early childhood indicate that the food most frequently responsible for this extreme food allergy is milk.[3]

According to the American Academy of Allergy, Asthma and Immunology (AAAAI), anaphylaxis is a life-threatening allergic reaction. It is a condition which affects several different parts of the body, and may proceed to unconsciousness and shock.

COMMON SIGNS OF ANAPHYLAXIS

Body area	Signs and Symptoms
Skin	Flushing, itching, or hives
Airway	Swelling of the throat, difficulty in talking or breathing
Digestive Tract	Nausea, vomiting, or diarrhea
Heart function	Reduced ability to pump blood, low blood pressure, increased pulse rate

Symptoms usually appear rapidly—sometimes within minutes of exposure to the allergen—and can be life threatening. Immediate medical attention is necessary when anaphylaxis occurs. Standard emergency treatment often includes an injection of epinephrine (adrenaline) to open up the airway and help reverse the reaction. Transportation to the nearest hospital is absolutely essential. The subject of anaphylactic reactions to foods is discussed in more detail in Chapter 18.

Table 4-1 is a summary of the more common symptoms of allergy in babies and young children.

Effects of Combined Allergies

Figure 4-1 is a graph providing a summary overview of the approximate occurrence of the various allergy symptoms with age.

As most allergies to foods are outgrown, the symptoms in the major organ systems may continue in response to allergens in the air and environment. However, a few food allergies do persist into adulthood in some people. The persistent allergies tend to be allergies to the most highly allergenic foods including peanuts, tree nuts, fish, shellfish, and, less frequently, egg, wheat,

Table 4-1
**SYMPTOMS THAT MAY INDICATE FOOD ALLERGY
IN THE BABY AND YOUNG CHILD**

Gastrointestinal tract

- Persistent colic
- Abdominal distress
- Frequent "spitting up"
- Nausea
- Vomiting
- Diarrhea
- Constipation

Skin

- Hives (urticaria)
- Facial reddening and swelling (angioedema)
- Swelling and reddening around the mouth
- Eczema
- Dry itchy skin
- Persistent diaper rash
- Redness around anus
- Redness on cheeks
- Reddened ears
- Rash of unknown origin
- Scratching and rubbing

Respiratory tract

- Nasal stuffiness
- Sneezing
- Nose rubbing
- Noisy breathing
- Persistent cough
- Wheezing
- Asthma
- Itchy, runny, reddened eyes
- Frequent earaches

Other

- "Feeding problems" (baby may forcibly reject food)
- Failure to gain weight (failure to thrive)
- Weight loss
- In extreme cases, involvement of all body systems in anaphylaxis. This can be life threatening.

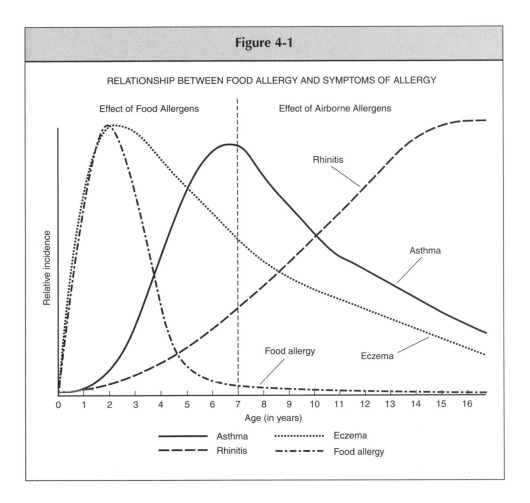

Figure 4-1

RELATIONSHIP BETWEEN FOOD ALLERGY AND SYMPTOMS OF ALLERGY

Effect of Food Allergens   Effect of Airborne Allergens

and other grains. These allergenic foods may be responsible for a severe or anaphylactic reaction.

You will see from the graph (Figure 4-1) that the major effects of food allergy occur in the first two years and then rapidly decline as the child begins to grow out of the early food allergies. You can also see from the graph that, as environmental and airborne allergies start to make their appearance at about 2 years of age, there is an overlap of allergies. This sometimes results in a combined effect involving both food allergies and environmental allergies between about 2 and 4 years of age. Do not be unduly concerned if your food-allergic child's symptoms seem to get worse at about the age of 2 years. IgE antibodies to airborne allergens, and the inflammatory mediators released in response, will add on to the mediators of food allergy. For a while your child's symptoms will appear more frequently and seem more severe. This will change over the next year or so as he or she outgrows their early allergies to foods.

INFANT COLIC AND ALLERGY

Colic is defined as a condition affecting healthy, well-fed infants, consisting of irritability and crying, which lasts for at least 3 hours a day and occurs more than 3 days a week. It consists of excessive and inconsolable crying, which seems to occur most often in the evening. Up to one third of infants under the age of 4 months experience some degree of colic. Although the cause of colic is still virtually unknown, it seems to be self-limiting and in most cases resolves by the age of 4 months.

A number of causes for colic have been proposed, none of which fit every situation. Most often food allergy or intolerance has been suggested and a variety of dietary strategies have been advised. Diet changes sometimes help. The most frequently suggested cause has been milk allergy, and elimination of milk and milk products from the diet of breast-feeding mothers has proven to be beneficial in a number of cases. For the formula-fed infant, some studies have shown that switching from a cow's–milk based formula to one that is based on soy has relieved the distress of a number of the colicky infants.

Transient lactose intolerance has also been investigated as a cause of colic. In one study, treating infant food with lactase reduced the symptoms in a significant number of cases.[4] The subject of lactose intolerance in the breast-fed baby is discussed in Chapter 8, Lactose Intolerance.

In other cases, feeding a hydrolyzed whey-based formula, or a casein-based formula that had been extensively hydrolyzed, seems to reduce the symptoms in many colicky babies.[5]

Other studies indicate that an overload of sugar, for example in apple juice, may have been a factor in causing the problem.

From the many studies on dietary triggers for infant colic, it would appear that food allergy or intolerance may be a contributing factor. However, it is probable that infant colic has multiple causes. No single dietary strategy is likely to improve the situation in all cases.

What Your Child's Symptoms Tell You

None of the symptoms discussed above are, by themselves, signs of food allergy. If your child is exhibiting any of the signs and symptoms discussed in this chapter, your first response should be to consult your doctor or pediatrician. The pediatrician will probably carry out appropriate tests, and may refer you to an allergy specialist. There are a number of ways that food allergy may be diagnosed; we shall discuss the diagnosis of food allergy in the next chapter.

References

1. Carroccio A, Iocono G. Review article: chronic constipation and food hypersensitivity — an intriguing relationship. *Alimentary Pharmacology & Therapeutics* 2006;24(9):1295-1304(10)

2. Joneja JMV. *Digestion, Diet and Disease: Irritable bowel syndrome and gastrointestinal function.* New Jersey: Rutgers University Press, 2004.

3. Pumphrey RS. Lessons for management of anaphylaxis from a study of fatal reactions. *Clinical and Experimental Allergy* 2000;30:1144-1150

4. Kanabar D, Randhawa M, Clayton P. Improvement of symptoms in infant colic following reduction of lactose load with lactase. *Journal of Human Nutrition & Dietetics* 2001;14(5):359-363

5. Jakobsson I, Lothe L, Ley D, Borschel MW. Effectiveness of casein hydrolysate feedings in infants with colic. *Acta Paediatric* 2000;89(1):18-21

CHAPTER 5

Diagnosis of Food Allergy

The most important step in the diagnosis of food allergy is obtaining a careful medical history. This is usually undertaken by your child's pediatrician, who will then decide whether a referral to a pediatric allergist is warranted.

An allergist usually relies on tests to determine whether your child has allergies. There are skin and blood tests for allergies caused by allergens such as pollens, animal dander, dust mites, mold spores, and other inhalants that cause respiratory allergies, including hay fever and asthma. These tests are considered fairly reliable and are routinely used in determining the most appropriate treatment for your child's allergies. However, because the tests for determining which foods may be responsible for symptoms are not reliable, many allergists do not perform tests for food allergies. If tests are carried out for food allergies, they always need to be followed by a direct challenge to determine their accuracy.

ALLERGY TESTS

There are few reliable laboratory tests available for the determination of specific foods responsible for the symptoms of food allergy. The tests used by allergists are designed to detect allergen-specific immunoglobulin E (IgE). These tests involve either applying an extract of the allergen to the child's skin and pricking or scratching the surface, to allow the allergen to come into contact with the underlying immune cells, or using immunological techniques to detect allergen-specific IgE antibodies in a sample of the child's blood. None of these tests alone is sufficiently accurate to identify the specific foods that are triggering a child's symptoms.

Tests for IgE antibody can be informative, but they carry limitations that make them unreliable as indicators of the precise foods responsible for the child's symptoms.[1] The tests detect only *sensitization* to the allergen (meaning that the child's immune system has formed IgE antibodies to the allergen), but they do not necessarily indicate that the child will develop symptoms when the food is eaten (allergic *expression*). A positive test correlates with reactions less than half of the time.[2] Positive test results are therefore *false positives* in some cases.[3]

Skin Tests

Skin tests involve the direct contact of an allergen with white blood cells, called mast cells, in the skin. Mast cells contain granules that release inflammatory mediators (reactive chemicals) when the allergen to which the child has produced IgE antibodies couples with these antibodies on the mast cell surface. The inflammatory mediators act on local tissues and produce the typical skin reaction (known as a wheal and flare) that indicates a positive reaction.

What to Expect When Your Child Undergoes a Skin Test

Several techniques are used for allergy skin testing, but research indicates that the most reliable is the *prick/puncture method.*[4]

Scratch tests are tests in which the skin is scratched and an allergen extract applied to the scarified skin. They are rarely used today.

Intradermal tests are tests in which the allergen extract is injected into the skin. They are frequently used for the diagnosis of inhalant allergies in adults. Inhalant allergies are those in which the allergen is airborne matter such as pollens, molds, dust mites, animal danders, and so on. However, intradermal tests are definitely not recommended for the diagnosis of food allergy because of the high number of false positive results and the danger of inducing a life-threatening anaphylactic reaction as the allergen encounters immune cells within the circulatory system. Intradermal testing should not be used in the diagnosis of food allergy in babies and children.

The Prick/Puncture Skin Test

Some allergy medicines, including over-the-counter antihistamines, may stop allergic reactions, so you should not give them to your child for a few days before the test. Talk to your doctor about discontinuing your child's allergy medicines prior to the test. If certain medications cannot be discontinued, even for a few days, the doctor or nurse may perform a separate *control test* to determine whether that particular drug interferes with the skin test results. The entire procedure will take about an hour. The allergen placement part of the test takes about 5 to 15 minutes. Once the placement is complete, you will have to wait about 15 or 20 minutes to see how your child's skin reacts.

The Procedure
The skin test procedure involves the following:

- First, a doctor or nurse will examine the skin on your child's forearm or back and clean it with alcohol.

- Areas of the cleaned skin are then marked with a pen to identify each allergen that will be tested.

- A drop of extract for each potential allergen is placed on the corresponding mark.

- A small disposable pricking device is then used to puncture the skin so that the extract can enter into the outer layer of the skin, called the epidermis. A number of devices can be used to apply the allergen, including 25- to 27-gauge hypodermic needles, metal lancets, plastic pricking devices, and bifurcated scarifiers.

- The skin prick is not a shot, and it does not cause bleeding.

To interpret prick tests properly, both positive and a negative control tests are needed:

- The negative control should be the fluid used for diluting the allergen extract (diluent). This measures nonspecific reactivity induced by the diluent or by the force or technique of the tester. If this negative test causes a wheal that is 0.12 inch (3 mm) or larger, the prick tests are difficult to interpret. In these cases, the tests are usually considered invalid.

- Positive controls are used to detect the skin's reactivity to histamine. The usual positive control is histamine phosphate (2.7 mg/mL, equivalent to 1 mg/mL of histamine base).

The test may be mildly irritating, but most children say it does not hurt too much. After the results are read, the doctor or nurse may apply a mild cortisone cream to relieve any excessive itching or pain at the sites of the skin pricks.

In a positive test, a wheal-and-flare reaction can be seen at the site of the puncture:

- The wheal (edema or blister) is a central raised area.

- The flare (erythema) is a flattened, reddened area extending outward from the central blister.

This reaction is caused by the release of inflammatory mediators, especially histamine, from mast cells in the skin. The allergen couples with IgE molecules attached to receptors on the mast cells' surfaces and triggers the release of the inflammatory mediators stored within the cells. Histamine acts on cells in the surrounding tissue, resulting in the local inflammation of the wheal and flare.

For specific allergens, a positive response is a wheal-and-flare reaction that is equal to or larger than that seen with a histamine control test and appears within 15 minutes after the prick. Although a large wheal-and-flare response might suggest a more marked hypersensitivity, significant clinical allergic symptoms may be seen in children who have only small wheal-and-flare reactions.

Several different scoring systems are used to record the skin test results and many allergists like to use their own methods. Some measure the size of both the wheal and the flare, usually grading the reaction from 1+ to 4+. Other allergists simply look for a positive response (a wheal of 0.12 inch [3 mm] or larger compared to the negative control).[5]

It is virtually impossible to quantify the exact amount of injected material used in prick tests. Therefore, the reliability of the test depends on the device used, the depth and force of the puncture device, the duration of force, the angle of the application device, and the stability of extracts.[6] Because of the impossibility of standardizing the test, the size of the wheal-and-flare reaction cannot be used as a measure of the severity of response (clinical reactivity) to the food when it is consumed. At best, the skin test is merely an indicator of the presence of allergen-specific IgE and the potential for clinical reactivity to the allergen.

Although small amounts of allergens are introduced into your child's system during the tests, allergists generally consider that, when performed properly, skin tests are safe. However, experts have recently begun to question this assumption.

Whole body (systemic) reactions to skin testing are extremely rare, although sometimes such things do happen. You should immediately call your child's doctor if your child develops symptoms such as the following soon after the test:

- Fever

- Lightheadedness

- Wheezing

- Shortness of breath

- Extensive rash

- Swelling of the face, lips, or mouth

- Difficulty swallowing

Skin Testing of Babies

Prick tests are sometimes carried out on children as young as 1 month of age, although they are rarely used in this age group. When they are used, the results are not considered to be very reliable. Children under the age of 2 or 3 years are more likely to have a negative skin test and a positive food challenge.[7] Allergen-induced skin test reactions are smaller in infants and young children than in adults. This is believed to be related to the lower levels of IgE and to the hyporeactivity of the infant's skin to histamine. Because data on the effect of age on skin reactivity to allergens are lacking, there are at present no age-related guidelines for what constitutes a positive reaction in babies.[8]

Skin tests cannot—and should not—be carried out on sites of active dermatitis or severe dermatographism (reddening and welting when the skin is scratched or exposed to heat or cold).

Reasons for a false positive test include the following:

- In skin testing, the positive reaction results from the relase of inflammatory mediators from white blood cells in the skin, called mast cells, that contain chemicals involved in the allergic reaction. The contact between the allergen (in the extract) and the "primed" mast cell results in the release of these chemicals, which act on local tissues. In false positive reactions, the release of these mediators may be provoked by factors (including physical contact with the pricking device) other than those that trigger their release in the digestive tract or other internal organs.[9]

- There may be differences in the form in which the allergen encounters the immune cells (for example, the extract may be from a raw food, but the food is normally eaten cooked, or the allergen may be derived from an unstable plant extract).

- Some commercial allergen extracts may contain small amounts of histamine,[10] which produces a reaction in the skin exactly like the histamine released from a skin mast cell.

On the other hand, false negative tests may occur, even if symptoms are induced when the child eats a particular food. False negatives may be caused by a variety of factors, including:

- The reaction is not based on the production of allergen-specific IgE.

- The wrong foods may have been tested.

- The test may not have been sensitive enough.

- The commercially prepared allergen extract may not contain any of the allergen[11] because the allergen has been changed or degraded during the extraction process.

Given these limitations, many allergists consider skin tests useful in determining whether or not a child has an IgE-mediated allergy but not accurate enough to be used for detecting the precise foods responsible for the reactions.

Note on Allergen Extracts Used in Skin Tests

Allergen extracts used by allergists in their offices and clinics are produced by a number of companies in the United States and other countries. Each is produced according to a set of guidelines developed by the manufacturer. The Food and Drug Administration (FDA) is currently working to improve standardization of allergen extract products made by different manufacturers.

Sterile aqueous stock solutions compose the vast majority of allergen extracts. A typical aqueous extract solution, as prepared by Bayer Laboratories, contains the active ingredients or allergens noted on the label (pollen, dander, molds, dust, etc.). The preservative is 50 percent V/V glycerin, and 0.4 percent phenol or, in a few instances where phenol cannot be used, 0.1 percent thimerosal. Additional ingredients include 0.5 percent sodium chloride and 0.275 percent sodium bicarbonate.

The perfect allergenic extract has been defined as one that contains all of the potential allergens in their native form, in the proper ratio, and with all irrelevant material removed. At the present time, there is a great deal of variability in the allergen extracts manufactured by different companies. Inevitably this leads to discrepancies in the results obtained by one allergy clinic compared to another. The FDA, working with the World Health Organization (WHO) and the International Union of Immunologic Societies, is in the process of developing procedures for establishing reference preparations for comparison (standardization[a]), but such standards are not in place at present.

Prick-in-Prick (Prick+Prick) Test

Another type of skin test is often used when the allergen is likely to become degraded and invalidate the test. It is called the prick+prick test. In this test, a

---

[a] "Standardization" refers to the quality of an extract product being comparable to an appropriate reference preparation of assured potency.

sterile needle is inserted into the fresh food (for example, an apple) and then used to prick the child's skin. This transfers the fresh food material directly, without any extraction or processing of the allergen. This test is principally used for identification of raw foods that might be responsible for oral allergy syndrome (see Chapter 21). However, because the sensitizing allergen is an airborne pollen and IgE reactions to the food itself may not be present, false positive and false negative reactions are common in this test.

Atopy Patch Test (APT)

A test that is beginning to be studied in the attempt to find a more predictable identifying marker for food allergens is the atopy patch test. Patch tests have been in use for many years for the identification of materials that cause a local reaction when they come into direct contact with the skin or mucous membranes. These materials include plant contact allergens, such as poison ivy; nickel; latex; materials in cosmetics; detergents; dyes; and other chemicals. Because these reactions are typically delayed, the patch stays in place for up to 72 hours.

The atopy patch test for foods was developed in an attempt to identify *late-phase reactions* that were not apparent in skin tests that typically reveal immediate-onset reactions (visible within about 15 minutes of the allergen being applied to the skin). Because the atopy patch test for foods is designed to identify a reaction that occurs after the food is ingested, a carrier solvent is necessary to transport the material across the outer skin layer (dermal barrier) to reach the immune cells within the skin tissues. Petrolatum (Vaseline) is most commonly used for this purpose.

In an atopy patch test, the allergen is suspended in the carrier substance as a coated patch and applied directly onto the child's skin (usually the back). The patch stays in place for up to 48 hours.[12] A reddened local area indicates a positive reaction. It is thought that this test allows identification not only of the immediate, IgE-mediated reactions, but also the delayed, possibly IgG-mediated reactions responsible for some types of food allergy. The test is most frequently used to identify food allergens as triggers in atopic eczema.

At the present time, this test lacks standardization, not only of the food allergen extracts used in the tests, but also of the type of suspension material employed and the technique itself. Some researchers have reported good results, but most agree that the "APT is time consuming and demands a highly experienced test evaluator"[13] before it can be used successfully. There is no indication that this test has any advantage over the skin and blood tests currently employed in food allergy diagnosis.

Blood Tests for Food Allergy

Blood tests for food allergy involve analysis of the patient's blood or of the straw-colored fluid that remains after blood has clotted, the blood serum. Various immunological techniques are used to detect antibodies in the blood or serum that have been formed in response to a specific food. In most cases, the tests detect allergen-specific IgE, which indicates the potential for allergy. In addition, the tests provide a measure of the total IgE level in the patient's blood—which gives a general idea of the likelihood that the child will be allergic—without specifying the exact allergens to which he or she has formed the antibodies.

Occasionally, other components are tested for in the blood, including other antibodies, such as IgG, and sometimes components of the complement system (see Glossary for an explanation). The most commonly employed testing technique is the radioallergosorbent test (RAST).

Because RAST and other blood tests are expensive in comparison to skin tests, blood tests are not used routinely in allergy diagnosis. They are usually reserved for situations in which skin testing is likely to be invalid, for example, when the child has skin conditions such as eczema, hives (urticaria), or reddening and welting when the skin is scratched or exposed to heat or cold (dermatographism). In most cases, a child's doctor, in consultation with the parents or caregiver, selects just a few allergens for the test. Usually, the major allergens (eggs, cow's milk, peanuts, soybeans, wheat, shellfish) are tested first, and then further tests are ordered based on the initial results. Sometimes mixtures of allergens are tested in the first instance (e.g., "vegetable mix," "fruit mix," "nut mix," "grain mix," etc.). If the mixture is positive, the doctor may then decide to test allergens within the mixture separately. For example, peanut, hazelnut, and walnut may be tested if the nut mix is positive or distinct vegetables if the vegetable mix is positive.

The RAST

A RAST requires blood to be drawn from your child and sent to a laboratory for analysis. The results will usually be reported 7 to 10 days (sometimes longer) after the blood is collected.

The RAST uses radioactive or enzyme markers to detect levels of IgE antibodies in the blood. Allergen in the test reagent binds to its own antibody (called homologous antibody) in the blood, forming a complex. The added radioactive substance then binds itself to the allergen-antibody complex in the patient's blood. The amount of radioactivity associated with the complex is reported as a numerical value.[14]

The Test Procedure

During the RAST, a blood sample is drawn. For most blood tests, the sample is drawn from a vein in a process called venipuncture. During a venipuncture, a health provider (usually a nurse or laboratory technician) wraps an elastic band around the upper arm to stop blood flow through the upper veins. This keeps the lower veins full of blood and less likely to collapse, making them ideal sites for drawing a sample.

The site chosen for withdrawing the blood is swabbed with alcohol. The needle is inserted into the vein. In some cases, the needle may have to be removed and inserted again, either to ensure that it is properly placed or in case the health provider cannot obtain enough blood from the original site. Your child may feel a brief sting as the needle is inserted, but discomfort is usually minor.

Once the needle is in place, a collection tube is attached and blood flows into it. Sometimes, more than one tube is collected. Once the required amount of blood has been obtained, the rubber band is removed. The needle also is removed from the vein, and a cotton ball or gauze pad is applied to the puncture site. Direct pressure is applied to the puncture spot for several minutes to help the blood clot, and a sterile bandage is placed over the site. The blood samples are then sent directly to the laboratory for analysis.

Usually, there are very few risks or side effects. Occasionally, bruising is reported at the injection site. This can be minimized by keeping direct pressure on the spot for several minutes after the needle has been removed.

Interpretation of the Results

The laboratory provides a numeric value for total IgE and for each allergen tested. Each laboratory has its own standards for "normal" levels of IgE, and a scale is provided for low, medium, and high levels.

As with any test for food allergy, the RAST may not be entirely accurate. This is because the level of antibody in the blood does not necessarily indicate the severity of the allergic reaction that occurs when the child actually eats the food. Sometimes, even low levels of IgE can be associated with a severe reaction, and occasionally, when the child eats a food to which higher levels of IgE have been recorded, there is no reaction. As with skin tests, the RAST is primarily used to predict the likelihood of a reaction. In general, the lower the level of allergen-specific IgE is, the less likely a reaction is to occur.

It is usually thought that, of all of the patients showing a suspected adverse reaction to a food, only half of them will have a positive specific IgE result, even if the doctor has chosen the right allergens for the test. For the other half of the patients, some other non-IgE mechanism may be causing their adverse reaction, in which case, of course, the specific IgE tests will be negative.

Other Blood Tests for Allergen-Specific IgE

There are other blood tests now available in some areas, using slightly different analytical techniques that may prove to be more effective at pinpointing specific antibody:allergen reactions or detecting other components in blood that may be involved in triggering an allergic response. Some of the more common of these include the following:

- Immuno Cap RAST, manufactured by Pharmacia. This is considered by some authorities to be the most sensitive of the RAST procedures currently in general use.[15]

- Fluorescent allergosorbent test (FAST). This blood test is similar to RAST, but it uses fluorescent instead of radioactive compounds to detect the allergen-antibody complexes in the blood. This makes the equipment suitable for use in an office (instead of a laboratory) and results can be delivered in about 6 hours.

- CAP-RAST FEIA. This blood test is similar to RAST, but it includes a method in which an added enzyme reacts with its substrate, linked to the allergen-antibody complex and detected with a compound that fluoresces. This process produces a visual method of analysis called a fluoro-enzyme immunoassay, which may increase the sensitivity of the RAST in determining reactivity to certain foods.

- Radio allergosorbent procedure (RASP). This blood test is a variant of the RAST. It usually includes a measurement of IgG complexes in addition to IgE. However, the role of IgG complexes in symptoms of allergy is not entirely clear in many cases; therefore, this test may not always provide valid results.

- Multiple antigen simultaneous test (MAST). This is a type of RAST that allows testing for 38 allergens at a time, whereas the RAST looks at only a single allergen per test. However, the MAST test has not yet been proven useful in the diagnosis of food allergy.

- Immunoassay capture test. This is one of the newest blood tests. The technique is used in the detection of specific antigens, especially in the diagnosis of infectious diseases. Essentially, it is an immunological technique in which monoclonal antibodies, specifically formed against the allergenic molecules in food, are used to capture the antigen. It uses the technique of a sandwich (antibody + antigen + antibody complex) enzyme-linked immunosorbent assay (ELISA) [see Glossary for information on the ELISA]. The ELISA measures the presence and level of the allergen-specific IgE that can be detected. Proponents of this technique say that the process used to make the child's blood and the test medium react can provide more accurate results than either skin tests or blood tests for the diagnosis of allergy. At the present time, this procedure is used mainly in research settings and is only in a developmental stage for the diagnosis of food allergies.

The Meaning of the Results of Blood Tests: General Comments

Test results are always evaluated in relation to the "normal range" for that test, as used in the laboratory performing the test. The range of values considered to be normal is the range of test results from the blood of normal, active, healthy people. At the present time, there are no standardized differences in values among adults, babies, and children or among different ethnic groups, although research is beginning to indicate that normal ranges may indeed vary based on age and racial background.

There are three important things to remember about allergy test results:

- IgE levels may indicate that an allergic response is taking place (the child has been sensitized to the allergen) but, if there are no physical symptoms experienced, the child does not have an allergy.

- If the IgE test is negative, there is still a small possibility that the child does have an allergy if he or she experiences symptoms after consuming the test food.

- The level of IgE present does not predict the potential severity of an allergic reaction in the child.

Many parents who are faced with a child's allergic symptoms are confused and frustrated by the apparent lack of definitive answers from conventional allergy testing. Understandably these parents look into alternative methods of diagnosis to find relief for their child's distress. Advice from well-meaning friends and searches on the Internet reveal a number of different types of protocols that promise amazing results from a variety of methods of diagnosis and treatment. Many of these pseudoscientific procedures sound very plausible, but, unfortunately, they may carry the risk of misdiagnosis, inappropriate treatment, and the potential for harm. Caution and diligence are strongly advised with respect to any diagnoses and treatments that are not scientifically validated by accepted methods of investigation.

The following are some of the most popular tests frequently used in the diagnosis of childhood food allergies:

- Cytotoxic tests

- ALCAT

- Applied kinesiology

- Electroacupuncture (Vega test)

Details of these tests and their possible value in practice are discussed later in this chapter.

Other tests such as the following, although popular in some circles, are rarely used in pediatric food allergy management:

- Provocation-neutralization procedures

- Reaginic pulse test

Subcutaneous provocation-neutralization testing may be defined as a technique for the diagnosis and treatment of allergic disease. For this test, a subcutaneous (beneath the skin) injection of an antigen of sufficient quantity is administered to elicit symptoms corresponding to the patient's complaints. This is followed by the immediate injection of weaker or stronger concentrations of the same antigen to relieve the provoked symptoms.

Sublingual provocation-neutralization testing consists of placing three drops of 1:100 (w/v) aqueous extracted and glycerinated allergenic extract under the tongue and waiting 10 minutes for the appearance of symptoms. When the physician is satisfied that the cause(s) of the symptoms has been determined, he or she then administers a neutralizing dose, usually three drops of a dilute solution (e.g., 1:300,000 w/v) of the same extract. The symptoms are expected to disappear in approximately the same sequence in which they appeared. If the neutralizing dose is given prior to a challenge (for example, the child eats a meal containing the offending food), the prevention of symptoms is also expected.

The reaginic pulse test involves taking the patient's pulse before and after ingestion of the suspect food. An increase in the pulse rate (usually an increase in excess of 10 beats per minute) is considered to be indicative of a positive reaction to the food.

The Cytotoxic Test

Cytotoxic testing is also called Bryan's test, the Metabolic Intolerance Test, or sensitivity testing. This test was popular during the early 1980s, especially in private clinics for alternative medicine. It was also used in the offices of some medical doctors. Advocates claimed that the test could determine sensitivity to food.

Description of the Test

Ten milliliters of the patient's blood are placed in a test tube and centrifuged to separate out the white cells (leukocytes). The cells are then mixed with plasma and sterile water and applied to a large number of microscope slides, each of which had been coated with a dried food extract such as that used by allergists for skin testing. The cells are examined under a microscope at various intervals over a 2-hour period to see whether they change shape or disintegrate. This is considered to be a sign of allergy to the particular food. The test results are used to explain the patient's symptoms and to design a "personalized diet program" that includes vitamins and minerals sold by those administering the test.

Critique of the Cytotoxic Test

The American Academy of Allergy, Asthma, and Immunology (AAAAI), the largest group of allergists in the United States, has concluded that cytotoxic testing is ineffective for diagnosis of food or inhalant allergies.[16] A position paper issued by the group reports:

- One study found that white cells from allergic patients reacted no differently when exposed to substances known to produce symptoms than when exposed to substances to which the patients were not sensitive.

- Another study found that cytotoxic test results did not correlate with allergic and other untoward reactions to foods and that the results were inconsistent when repeated in the same patient.

- In a double-blind controlled study, cytotoxic tests were frequently positive for foods that produced no clinical symptoms, and reactions to foods that did produce symptoms were negative.

- Another double-blind study found that the test results in the same patient varied daily.

In 1985, the FDA issued a Compliance Policy Guide stating that cytotoxic testing kits could not be legally marketed without FDA approval and that the agency would consider regulatory action if test kits were marketed in violation.[17]

These actions greatly reduced the marketing of cytotoxic testing, but some practitioners still use the test.

Antigen Leukocyte Cellular Antibody Test (ALCAT)

The ALCAT is a patented test that measures the blood cell reactions to a foreign substance under conditions that attempt to mimic what actually happens when the food is consumed in real life.

Description of the Test

White blood cells extracted from a sample of the patient's blood are incubated at body temperature with extracts of foods, molds, food colorings, chemicals, and certain medications.

The blood samples are taken in a doctor's office or laboratory and shipped to the testing laboratory, where the blood is diluted with 1:5 buffer, and 500 mL are added to each freeze-dried test extract on nylon discs in Coulter-type cuvettes.

Following 45 minutes of incubation (at 98.6°F [37°C]) with constant agitation, the cuvettes are incubated for a further 45 minutes (at room temperature). The red cells are then broken apart (lysed) by adding 16 mL of Isotone II containing 0.5 percent alkalyse to each cuvette. This process removes the red cells, but leaves the white cells intact.

The samples are then put through a modified cell counter (Coulter counter) every 30 seconds, with one control for every 10 test cuvettes. The counter is linked to a computer program that records the size and numbers of the white blood cells in each test sample. Changes in the size of the cells (smaller or larger) and increase or decrease in the numbers of cells in the sample are compared to the "Master Control" (baseline) graph. Deviations from the standard are evaluated in determining the results, on which a diagnosis is based. A maximum of 100 substances can be tested, but usually a battery of 50 foods is used.

Critiques of the ALCAT

Proponents of the ALCAT claim that this method can detect immediate reactions to foods as well as reactions delayed for hours or days. They claim that the elimination and challenge method (the "Gold Standard" of food allergy diagnosis) of detecting culprit foods and additives takes weeks or months, whereas the ALCAT method can provide valid answers in a matter of hours.

Although some practitioners have found this method helpful in diagnosis, many consider the technique to be unproven and, as such, to have the potential to lead to misleading diagnoses and treatments.[18] This is of particular concern when babies and young children are the patients.

Applied Kinesiology

Applied kinesiology (AK) is the term most commonly used to identify a system of muscle testing and therapy. It was initiated in 1964 by George J. Goodheart, Jr. Its basic notion is that every organ dysfunction is accompanied by a specific muscle weakness, which enables diseases to be diagnosed through muscle-testing procedures. AK proponents claim that nutritional deficiencies, allergies, and other adverse reactions to foods or nutrients can be detected by this method.

Description of the Test

Most commonly, the patient holds the test material, usually contained in a vial or test tube, close to the body. The practitioner tests the muscle strength of the patient holding the vial by pressing down on the outstretched arm. Apparently, the food or nutrient in the vial is thought to have an immediate effect: "good" substances make specific muscles stronger, but "bad" substances cause weaknesses that indicate problems. Thus, if the patient is able to resist the downward pressure of the practitioner, the muscle is strong, and the test substance has no adverse effect. If the patient is unable to resist the pressure, the substance is presumed to be a cause of problems. When AK is used in the diagnosis of allergy, the food is considered to be an allergen.

For babies and small children, a surrogate method is used. The baby or child is held by an adult. The vial containing the test substance is placed in the child's sock or other clothing so that it is in close proximity to the body. The arm strength of the adult holding the child is then tested by the practitioner.

Critique of Applied Kinesiology Test

Several controlled trials were designed to validate AK testing, particularly with regard to the claim for its use in detecting nutritional deficiencies. Some studies found no difference in muscle response from one substance to another; others found no difference between the results with test substances and with placebos. One study, for example, found that three practitioners testing 11 subjects made significantly different assessments. Their diagnoses of nutritional deficiencies did not correspond to the nutrient levels obtained by blood serum analysis, and the responses to nutrient substances did not significantly differ from responses to placebos.[19] Another study showed that suggestion can influence the outcome of muscle testing.[20]

Detractors of the method think that differences from one test to another may be due to suggestibility; variations in the amount of force, leverage, or follow-through involved; and/or muscle fatigue.[21] Distraction can also play a role: for example, touching another part of the body just before pulling down the arm may cause the patient to focus less on resisting. A sudden slight upward movement can cause a *set* muscle to relax so that it can be immediately pulled downward. Apparently, when this is done quickly, the person being tested is unlikely to detect the upward motion.

Electrodermal Diagnosis: Electroacupuncture (The Vega Test)

Some physicians, dentists, naturopaths, and chiropractors use electrodiagnostic devices to help select the treatment they prescribe, which usually includes homeopathic products. These practitioners claim that they can determine the cause of any disease by detecting the "energy imbalance" causing the problem.

The first electrodiagnostic device was developed by Reinhold Voll, a German physician who had been engaged in acupuncture practice in the 1950s. In 1958, he combined Chinese acupuncture theory with galvanic skin differentials to produce his system. About 10 years later, one of his students, another German physician named Helmut Schimmel, simplified the diagnostic system, made small modifications to the equipment, and went on to help create the first model of the Vega test. Proponents claim these devices measure disturbances in the body's flow of electromagnetic energy along acupuncture meridians.

Description of the Test

The Vega test device emits a tiny direct electric current that flows through a wire from the device to a brass cylinder, covered by moist gauze, which the patient holds in one hand. A second wire is connected from the device to a probe, which the operator touches to acupuncture points on the patient's other hand or foot. This completes a low-voltage circuit and the device registers the flow of current. A galvanometer registers a response, or a bar rises on the right side of a computer screen, accompanied by a sound. The reading supposedly determines the status of various organs of the body.

After the patient's problems are diagnosed, glass ampoules containing homeopathic solutions are usually placed in a holder connected to the circuit, and the tests are repeated to determine whether they are suitable for correcting the imbalances.

Critique of Electroacupuncture Tests

No randomized, well-designed controlled trials have been able to validate the results of Vega test devices in diagnosis of allergies, nutrient deficiencies, or other documented illnesses for which the devices are claimed to function. There have been numerous malpractice suits against practitioners who have caused harm in using the devices for incorrect diagnoses.

Traditional medical practitioners strongly condemn the use of the devices for diagnosis and treatment. A Position Statement from the Australian College of Allergy states:

> *"Vega testing (the Vega test method) is an unorthodox method of diagnosing allergic and other diseases. It has no established scientific basis and there are no controlled trials to support its usefulness. Vega testing may lead to inappropriate treatment and expense to the patient and community."*[22]

Other Tests

The following immunologic test procedures have occasionally been misused:

- Measurements of circulating antigen-specific IgG antibodies

- Serum immunoglobulin concentrations
- Levels of complement components
- Flow cytometry

These tests are not helpful for diagnosis of specific IgE-mediated allergic disease, but they may be useful in the detection of other immunologic processes.

References

1. Joneja JM. Food allergy testing: Problems in identification of allergenic foods. *Canadian Journal of Dietetic Practice and Research* 1999;60(4):222–226.

2. Sampson HA. Food allergy. Part 1: Immunopathogenesis and clinical disorders. *Journal of Allergy and Clinical Immunology* 1999;103:717–728.

3. Sicherer SH, Munoz-Furlong A, Murphy R, Wood RA, Sampson HA. Symposium: Pediatric food allergy. *Pediatrics* 2003;111(6):1591–1594.

4. Sampson HA. Food allergy. Part 2: Diagnosis and management. *Journal of Allergy and Clinical Immunology* 1999;103:981–989.

5. Bock SA. Diagnostic evaluation. *Pediatrics* 2003;111(6):1638–1644.

6. Bernstein IL, Storms WW. Summary statement of practice parameters for allergy diagnostic testing. *Annals of Allergy, Asthma, and Immunology* 1995;75(Pt 2):543–625.

7. Bock SA. In vivo diagnosis: Skin testing and oral challenge procedures. In: *Food Allergy: Adverse Reactions to Foods and Food Additives.* 2nd edition. Oxford, London, Cambridge: Blackwell Science, 1997: 11–16; 151–166; 250.

8. David TJ. *Food and Food Additive Intolerance in Childhood.* Oxford: Blackwell Scientific Publications, 1993; 249, 264, 265.

9. Barrett KE. Mast cells, basophils and immunoglobulin E. In: Metcalfe DD, Sampson HA, and Simon RA (eds) *Food Allergy: Adverse Reactions to Foods and*

Food Additives. 2nd edition. Oxford, London, Cambridge: Blackwell Science, 1997: 27–48.

10. Williams PB, Nolte H, Dolen WQK, Koepke JW, Selner JC. The histamine content of allergen extracts. *Journal of Allergy and Clinical Immunology* 1992;89(3):738–745.

11. Bock SA. In vivo diagnosis: Skin testing and oral challenge procedures. In: *Food Allergy: Adverse Reactions to Foods and Food Additives*. 2nd edition. Oxford, London, Cambridge: Blackwell Science, 1997: 11–16; 151–166; 250.

12. Rancé F. What is the optimal occlusion time for the atopy patch test in the diagnosis of food allergies in children with atopic dermatitis? *Pediatric Allergy and Immunology* 2004;15(1)93.

13. Mehl A, Rolinck-Werninghaus C, Staden U, Verstege A, Wahn U, Beyer K, Niggemann B. The atopy patch tests in the diagnostic workup of suspected food-related symptoms in children. *Journal of Allergy and Clinical Immunology* 2006;118(4):923–929.

14. Joneja JMV, Bielory L. *Understanding Allergy, Sensitivity and Immunity: A Comprehensive Guide*. New Brunswick, NJ: Rutgers University Press, 1990. Reprinted 1994, pp. 183–185.

15. Szeinbach SL, Barnes JH, Sullivan TJ, Williams PB. Precision and accuracy of commercial laboratories' ability to classify positive and/or negative allergen-specific IgE results. *Annals of Allergy, Asthma, and Immunology* 2001;86(4):373–381.

16. American Academy of Allergy: Position statements—Controversial techniques. *Journal of Allergy and Clinical Immunology* 67:333–338, 1980. Reaffirmed in 1984.

17. Cytotoxic testing for allergic diseases. FDA Compliance Policy Guide 7124.27, 3/19/85.

18. Wuthrich B. Unproven techniques in allergy diagnosis. *Journal of Investigative Allergology and Clinical Immunology* 2005;15(2):86–90.

19. Kenny JJ, Clemens R, Forsythe KD. Applied kinesiology unreliable for assessing nutrient status. *Journal of the American Dietetic Association* 1988;88:698–704.

20. Barrett S. Applied kinesiology for "allergies" and "nutrient deficiencies." http://www.quackwatch.org/01QuackeryRelatedTopics/Tests/ak.html

21. American Academy of Allergy: Position statements—Controversial techniques.

22. Katelaris CH, Weiner JM, Heddle RJ, Stuckey MS, Yan KW. Vega testing in the diagnosis of allergic conditions. *Medical Journal of Australia* 1991;115:113–114.

CHAPTER 6

Detecting Allergenic Foods: Elimination and Challenge

This chapter provides you with the information you need to ascertain exactly which foods are responsible for your child's food allergies. Determination of the foods responsible for clinical symptoms requires elimination of the culprit foods for a trial period in which the symptoms should disappear. This is followed by careful challenge of each individual food component in a precisely selected and controlled fashion so that its effects on the body can be monitored. This is the only way in which the role of foods in allergy can be determined accurately.

The elimination and challenge process may be used to confirm or refute any allergy tests. This process may also be used to establish the most appropriate therapeutic diet in the management of specific food-related conditions. The process may appear time-consuming and tedious, but the exercise is definitely worthwhile. It will provide you with invaluable information about precisely how your child reacts to foods. Every child is unique, and the diet that works for one will not be appropriate for another.

This process may sometimes involve quite extreme dietary changes for a short period. As a result, it is best carried out with the help of a professional trained in the field. Ideally, you will work with your child's doctor and a qualified, registered dietitian so that any risk of severe reactions and unsafe diets can be dealt with quickly. For mild, chronic types of symptoms, you may be able to carry out the process yourself. However, involving a health care professional is always the best and safest route to follow.

The following warnings cannot be stressed strongly enough:

If you have any cause to suspect that your child has had a severe or ana-phylactic reaction to a food, challenge tests should be undertaken *only* under medical supervision in a suitably equipped facility.

Never challenge on your own a food that has caused a severe reaction in the past, elicited a strong reaction on a skin test, or resulted in a high level of IgE on your child's blood test!

Any food that has been avoided for a long period (6 months or more) because of a previous reaction should always be rechallenged under the supervision of a qualified medical practitioner. Reactions after long absti-nence tend to be more severe than when the food has been eaten regular-ly.

Many pediatric allergists strongly recommend challenging the most highly allergenic foods *only* under medical supervision. The most highly aller-genic foods include:

Milk	Peanuts	Shellfish
Eggs	Tree nuts	Fish
	Soy	

The elimination and challenge process requires three stages or steps. The first stage of the detection process starts with an elimination diet. Elimination diets are designed to remove all of the food components that could be responsible for the symptoms. It is useful to keep a careful food and symptom record for your child. If the child is a baby being breast-fed, a record of the mother's food intake is also important because foods being consumed by the breast-feeding mother could be responsible for the baby's food allergy symptoms.

Next follows the challenge phase. In this phase, each individual food component is reintroduced in such a way that you can monitor your child's response not only to the component itself but also to the specific dose of the component that triggers his or her symptoms.

Once the culprit foods have been detected, a diet is developed. This diet will avoid all of the offending foods and provide complete balanced nutrition from alternative sources. It is absolutely crucial that a child is provided with all of the nutrients that he or she requires during this critical stage of growth and development. Deficiencies in essential nutrients at this stage could have far-reaching adverse effects. In extreme cases, these effects can persist for life.

STEP 1: ELIMINATION DIETS

The aim of any elimination diet is to remove the food components that are causing or worsening the clinical symptoms of concern. Elimination diets are designed to set the stage for subsequent determination of the culprit food components. They do this by rendering the allergic person symptom-free. Then the specific reaction triggers may elicit noticeable, and sometimes measurable, symptoms. In general, the elimination phase of the management program utilizes diets of three types:

1. Selective elimination diets

2. Few foods elimination diets

3. Elemental diets

Each of the diets has a specific function in the management of food sensitivity.

Choosing the Most Appropriate Elimination Diet

In order to determine which elimination diet is the most appropriate for your child, several pieces of information are required:

*   A careful *medical history*. It is especially important to record any *anaphylactic reactions* suspected to be due to food.

*   Exclusion of *any other cause* for the symptoms. This should be determined by diagnostic tests and procedures carried out by your child's doctor.

- Results of any *allergy tests* previously carried out by qualified practitioners.

- A careful record of all foods, beverages, supplements, and medications ingested by your child during a 7-day period. Details of symptoms experienced during this time should also be included. This record is called an exposure diary.

Exposure Diary

Record the following information each day, for a minimum of 7 days:

- All foods, beverages, medications, and supplements ingested

- Approximate quantities of each (teaspoons, tablespoons, cups, ounces grams)

- Composition of compound dishes and drinks (ingredient list)

- The time at which each was consumed

- All symptoms experienced, graded according to severity: 1 (mild); 2 (mild to moderate); 3 (moderate); and 4 (severe)

- Time of onset of the symptoms

- How long the symptoms last and whether medications were taken to control the symptoms

- Status on waking in the morning (Symptom-free? Type and severity of any symptoms)

- If sleep was disturbed during the night, indicate whether this was due to specific symptoms

The sample charts provided in Table 6.1 (see the end of this chapter) are for recording everything consumed and for recording symptoms. By comparing the completed charts, side by side, it will become clearer which foods to suspect as potential triggers for a child's reactions. This is particularly evident when the response is immediate (within an hour or less of ingestion) and when the reaction occurs every time a specific food, beverage, or supplement is consumed.

Exposure Diary for a Breast-Fed Baby

When a baby is breast-fed, it is important to record not only the baby's food and liquid intake, but also that of the breast-feeding mother. Food components from the mother's diet will be present in her breast milk. The breast milk will therefore be a source of potential food allergens if the baby has already been sensitized to them (see Chapter 5 for details).

The sample charts at the end of this chapter provide a separate record for the mother's and the baby's intake. So, for the breast-fed baby, you should have three charts:

1. Baby's intake. If the baby is exclusively breast-fed, this chart will be a record of the times and duration of nursing. If the baby is eating some solid foods, this will include time of consumption and quantities of each food.

2. Baby's symptoms: time of onset, severity, and duration

3. Mother's diet record: foods, beverages, supplements, and medications, including times of consumption and approximate quantities of each

The Elimination Diet

Based on an analysis of the records for both food intake and symptoms, we can develop an appropriate elimination diet. This diet will exclude all of the suspected foods and take into account the following information:

*   The child's detailed medical history

*   Analysis of the exposure diaries for both baby and mother

*   Results of any allergy tests

*   Foods that you suspect may be a cause of your child's symptoms

The three types of elimination diet each have a place in the determination of the offending foods:

1. Selective elimination diets: One food, or a small number of specific foods, is eliminated for a specified period. For example, it might be a milk-free diet, egg-free diet, wheat-free diet, or a combination of these (see Chapters 7 to 16).

2. Few foods elimination diets (sometimes referred to as oligo-antigenic diets): Only a few (usually fewer than ten) foods are allowed for a specified period.

3. Elemental diets: Only an amino acid-based formula is allowed for the duration of the elimination phase. We usually use an extensively hydrolyzed formula (EHF), such as Nutramigen®, for babies and young children.

Selective Elimination Diets

Selective elimination diets are usually used when ingestion of a specific food causes a sudden acute response and an IgE-mediated hypersensitivity reaction is suggested by skin or blood tests for a food-specific antibody.

For children who are eating a range of foods, we select the foods for elimination based on the results of allergy tests. We also select the foods that seem to be followed by an immediate development of symptoms. For breast-fed babies, the foods we select as suspects in the mother's diet are those that she consumed from 2 to 6 hours prior to the development of symptoms in her baby.

Selective elimination diets may also be used for identification of specific food triggers in chronic allergic disease, such as eczema (atopic dermatitis), hyperactivity, and the trial gluten/casein-free diet for autism. In these cases, if the symptoms persist after specific foods have been eliminated, the assumption can be made that the foods avoided are not an important part of the reaction.

Selective diets in children are normally followed for 4 weeks. This allows sufficient time for recovery from the initial withdrawal symptoms (if any) and, in most cases, the disappearance of all of the symptoms that are due to food components. It also allows sufficient time for both the parents and the child to adapt to the diet, both physiologically and psychologically.

The breast-feeding mother should follow the elimination diet for 4 weeks, looking for improvement in her baby's symptoms. If the baby is consuming some solid foods in addition to breast milk, the suspect foods will be eliminated from the baby's diet and from that of the mother for the specified period.

Carefully constructed selective elimination diets are nutritionally adequate. No risk is associated with adherence to the diet for the 4-week trial. Taking into consideration the immunological response, 4 weeks of freedom from exposure to an allergen is also a suitable time for challenge with the offending allergen. This interval of freedom allows symptom remission. However, the level of antigen-specific IgE will not be reduced. As a result, in an IgE-mediated allergic reaction, challenge will elicit a clear and sometimes enhanced response.

Selective elimination diets are particularly useful in several situations:

- When specific foods need to be eliminated: This is usually done to confirm the accuracy of allergy tests such as skin tests, food-specific antibody tests (e.g., RAST or ELISA), and others (see Chapter 5).

- When food allergy is suspected as a factor in conditions such as atopic eczema, autism, hyperactivity, and asthma: In this case, there is no other direct evidence of food allergy.

- Therapeutic diets: These diets are used when food components are known or suspected to be the major factor in the etiology of defined conditions, but allergy to a specific food is not the cause, for example, celiac disease or food protein enteropathies (see Chapter 24).

Specific Food Restrictions

The elimination of specific foods in preparation for challenge, or when the culprit food component has been definitively identified, is a relatively straightforward process. It is a good idea to become familiar with the food restrictions before starting the elimination process. Begin with the following 3 important written lists:

1. A listing of the foods that must be avoided and manufactured foods that commonly contain the subject food.

2. A comprehensive list of the terms that would identify the food in an ingredient list or on a food label.

3. Alternative food sources of all of the nutrients that may be deficient when the subject food is eliminated. This is necessary to reduce the risk of nutrient deficiency. If easily accessible food sources are limited, appropriate and specific supplements should be found.

Specific examples of selective elimination diets include those that are free from the following foods:

- Milk (Chapter 7)

- Egg (Chapter 9)

- Peanut (Chapter 10)

- Soy (Chapter 11)

- Tree nuts (Chapter 12)

- Fish (Chapter 15)

- Shellfish (Chapter 15)

- Wheat (Chapter 13)

- Corn (Chapter 14)

A single food can be eliminated if it is suspected to be the cause of the child's symptoms. Use the charts provided in each chapter that discusses that food. Also, ensure that your child is eating all of the allowed foods.

In many cases, you will suspect more than one food as the trigger for your child's allergies. Look at each of the chapters on the suspect foods. Then compile a list of allowed foods by combining the instructions from each of the relevant charts.

There is no point in removing a single food if you suspect more than one food. The symptoms triggered by the remaining offending food(s) will still occur and mask any benefit from exclusion of the single food. If you suspect several of the most allergenic foods, use the Top Ten Allergens instructions in Chapter 16. Subsequent reintroduction of each food will show you which foods are triggering your child's symptoms.

You may be trying to deal with a condition that involves both food and environmental or airborne allergens. In that case, use the diets in Chapters 19 to 23. They are free from the foods and food additives that may be associated with specific conditions.

Selective elimination diets are designed to remove all suspect allergens and intolerance triggers. They do, however, include all of the foods that are not involved in the clinical condition or that have tested negative on the diagnostic tests. If older children are to be on an elimination diet, it is wise to put forbidden foods in places that are not easily reached. Parents of defiant youngsters have been known to install locks on cupboards and luggage straps on refrigerators and freezers.

Additional instructions for management of selective elimination diets for specific foods (and details and discussion of therapeutic diets) can be found in Reference 1.[1]

Nutritional Adequacy of Selective Elimination Diets

A child's nutritional needs can be adequately supplied by a selective elimination diet if it incorporates alternative foods that are nutritionally equivalent to those removed. The child should never lose weight or fail to obtain all of his or her essential nutritional requirements on a selective elimination diet. If the allowed foods do not provide all of the nutrients required, use defined amounts of specified brands of appropriate dietary supplements.

The need for nutrient supplements is determined by the foods being eliminated from the diet. Details of the micronutrients (vitamins and minerals) associated with each of the foods most frequently associated with allergy are provided in Appendix E. However, in most cases, following the list of allowed foods in each of the appropriate chapters will be quite sufficient for providing all of the nutrients required during the 4-week trial.

Duration of the Selective Elimination Diet

The selective elimination diet is usually followed for 4 weeks. If the symptoms have not disappeared or greatly decreased after 4 weeks, either allergens or intolerance factors remain in the child's diet or the symptoms are unrelated to foods.

To determine whether foods in the elimination diet are responsible for the remaining symptoms, you should keep another exposure diary for 5 to 7 days while continuing with the elimination diet. Analysis of this second exposure diary should indicate if other foods or chemicals could be causing the remaining symptoms. A further elimination of foods can be carried out for 2 weeks or more if indicated by the second food exposure diary. The new diet should be followed no longer than 2 weeks, and an exposure diary should be kept for the second week of the diet.

Follow-Up to the Selective Elimination Diet

Following the 4 weeks (or 6 weeks, if extra foods are eliminated for an additional 2 weeks) on the selective elimination diet, the challenge phase begins. Even if the symptoms have improved only moderately, a specific challenge of food components may reveal adverse reactions that are not noticeable when the food is eaten frequently. Some practitioners refer to this as the unmasking of a hidden food allergy.

Few Foods Elimination Diet

Sometimes it is very difficult to determine which foods should be excluded on a selective elimination diet. There may be multiple symptoms that do not fit into any perceivable pattern of reactivity that would suggest a reaction to food allergens. Sometimes there are no indicators of food additive intolerance or sensitivity to natural components of foods. In these cases, a few foods elimination diet is useful. Such diets are particularly valuable in the management of chronic allergic conditions.

A few foods elimination diet (oligo-antigenic diet) differs from a selective elimination diet in that only a small number of foods are allowed. These are the foods considered to be the least likely to trigger an allergic reaction. Such diets are indicated when there are many symptoms with no clear relationship to specific foods.

Because an oligo-antigenic diet is not nutritionally complete, it should never be followed for more than 14 days. Usually, a period of 7 to 10 days is sufficient to show results.

Young children are especially vulnerable to nutritional deficiency because all nutrients are needed in the years of maximal growth. It is particularly important that supervision of the elimination diet should include careful and frequent evaluation. This evaluation ensures that the child's nutritional needs are being met at each stage of the process of determining the allergenic foods. For this reason, a few foods elimination diet is rarely recommended before the child enters puberty. If it is really necessary for purposes of identifying extremely extensive food allergy, the few foods elimination diet should not be followed for longer than 7 days for children under the age of 13 years. The diet also should be administered under the supervision of a suitably qualified health care practitioner. In most cases, simply eliminating the Top Ten Allergens (Chapter 16) and feeding the allowed foods on that diet will achieve remission of the child's most important symptoms and avoid the risk of any nutritional deficiency.

Use of Supplemental Formulas

In many cases, an EHF casein-based formula, such as Nuramigen®, can be used to replace the deficient nutrients. However, most children will need time to get used to the rather unusual taste of these types of formulas. In the rare cases in which EHFs are not tolerated, an elemental formula such as Neocate® (SHS) or Neocate® Junior might be a good alternative. For the breast-feeding mother, an elemental formula, such as Tolerex®, will supply the deficient nutrients. Again, a period of adjustment is wise due to the unusual taste and the change in osmotic pressure in the large bowel (which at first might lead to mild stomach upset).

A role for foods in the etiology of the child's symptoms should become apparent if symptoms disappear or improve significantly within this period. Avoid extending the few foods elimination diet beyond 14 days if the symptoms remain unchanged. A longer period on the diet in this case is a fruitless exercise and can be detrimental to the child's health. The child's immune system could become depressed on this semi-starvation regimen.

If the symptoms do not clear up within 7 to 10 days, two assumptions for the lack of response can be considered:

1. One or more of the foods included in the diet are allergenic for the child.

2. Foods are not contributing to the child's symptoms.

To confirm assumption 1, replace each food with one from the same food group and continue the elimination diet for 4 or 5 days more.

To confirm assumption 2, initiate a sequential incremental dose challenge for each restricted food (see Chapter 7).

Foods Allowed

There are many diets in use that are called Few Foods Elimination Diets. Each practitioner tends to favor a particular diet. The Few Foods Elimination Diet provided here includes foods that consistently prove to be low in allergenicity for the majority of children. Adjustments must be made for individuals with unusual reactions who might respond adversely to one or more of the foods included. The most effective oligo-antigenic diets are individualized for each child. This is done because the persistence of symptoms could be due to one or more foods left in the diet. It is important that the foods selected are ones to which the child has shown no evidence of reactivity in the past. The diet contains no food additives, flavor enhancers, or modifiers. As a result, both allergens and chemical food additives are minimized or eliminated.

General Instructions for the Few Foods Elimination Diet

*   It is wise to begin the diet trial during a quiet social season (i.e., not at Christmas, Chanukah, or other religious holidays or around birthday

parties, weddings, or other important celebrations). If there is a social event during this diet, take your own food or hold the party in your home so that appropriate foods are available for you and your child at all times.

- It will be necessary to shop ahead, having plenty of appropriate foods on hand. The diet may be somewhat boring, but there is no need to go hungry. It is important that you and your child remain healthy and as well-nourished as possible while investigating specific responses to foods.

- The meals are quite simple, without spices, butter, or condiments.

- As many fresh food sources as possible should be used. Frozen food is the next best alternative.

- Keep a diary of your child's intake and symptoms during the entire 7 to 10 days that he or she is following this diet.

- Food should be washed and cooked with distilled water only. Tap water may contain contaminants that could cause reactions.

- The following things should be avoided:

  – Chewing gum
  – Over-the-counter medications (unless essential)
  – Candies and other non-food treats
  – Coffee
  – Tea (including herbal tea)
  – Diet drinks
  – Mouthwash

- Necessary prescription medications should be continued. Consult your doctor about the advisability of discontinuing any prescribed medication.

FOODS ALLOWED ON THE FEW FOODS ELIMINATION DIET		
Food Category	**Food**	**Specific Food Items**
Meat and Alternatives	Lamb Turkey Chicken	If any of these meats are known to cause a reaction, choose another that has always seemed safe.
Grains	Rice Tapioca Millet	Whole grains, flours, and pure cereals made from these grains
Vegetables	Squash	All kinds, including: • Acorn • Butternut • Chayote • Hubbard • Winter squash • Pattypan • Spaghetti squash • Yellow squash • Summer squash • Crookneck • Zucchini • Pure infant squash in jars
	Parsnips Sweet potatoes	• Pure Infant Sweet Potatoes in Jars
	Yams Lettuce	Iceberg (head lettuce) is the least tolerated of the lettuces. Try other varieties.
Fruits	Pears	Pure bottled pear juice Pure infant pears in jars
	Peaches	Infant peaches in jars Pure peach juice

FOODS ALLOWED ON THE FEW FOODS ELIMINATION DIET

Food Category	Food	Specific Food Items
	Fruits	If any of the suggested fruits are suspects, replace them with those that the child has eaten without symptoms in the past.
Oils	Canola oil Safflower oil	
Condiments	Sea salt	
Desserts	Pudding made from tapioca beads or pearls or rice; fruit and fruit juice of of allowed fruits	
	Agar-agar (seaweed) may be used as a thickener.	
Beverages	Distilled water Juice from the allowed fruits and vegetables: For your child, dilute 1:1 with distilled water.	Use **glass** bottles only. Distilled water is available in drug stores. (Take your own container to be filled; it is less expensive and most drug stores only supply plastic bottles.)

Recipes and meal planning for a sample of the Few Foods Elimination Diet are provided in Reference 1.

Elemental Diets

Sometimes allergy to multiple foods is suspected and either selective or few foods elimination diets have failed to resolve a child's symptoms. In that case, an EHF casein-based formula alone for a short period (about 7 days) should determine whether the child's symptoms are food related. An elemental diet supplies calories and all of the essential macro- and micronutrients in the form of an amino-acid based formula. Such diets are easy to maintain in infancy, but more difficult as children become older. Unless they have become used to the formula in infancy, children tend to dislike the unusual taste at first. Manufacturers can add flavoring to elemental formulas, but this adds the risk of adverse reactions to the chemicals in the flavoring compounds. Some children like the formula when allowed fruit or fruit juice is added to it. For example, peaches or pears can be blended into the formula.

Elemental formulas are used only in rare cases when all other elimination diets have failed to resolve symptoms but the suspicion of an allergic etiology for the child's illness remains high.

There are a number of predigested (hydrolized) and elemental formulas available. None should be used without the knowledge and approval of your child's doctor, and none should be continued for any prolonged period. Hydrolyzed casein formulas include Nutramigen™, Similac Alimentum™, and Enfamil Pregestimil™; if these are not tolerated, the elemental formula Neocate™, or Neocate Junior™, should be tried. The suitability of a specific formula for an individual child should be ascertained by a physician. The number of daily calories supplied by the formula must be calculated for each child individually so that the required quantity of formula is consumed. In addition, the precise composition of each formula should be confirmed by the manufacturer, because the ingredients are sometimes changed without notice.

Expected Results of the Elimination Diet
Here is what you might expect to see during the elimination diet:

- If all or most of your child's major reaction triggers have been excluded, he or she may actually feel *worse*, in unusual cases, on days 2 through 4 of the elimination diet. Theoretically, this has been explained as a condition of antibody excess, causing a condition known as serum sickness.

- By days 5 through 7 of exclusion, your child should definitely appear to be noticeably better if the allergens and intolerance triggers responsible for his or her symptoms have actually been eliminated.

- Your child's symptoms should have improved significantly after 10 to 14 days of exclusion on the selective elimination diet. If all allergens and antagonistic foods have been eliminated, all symptoms should have disappeared by the end of 3 weeks.

- If substitution of alternative foods for excluded nutrients is adequate, your child will not lose any weight in the 2 or 4 weeks of the elimination diet.

- If your child's symptoms have not improved significantly, it is likely that he or she is still consuming unidentified allergens or intolerance factors. Or it may be that foods are not the cause of the symptoms.

- The duration of the initial elimination phase will depend on the type of symptoms being managed. For example, reactions that appear only intermittently at widely spaced intervals or that may be due to delayed reactions may require a longer elimination phase. When the reaction is in the skin—for example, in the case of eczema—symptom remission may not be apparent immediately because it takes time for the skin to begin healing. However, signs of improvement include less reddening and overt inflammation, as well as the fact that the child is no longer scratching. Gastrointestinal symptoms, on the other hand, will usually respond promptly to appropriate dietary measures. Improvement can be experienced within a few days, if not immediately.

- An elimination diet should never be followed for longer than 10 to 14 days if there is any danger of nutritional deficiency (such as may occur on the few foods elimination diet). Never extend the few foods elimination for longer than 7 days for a child under the age of 13 years.

- Keep another food and symptoms record for the last week of your child's elimination diet phase. This will show you clearly whether his or her symptoms have improved. If symptoms still persist, a clear pattern of occurrence might be obvious. That pattern could point to a specific food trigger that can be avoided for a further trial period.

- Further elimination of foods can be carried out, in addition to the original list, for another 2 weeks, based on analysis of the second exposure diary.

- A sequential incremental dose challenge should be started (see Chapter 7) at the end of 7 days on the few foods elimination diet and the elemental diet, or at the end of 4 weeks on a selective elimination diet (6 weeks if more foods have been eliminated for 2 weeks after the original 4 weeks).

- Even if your child does not seem to have improved a great deal, specific challenge of food components sometimes reveals adverse reactions that are not noticeable when the food is eaten continuously.

Reasons for Failure in Following an Elimination Diet (Why You Might Give Up)

There are several key reasons why a child or the child's parents might not comply with the dietary restrictions. These reasons include the following:

- The parents may have insufficient knowledge or understanding about restrictions and why they are necessary.

- The child rebels against the restrictions. In this case, try to adjust the allowed foods to take into account your child's normal selection of foods, keeping in mind preferences in taste, texture, and form of the food (e.g., finger foods rather than those requiring a knife and fork; softer or firmer texture; liquid rather than dry). Your child will be unlikely to follow a diet that is drastically different from his or her normal way of eating. One alternative in this case is to go over the original exposure diary again and insert substitute foods rather than trying to develop a totally new diet from scratch.

- The diet fails to reduce or abolish symptoms. This can be due to a number of factors:
    - The diet is frequently abandoned during the first 2 to 4 days if parents forget about the possibility that symptoms may seem a little worse during this period.
    - The diet may have improved the symptoms for which food components are responsible, but the remaining symptoms are caused by factors other than foods. In this case, the symptoms will not improve by dietary manipulation.
    - Sources of the allergenic foods remain in the diet. Make sure that you are well-informed about hidden sources of the food and that you are familiar with all the terms that can indicate the presence of the food on ingredient labels. Reread the chapters on specific food restrictions. Lists of terms are provided under each food category.
    - Some of the restricted ingredients might have been introduced during manufacture or serving of the allowed foods. For example, utensils or equipment may have been contaminated in the processing of several different foods without adequate cleaning between batches. This is a particular problem with ice cream and with bakery products such as cookies.

- Excessive expectations of the diet have not been met (perhaps a total cure was expected rather than mere improvement).

- The diet is no longer needed because the symptoms abated spontaneously or the child grew out of the symptoms.

- Cost should not be an important element in failing to adhere to a diet. Most of the initial elimination diets are only followed for a short period, and the savings from eliminated foods usually offset the cost of substitute foods. A few comparison studies show no significant difference in cost between the regular diet and the elimination diet except when expensive elemental food replacements and supplements have been prescribed.

Follow-Up to the Elimination Diet

Following the elimination diet, sequential incremental dose challenge should be initiated in order to identify the specific food(s) responsible for the child's reactions. When the culprit food components have been identified, a selective elimination diet, now referred to as a maintenance diet, can be continued as long as necessary, without incurring any nutritional risk.

Note on Therapeutic Diets

The information previously provided is designed for the management of the diet when food allergy and intolerance are the suggested causes of a child's symptoms. However, another type of selective elimination diet is used when a diagnosis has been made and the cause of the condition has been identified as a food component. Treatment for these conditions is strict avoidance of the causative food component. Carefully designed therapeutic diets are essential in the management of the child's condition.

Therapeutic diets are usually classified into different categories, depending on the conditions for which they are used:

- Inborn errors of metabolism of various types such as the following:
  - Errors in carbohydrate metabolism, such as galactosemia, hereditary fructose intolerance, and glycogen storage diseases
  - Errors in amino acid metabolism, including the well-known phenylketonuria, in which dietary phenylalanine must be restricted
  - Anomalies in lipid metabolism, particularly hyperlipoproteinemia, probably the most frequently encountered example

- Metabolic anomalies that are more commonly referred to as food intolerances. Examples include several types of disaccharide deficiency:
  - Lactose intolerance, caused by a deficiency in the enzyme lactase
  - Sucrose intolerance, usually a congenital condition caused by a deficiency in the production of sucrase
  - Fructose malabsorption
  - Glucose-galactose intolerance

- Conditions in which food components need to be restricted, although their role in the etiology of the disease is as yet undefined. These conditions include:
  - Gluten-sensitive enteropathy (celiac disease), in which all gluten-containing foods need to be avoided

- Cow's milk protein enteropathy, or soy protein enteropathy, most frequently seen in young infants, in which all cow's milk proteins or soy proteins need to be excluded

Different therapeutic diets are used when specific food components are suspected to be a cause or exacerbating factor in a clinical condition for which all other causes have been ruled out. Most of the diets in this category should probably be considered experimental. Further research may confirm their utility and, possibly, define the physiological mechanism by which the suspect food component has an adverse impact. Therapeutic elimination diets have been utilized successfully in the management of conditions such as the following:

- Idiopathic urticaria and angioedema, in which dietary sources of histamine are restricted

- Irritable bowel syndrome, in which the foods are modified to promote digestion and absorption in the small intestine and to reduce the residue of undigested food passing into the colon where it acts as a substrate for microbial fermentation

- Migraine headache, in which biogenic amines such as histamine, tyramine, phenylethylamine, and octopamine are restricted

Therapeutic diets are designed to remove all suspect allergens and intolerance triggers. But they include all foods that are not involved in the clinical condition or that have tested negative on the diagnostic tests.

STEP 2: CHALLENGE PHASE: REINTRODUCTION OF FOODS

When the elimination test diet has been completed, the next step in the identification of the foods and food additives associated with adverse reactions is to reintroduce each component individually. The reintroduction is done so that those foods responsible for symptoms can be clearly identified. This is achieved by careful challenge with precise quantities of each food component and careful monitoring of symptom development. During this process, it is important to look for immediate reactions (within a 4-hour period) or delayed reactions (from 1 to 4 days) following ingestion.

The three basic types of food challenges employed by food allergy practitioners involve different methodologies:

1. Double-blind placebo-controlled food challenge (DBPCFC) is usually employed in research studies or specialized clinics. Neither the child nor the challenge supervisor knows the identity of the test food component. Each test is compared to the child's reaction to a placebo (usually glucose powder) enclosed within a gelatin capsule similar to that of the food.

2. Single-blind food challenge in an office setting is usually supervised by a physician or, more commonly, a dietitian or nurse. The child is unaware of the identity of the food. The supervisor knows which food is being challenged. The food is disguised in another stronger-tasting food.

3. Open food challenge is most frequently carried out at home. The child is aware of the identity of the food and the quantity being consumed in each test.

Double-Blind Placebo-Controlled Food Challenge

The DBPCFC is regarded as the gold standard by most traditional allergists. It is always conducted by a clinician. In this procedure, neither the child nor the supervisor of the challenge knows the identity of the food:

- The food is lyophilized (freeze-dried) and, in the powder form, is enclosed in a gelatin capsule.

- A placebo, usually glucose powder, is enclosed within a similar capsule and is used as a negative control.

For IgE-mediated reactions, the method of administration tends to vary from clinic to clinic. Two examples reported in the literature are as follows (others may be obtained from published data).[2,3]

Method 1

IgE-Mediated Reactions

The challenge is administered in the fasting state, starting with a dose unlikely to provoke symptoms (very small amounts [0.0008 to 0.0178 ounce or 25 to 500 milligrams] of lyophilized food).

- The dose is usually doubled every 15 to 60 minutes; the interval between doses is dictated by the reported course of the child's symptoms.

- The child is usually observed for the development of symptoms for 2 hours after the feeding.

- If the child tolerates 0.3527 ounce (10 grams) of lyophilized food (equivalent to about one egg white, or one 4-oz glass of milk), clinical reactivity is considered to be unlikely.

- In most IgE-mediated disorders, challenges to new foods may be conducted every 1 to 2 days.

Non-IgE-Mediated Reactions:

- In dietary protein-induced enterocolitis, for example, allergen challenges require very small amounts of food (up to 0.010 to 0.021 ounce [0.3 to 0.6 gram] of food per kilogram of body weight) given in 1 or 2 doses. The patient is usually observed for 24 to 48 hours for the development of symptoms.

- In eosinophilic gastroenteritis, several feedings over a 1- to 3-day period may be required to elicit symptoms; the patient is observed for up to 4 days for the development of symptoms.

- With most non-IgE-mediated reactions, challenges need to be at least 3 to 5 days apart.

Method 2

- For the test dose, very small amounts (0.082 to 0.3527 ounce[8 to 10 grams]) of the dry (lyophilized) food, 0.4226 cup (100 milliliters) of wet food, or double these quantities for meat or fish are used.

- The dose is consumed at 10- to 15-minute intervals over a total of 90 minutes.

- A meal-sized portion of the food is consumed a few hours later.

- Symptoms are recorded and assessments are made for reactions in the skin, gastrointestinal tract, and respiratory tract.

- Challenges are terminated when a reaction becomes apparent.

However, all negative challenges need to be confirmed by an open feeding under observation. In this way, false-negative responses can be ruled out.

Occasionally, a child reacts adversely to the gelatin of the capsule rather than the food itself. This false-positive reaction needs to be considered when a child reacts to all of the foods in a challenge test. Reactivity to only one or two foods is the most common result of DBPCFC (as opposed to intolerance reactions) for allergy.

DBPCFC are expensive and labor-intensive. For this reason, most are conducted either in a research setting or in specialized facilities such as allergy clinics or hospitals. These tests are performed only when knowing the identity of the culprit food is extremely important for the health of the patient. DBPCFC are usually unnecessary for very young children, who would not recognize the food in an open food challenge, or for older children, who would not recognize the food if it were disguised in a stronger-tasting carrier food.

Single-Blind Food Challenge

In this method of challenge, the suspect allergen is known to the supervisor, but unknown to the patient. The food is disguised in a strongly flavored food such as:

- Fruit juice (cranberry, apple, or grape)

- Infant formulas for babies and children

- Elemental formulas, appropriate for children or adults

- Meat patties

- Cereals

- Added ingredients with strong flavors such as mint, fish, or garlic
- Lentil soup

Most IgE-mediated reactions and those resulting in severe allergic symptoms are conducted under medical supervision in appropriately equipped facilities. The majority of anaphylactic reactions to foods are not challenged. This is because it is frequently possible to identify the food responsible, based on the child's medical history. If such challenges are necessary, they should only be conducted under the strictest medical supervision with appropriately qualified and equipped personnel in attendance.

Open Food Challenge: Sequential Incremental Dose Challenge (SIDC)

Many adverse reactions to foods are not severe reactions. In these cases, challenges can be safely carried out at home. The methods described here for identifying foods that trigger adverse reactions would be more appropriately considered re-introduction rather than challenge. These re-introductions would be carried out on foods that the child has eaten in the past and displayed only a mild reaction, if any. They are not deemed likely to cause a severe reaction.

Unnecessary restriction of foods can be extremely detrimental to a child's nutritional health and emotional and social well-being. It is therefore very important that the foods responsible for adverse reactions be correctly identified, even though they do not threaten the child's life. They do threaten his or her quality of life, which can be very important for a young person.[4]

In many types of foods, there are several different components that can be challenged individually. It's best to separate those that can be tolerated from those that need to be avoided. As a result, a child's diet can be liberalized to include those that are safe. This provides a wider range of food choices and ensures a more complete nutritional intake. A person's reactions may be to a component of a food, but not the whole food. Lactose intolerance is a well-known example of this. With lactose intolerance, only the milk sugar (lactose) needs to be avoided; the milk proteins are tolerated, so lactose-free milk and its products can be included in the diet to supply many essential nutrients. A similar liberalization of dietary restrictions can be achieved when individual food components are re-introduced separately. For example, in milk allergy or intolerance, a challenge with casein, whey, or lactose individually will determine a child's reactivity to each one of these components. Those that cause a reaction will be avoided; those that are tolerated can be included in the regular diet.

Details of the SIDC protocols are provided below and in Appendix D. The initial diet—selective elimination diet, few foods elimination diet, or elemental formula—is continued for the duration of the challenge phase of the program. Foods are not added back into to the diet until all of the foods within a category have been tested separately. This is the preferred procedure, even if they produce no reaction during the challenge. This is to ensure that the quantity of each food component is consistent with the test directives. If foods are added back as they are tolerated, the quantity of a single component will be increased by inclusion of previously tested and tolerated foods containing that component. For example, during testing for milk components, Test 1 for casein proteins may be tolerated. In that case, including cheese in the diet during the subsequent challenges will increase the quantity of casein in each test.

These instructions are designed to allow re-introduction of increasing doses of the test components. As a result, an idea of the child's limit of tolerance (quantity to which he or she does not react) can be determined, as well as the safety of individual food components.

Detailed instructions for re-introducing each individual food component in sequence are provided in Appendix D.

The selective or few foods elimination diet continues for all meals throughout the testing period. An initial screening challenge provides a measure of safety:

- Before offering the food for consumption, rub a little of the food on the child's cheek and monitor for about 20 minutes for signs of a reaction, such as reddening or irritation.

If there is no reaction:

- Apply a small quantity of the food on the outer border of the child's lower lip.

- Observe the area for 30 minutes for the development of a local reaction.

**GENERAL INSTRUCTIONS FOR THE SIDC
FOR A CHILD EATING SOLID FOODS**

Certain foods should only be challenged under medical supervision in a facility equipped for resuscitation:

- **Any food that have caused an anaphylactic reaction**

- **Any foods that have been suspected to be the trigger for an anaphylactic reaction**

- **Any foods that have been or are suspected to be the cause of a severe allergic reaction (especially in an asthmatic child)**

If a food has been avoided for 6 months or more, it should only be challenged under medical supervision.

Some allergists insist that the most highly allergenic foods should never be challenged except under medical supervision. These foods include:

Peanuts	**Milk**	**Shellfish**
Tree nuts	**Eggs**	**Fish**
	Soy	

- Signs of a positive reaction are the following:
  - Swelling, reddening, or irritation at the site of application
  - Development of a rash of the cheek and/or chin
  - Rubbing of the site by a young child, indicating irritation
  - Rhinitis or conjunctivitis
  - A systemic reaction

- If there is no sign of a reaction in either of the tests, give the child a small quantity of the food three times on the test day at intervals of 4 hours and carefully monitor him or her for the development of symptoms in the following way:

- The symptoms that develop will be the same as those that you have seen in the past. However, the intensity or severity may be significantly increased. Any symptoms not previously experienced are unlikely to be due to the food. An unrelated cause should be investigated.

- If symptoms develop at any time, consumption of the food component being tested stops immediately. Continue the basic elimination diet until the symptoms subside completely. Testing of the next food in the sequence can commence 48 hours after the symptoms have stopped. This interval allows sufficient time for all of the reactive food to be eliminated from your child's body before another food is introduced.

- If the test food does not cause an immediate reaction on day 1 of its introduction, the next day (day 2) is a monitoring day for delayed reactions. The basic elimination diet is eaten at each meal, but none of the test food is eaten during day 2. Symptoms that appear on day 2 are usually due to a delayed reaction to a food or to a nonimmune-mediated reaction to a food additive.

- If no symptoms develop on days 1 or 2 of the test, the food can be considered safe. Proceed to the next food component in the sequence.

- Under most circumstances, a 2-day period is adequate for reactions to the test food to become apparent. However, occasionally it is unclear whether the symptoms were due to the food or to some unrelated event. Or the reaction may be extremely mild. In such cases, give your child the same food on day 3 in larger quantities than on day 1, again in 3 increasing doses. Day 4 would then become a second monitoring day for delayed reactions. If the test food is responsible for the reaction, the symptoms will increase in severity on both day 3 and day 4. If the food is not responsible, the symptoms will diminish or remain unchanged over days 3 and 4.

- The individual foods to be tested, the sequence of testing, and the recommended dosages are provided in Appendix D.

- The food category selected for each test is an individual choice. However, when one category of food is selected, each test in the category should be followed in the prescribed sequence. This is suggested so that the maximum amount of information about the child's pattern of reactivity can be gleaned from the results.

Challenge Phase for the
Breast-Feeding Mother and Infant

After avoiding the suspect foods for 4 weeks, the breast-feeding mother should determine which of the foods triggers symptoms in her infant. There is no advantage in consuming increasing doses of the food, as recommended for a direct challenge. There is no way to determine the quantity that reaches the breast milk in relation to the amount consumed. Therefore, the mother should consume a large quantity of the food or beverage (at least a serving and as much more as she can tolerate). Then she should monitor her baby's reactions for up to 6 hours afterward. In most cases, the baby will show symptoms from 2 to 6 hours after the mother has consumed the food. It is a good idea to repeat this procedure at least three times to confirm the results. Of course, a mother who is allergic to any of the foods herself should not consume them, even to confirm or refute an allergy in her baby.

Suggested quantities of individual foods that mother should consume to determine allergic reactivity in her baby:

- A cup or more of whole milk

- Three or more eggs (make them into an omelette if you wish)

- Half a cup or more of peanuts or nuts of any individual type

- Two or more slices of whole wheat bread (toasted if you prefer) to test for wheat allergy

- Half a cup of tofu (tastes best fried in oil) to test soy allergy

- Three or more ounces of any fish

- Three or more ounces of meat

STEP 3: MAINTENANCE DIET

When you have determined your child's allergenic foods, the next step is to develop a maintenance diet that you and your child can live with for the long term. It must contain all of the nutrients that your child needs for growth and development during this critical stage of his or her life. But it must also contain foods that your child enjoys, as well as those that he or she regards as treats for celebrations such as birthdays, Christmas, Chanukah, and other holidays. It is important that food allergy is not a central issue for the child and the family. It should be considered as only a mild irritant, one that needs to be dealt with responsibly, but not as the focus of life.

Appendix E will provide you with the information you need to develop an acceptable diet for your child. If the child is old enough, include him or her in the process of diet design, and get the child to help with recipe and meal preparation so that it becomes a pleasurable, not burdensome, process for everyone. Enlist the help of grandparents, aunts, and uncles, and make the meal planning a family affair to which everyone can contribute. Grandparents in particular love making special foods for their grandchildren. Most of them find it particularly rewarding when they can come up with new and different recipes to delight the child and the whole family.

In managing the diet of allergic children, I am frequently reminded of a particularly delightful way that one family solved the problem of a restricted diet for their 3-year-old. They were going for a 4-week camping holiday— exactly the right length of time to carry out an elimination diet. You might think that camping would have posed a greater problem in finding alternative foods than cooking at home. But this was a resourceful family! They successfully cooked all of the allowed foods on a campfire (with careful pre-trip planning) and told the children that they were eating special camp meals. The whole family loved the meals, and the child was symptom-free for the entire holiday. Now the children frequently request camp foods, which they regard as special treats, at home.

Maintenance Diets for the Breast-Feeding Mother

Once the breast-feeding mother has determined which foods cause symptoms in her baby, she will need to avoid them as long as she is breast-feeding. It is very important that she consume a nutritionally complete, well-balanced diet to maintain her own health. Of course, her breast milk will always be nutritionally complete for her baby's needs. But, if the mother is not consuming a nutritionally adequate diet, the deficient nutrients will be taken from her own body. This is not good for the mother. Use the information and nutrient tables in Appendix E to formulate an acceptable, enjoyable diet.

Table 6-1

INSTRUCTIONS FOR COMPLETING THE FOOD AND SYMPTOM RECORD FOR A BABY UNDER 3 YEARS OF AGE

1. Write down everything your child eats, drinks, takes as medication and supplement on the Food record. Record each as your child consumes it—try not to complete this record in retrospect (i.e. as you remember it).

2. Record the time your child consumes each item.

3. If dishes include several different ingredients, write down as many of the ingredients as you know.

4. Estimate the amount of each food that your child actually consumed, not the amount offered, and include it in the chart.

5. For ease of recording, write down the medications that your child takes regularly on a separate sheet of paper, and indicate their consumption on the chart with a number or letter that you assign to that medication. Do the same for supplements that your child takes regularly.

6. If your child takes a medication only occasionally write it on the chart as he or she takes it.

7. Complete your child's symptom record at the same time as you complete his or her food record. Enter the same times as in the food record, and record your child's symptoms in relation to those times.

8. Try to rate your child's symptom on a scale of 1 to 4. 1 is mild; 2 is mild to moderate; 3 is moderate to severe; 4 is the most severe.

9. Write down the time of onset of your child's symptom, and the approximate time that it ends.

10. Include any unusual events that might affect your child's symptoms; for example: unusually strenuous exercize; pollen, dust, mold, or animal dander exposure resulting in symptoms of hay fever or asthma; consumption of unknown foods given by babysitters, at a party or family gathering, or when in the care of another person away from home.

Table 6-1 (continued)

INSTRUCTIONS FOR COMPLETING THE FOOD AND SYMPTOM RECORD FOR A BABY UNDER 3 YEARS OF AGE

BREAST-FED BABIES

11.   Follow the guidelines above.

12.   The record may have to be extended into the night—indicate night feedings and symptoms after "dinner" on the record.

13.   Estimate the length of time of nursing for each feeding and write it in the appropriate time slot.

14.   Complete a second food record for mother to cover the same 7-day period.

FORMULA-FED BABIES

15.   Record the name and type of formula (milk-based, soy-based, partial or extensively hydrolysed milk proteins) and the amount consumed (not the amount offered).

BABY'S FOOD RECORD:

Name_____

Age_____ Start Date_____

	Day 1	Day 2	Day 3	Day 4	Day 5	Day 6	Day 7
Breakfast *Time:*							
Medications							
Supplements							
Snack *Time:*							
Lunch *Time:*							
Medications							
Supplements							
Snack *Time:*							
Dinner (Supper) *Time:*							
Medications							
Supplements							
Snack *Time:*							
Medications							

BABY'S SYMPTOM RECORD:

Name_____

Age_____   Start Date_____

	Day 1	Day 2	Day 3	Day 4	Day 5	Day 6	Day 7
Breakfast *Time:*							
Medications							
Supplements							
Snack *Time:*							
Lunch *Time:*							
Medications							
Supplements							
Snack *Time:*							
Dinner (Supper) *Time:*							
Medications							
Supplements							
Snack *Time:*							
Medications							

MOTHER'S FOOD RECORD:

Name_____

Age_____   Start Date_____

	Day 1	Day 2	Day 3	Day 4	Day 5	Day 6	Day 7
Breakfast *Time:*							
Medications							
Supplements							
Snack *Time:*							
Lunch *Time:*							
Medications							
Supplements							
Snack *Time:*							
Dinner (Supper) *Time:*							
Medications							
Supplements							
Snack *Time:*							
Medications							

References

1. Joneja, JMV. *Dealing with Food Allergies: A Practical Guide to Detecting Culprit Foods and Eating a Healthy, Enjoyable Diet.* Boulder, CO: Bull Publishing Company, 2003.

2. Sampson HA. Food Allergy Part 2. Diagnosis and management. *Journal of Allergy and Clinical Immunology* 1999;103(6):981–989.

3. Sicherer SH. Food allergy: When and how to perform oral food challenges. *Pediatric Allergy and Immunology* 1999;10:226–234.

4. Sicherer SH, Noone SA, Munoz-Furlong A. The impact of childhood food allergy on quality of life. *Annals of Allergy, Asthma and Immunology* 2001;87(6):461–464.

CHAPTER 7

Milk Allergy

Cow's milk is the most frequently encountered food allergen in infancy, and milk allergy is often the earliest indicator that a baby is atopic. Precise figures of the incidence of cow's milk allergy (CMA) are hard to find because of the difficulties in obtaining an accurate diagnosis, differences in the populations used for research studies, and disagreement about the symptoms (clinical criteria) for the condition. All studies agree, however, that CMA is most prevalent in early childhood with an incidence of 2 to 7.5 percent being reported. About 80 to 90 percent of children outgrow early CMA by the age of 5 years, and the incidence of CMA in adults is reported to be only about 0.1 to 0.5 percent of the population.[1]

Milk is an extremely complex food with multiple proteins. Many of its proteins have the capacity to act as allergens and to elicit immunological responses in sensitized individuals. To increase the complexity of CMA, different individuals react to different proteins. There can be considerable differences in the immunological response to each different protein, resulting in several quite distinct clinical presentations of CMA. These factors often lead to problems for doctors in diagnosing the condition in babies and children.

Several practitioners have attempted to classify CMA, on the basis of immunological mechanism and clinical presentation, to aid in diagnosis. A 1995 report identified three distinct types of infant CMA with different symptoms and laboratory findings.[2]

FACTS ABOUT COW'S MILK AND ALLERGY

- More than 25 proteins in cow's milk can induce antibody production in humans.

- The most important allergens are beta-lactoglobulin (in whey); alpha-, beta-, and kappa-casein; and bovine serum albumin.

- Clinical reactions have been documented for all of the major antigens in cow's milk.

Group 1

- Symptoms developed within minutes of ingestion of small volumes of cow's milk.

- Symptoms included hives, tissue swelling (angioedema), eczema, and gastrointestinal and respiratory symptoms that were part of a generalized anaphylactic reaction varying in severity from child to child.

- Skin prick tests to milk allergen were positive.

Group 2

- Symptoms were confined to the digestive tract.

- Vomiting and/or diarrhea developed several hours after ingestion of modest volumes of cow's milk.

- Skin prick tests to milk allergen were mostly negative.

- This group was described as suffering from cow's milk protein enteropathy.

Group 3

- Symptoms developed in the gastrointestinal tract more than 20 hours after ingesting large volumes of milk.

- Sometimes symptoms in the gastrointestinal tract were accompanied by respiratory symptoms and eczema.

- Skin prick tests to milk allergen were less marked than for the patients in Group 1 and usually occurred only in those children with eczema.

This report highlights some important factors in CMA diagnosis:

- Symptoms can develop from minutes after ingestion of cow's milk to up to 20 hours later.

- Skin prick tests are of very limited value in diagnosing the condition.

- The prevalence of gastrointestinal symptoms makes the distinction between CMA and lactose intolerance difficult to determine on clinical signs alone. [Lactose intolerance is discussed as a separate condition in Chapter 8.]

SYMPTOMS OF MILK ALLERGY

Most often, symptoms appear in the skin—where eczema, hives, and swelling (angioedema) may occur—and in the gastrointestinal tract, with abdominal bloating, pain, gas, diarrhea, constipation, nausea, vomiting, and, occasionally, blood in the stool (occult blood). In some individuals, upper respiratory tract symptoms and asthma may be caused or worsened when milk or dairy products are consumed.

Blood in the stool, often difficult to see because it is hidden within the feces (called occult blood loss), associated with CMA can be a cause of iron-deficiency anemia. This is especially the case in children, because blood is the most important source of iron in the body.

Another effect of CMA that is currently being investigated in children is the inability to fall asleep and trouble with restless, disturbed sleep.

In an infant, inadequate growth and weight gain (failure to thrive) may be a result of CMA. The allergic reaction results in inflammation in the intestines, and absorption of nutrients may be impaired as a result of damage to the transport mechanisms that reside in the intestinal cells.

Although very rare, CMA can be a cause of fatal anaphylaxis in very young children. In 2000, a study from the United Kingdom[3] reported 8 fatal cases of anaphylaxis from food allergy in children under the age of 16 in the 10 years from 1990 to 2000. Four children died from CMA, and one from the inappropriate use of injectable adrenalin to treat a mild reaction to a food. None died from eating peanuts. This report emphasizes the fact that CMA in early childhood cannot be taken lightly but should always be treated with the utmost care and caution.

The diagnosis of CMA is not a simple matter. Any adverse reaction experienced after drinking milk is often ascribed to CMA. However, when the symptoms are localized in the gastrointestinal tract, the problem may be lactose intolerance, not an immunologically mediated allergy to milk proteins. It is important to differentiate between lactose intolerance (lactase deficiency) and CMA because some symptoms, such as abdominal pain, diarrhea, and vomiting, may be common to both conditions. However, CMA can cause inflammation of the gastrointestinal tract and then trigger a lactase deficiency, so it is possible for both conditions to exist together. Symptoms in other organ systems, such as the respiratory tract and the skin, are never symptoms of lactose intolerance. If these occur as a result of drinking milk, it is clear that CMA is also a problem. Management of lactose intolerance is discussed in further detail in Chapter 8.

ADVERSE REACTIONS TO MILK

Milk allergy is caused by an immune reaction against milk proteins. More than 25 distinct proteins are identifiable, and any number of these may trigger an immune response.

Lactose intolerance is due to an inability of the body to produce sufficient quantities of the digestive enzyme, called lactase, which splits lactose into its constituent single sugars (monosaccharides): glucose and galactose.

BIOLOGICAL MECHANISMS OF CMA

CMA results when antibodies against milk allergens are produced by the immune system. (See Chapter 1 for a discussion of the immune system and allergy.)

- Milk allergens are proteins; more than 25 distinct milk proteins have been identified in the various fractions of milk. The fractions include casein, whey, serum, and certain additional ingredients (see Table 7.1).

- Most milk-allergic individuals (children and adults) react to more than one milk protein.

- The potential of individual milk proteins to cause allergy has been studied by skin tests and oral challenge. However, the results obtained from the two types of test often do not agree.

- Casein proteins produce the highest number of positive skin tests in children with CMA, whereas beta-lactoglobulin produces the highest number of positive oral challenges.

Table 7-1
INDIVIDUAL PROTEINS IN COW'S MILK

Caseins	**Whey Proteins**
Alpha Caseins	Beta-Lactoglobulin
Alpha S1	Alpha-Lactoglobulin
Alpha S2	Proteose peptones
Beta-Caseins	
Kappa-Caseins	
Gamma-Caseins	
Serum Proteins	**Others**
Albumin	Lactoferrin
Immunoglobulins	Lactoperoxidase
	Alkaline phosphatase
	Catalase

Heat will change the nature of some milk proteins (heat-labile proteins), but others remain unaffected (heat-stable proteins). Serum proteins, beta-lactoglobulin, and alpha-lactalbumin are the most labile and are readily decomposed by heat. The caseins are the most heat stable. This means that people who are only allergic to the heat-labile proteins will be able to consume boiled or cooked milk, but those who are allergic to heat-stable proteins will not be able to consume either one.

Antibodies produced against milk proteins may be IgE, IgM, IgG, or sometimes IgA (see Chapter 1, p. 14 for a discussion of antibodies). Coupling of the milk protein antigen with its matching (homologous) antibody leads to the release of inflammatory mediators, which act directly on body tissues and cause inflammation. The tissues may be in the digestive tract, the skin, or the respiratory tract. Symptoms typical of allergy result in the affected tissues.

CMA is much more common in young infants and children than in adults. It is considered a condition of childhood rather than of adulthood. More than 90 percent of cases of IgE-mediated allergy occur within the first year of life. The majority of these occur within the first 6 months. However, in most cases, IgE-mediated CMA is outgrown by the age of 18 months to 2 years due to the maturing of both the immune system and the lining of the digestive tract.

In order to manage adverse reactions to cow's milk constituents successfully—whether the problem is an IgE-mediated allergy to cow's milk proteins or an inability to tolerate lactose—a diet free from all sources of milk proteins and lactose is necessary, at least initially. When the culprit components have been identified by appropriate challenge, the tolerated milk fractions can be re-introduced and the diet can be liberalized.

FEEDING THE MILK-ALLERGIC INFANT

There are several options for feeding the baby who is allergic to milk. Following is a discussion of these options and the steps needed to provide a nutritionally complete diet for the baby.

Mother's Milk

Without question, the best nutrition for the new-born baby and young infant is the mother's breast milk. A baby will never be allergic to mother's milk but may react to allergenic proteins that gain access to her milk from her diet. If the baby is definitely showing signs of allergy and is being exclusively breast-fed, the mother's diet must be investigated for the presence of allergenic foods to which her baby is reacting.

When CMA is suspected or proven to be a cause of the baby's symptoms, it is essential for the mother to remove all sources of milk from her own diet while she is breast-feeding. Molecules of milk from the maternal diet pass readily into her milk and will cause distress in her baby. Mothers should carefully follow the milk-free diet given in Table 7.2. They should also make sure to take supplemental calcium and vitamin D in addition to any vitamin and mineral supplements they are taking, as long as their diet remains milk-free.

Detecting CMA in the Breast-Fed Baby

If an exclusively breast-fed baby is exhibiting the type of symptoms previously discussed, the mother will inevitably question whether foods in her diet are responsible. Of course, the first thing she must do is consult her baby's doctor to rule out any other cause for the symptoms. Then the doctor will probably guide her in determining whether her baby's symptoms could be due to food allergy.

The most common allergenic foods that seem to cause symptoms at this early stage of life are eggs and milk. The mother should avoid these, and any other foods suspected to be causing a reaction in her infant, for a period of not less than 4 weeks to determine whether these are the cause of the baby's symptoms. (See Chapter 6 for detailed instructions for elimination and challenge to detect food allergy in the breast-fed baby.) Mothers should follow the milk-free diet given in Table 7.5 and the egg-free diet (Chapter 9) and exclude any other food that they suspect for 4 weeks while continuing to breast-feed their baby. Most important, they should be sure to obtain complete balanced nutrition from alternative sources while following these restrictions. Each of the diet plans in this book provides many alternatives to ensure that there will be no risk of a nutritional deficiency, as long as the directives are followed closely and completely.

After 4 weeks, mothers should consume each food individually and then monitor the baby's reactions from 2 to 6 hours after the mothers eat the food. Mothers should eat a good quantity to ensure that enough of the food molecules pass into the breast milk to trigger a response in the baby. This means at least one serving (more if they can) of each food that they have been avoiding (of course, as long as they are not allergic to it!). To determine whether the baby is allergic to milk, for example, mothers should drink a cup or more of whole milk.

If the baby reacts adversely to the food that the mothers have been avoiding, they will need to continue to avoid that particular food as long as they are breast-feeding their baby.

This is also a good way to determine whether the baby is still allergic to a food after the mothers have avoided it for 4 or 6 months. Sometimes babies outgrow their food allergies early. Then both mother and baby can relax their food restrictions, to the relief of all concerned.

Feeding the Lactose-Intolerant Baby

If the breast-fed baby is lactose intolerant (usually a temporary condition following intestinal infection at this age), mothers can continue to breast-feed, or pump their milk and treat it with lactase enzyme, until the baby's symptoms stop. (Details concerning feeding the lactose-intolerant infant are provided in Chapter 8, Lactose Intolerance.) There is no point in mothers' eliminating milk and milk products from their diet to treat lactose intolerance in the baby, because their breast milk will contain 6 percent lactose (w/v) regardless of whether or not they consume cow's milk.

Milk-Free Infant Formulas

Extensively hydrolyzed formulas (EHF) are the best alternative to milk-based formulas if the baby cannot be breast-fed. Hydrolyzed casein formulas (such as Similac® Alimentum [Abbott Nutrition], Nutramigen® or Enfamil Pregestimil® [Mead-Johnson]), or extensively hydrolyzed whey formulas (such as Profylac and Hypolac [Arla Foods] available in Europe) are usually tolerated by the milk-allergic infant. In these formulas, the proteins have been broken down into constituent amino acids and peptides too small to be allergenic. The biggest disadvantage of these formulas is their high cost.

If there is no resolution of symptoms on the EHF, an elemental amino acid formula (such as Neocate® [SHS]) might be the next step in managing the baby's condition. Your doctor or registered dietitian will discuss the need for this formula with you; its high cost may be a problem for some families.

Partially hydrolyzed milk-based formulas (PHF) (such as partially hydrolyzed whey [GoodStart from Nestlé]) are not suitable for infants with suspected or diagnosed cow's milk protein hypersensitivity. These formulas are suitable for babies who have no signs of CMA. Recent studies suggest that these types of formula may be effective, however, in reducing the risk of a non-allergic baby developing milk allergy.[4]

Introducing a Formula to the Breast-Fed Baby

The change from nursing at the breast to sucking on a nipple can, at first, be confusing to the exclusively breast-fed baby. But, eventually, all babies will adjust. However, mothers who wish to continue breast-feeding at the same time as supplementing with a formula often prefer to give the formula in a nursing cup rather than using a feeding bottle. Babies use less energy in feeding from a bottle compared with extracting milk from a breast, so, over time, they reject the breast for the easier option. Using a cup for the formula avoids this problem.

Adapting to the change in taste of the formula compared to breast milk requires further adjustment. This is particularly demanding when giving an EHF to the milk-allergic baby; the hydrolysis process radically changes the taste of milk. Nevertheless, over time, all babies will accept the taste. Taste preferences are not well-established at such an early age, and, even if the parents find the taste of the hydrolyzed formula unappealing, babies have no such prejudices. Adult distaste is not a reason to withhold the formula from a baby who would benefit from it!

A further difference between an extensively hydrolyzed formula, a cow's milk-based formula, and breast milk is the osmotic pressure of the EHF. EHFs require adaptation of the digestive tract to avoid the transient abdominal distress that accompanies a sharp change in osmotic pressure within the colon. With a previously breast-fed baby, this is best achieved by gradually introducing the formula over time. The following replacement schedule seems to work well:

- Replace one nursing per day with formula for a week; mix with breast milk for the first day or two to allow the baby to adjust to the change in taste.

- Replace two nursings per day with formula for the next week.

- Continue replacing one extra nursing period with formula per week until all feedings are replaced with formula, without mixing with breast milk.

For a baby fed with cow's milk-based formula, start by diluting the EHF by half with sterile (boiled and cooled) water. Then gradually increase the strength of the formula over 1 week (or 2 weeks if the baby is fussy) until the baby is taking the EHF at full strength.

Infants should continue the hydrolysate or amino acid formula (or soy-based formula, if a soy protein allergy or intolerance has been ruled out) until they are eating a range of solid foods sufficient to supply all of their nutritional needs. After the age of 12 months, or when they are eating a good range of solid foods, milk-allergic children may do well on milk substitutes (for example, fortified soy or rice milks) and other calcium-fortified foods, if allergy to these foods is not suspected.

SOY AND THE ALLERGIC BABY

- About 50 percent of babies with IgE-mediated CMA develop an allergy to soy.

- In addition, soy can cause a non-IgE mediated response (intolerance) that is separate and distinct from allergy. The effects are localized in the digestive tract, where symptoms such as colicky pain, abdominal bloating, gas, and diarrhea are apparent. This is sometimes referred to as soy enteropathy.

THE MILK-FREE DIET

All milk and milk-containing foods must be avoided. These foods include liquid and evaporated milks, fermented milks (yogurt, buttermilk), all cheeses (hard cheeses, cottage cheese, cream cheese), ice cream, ice milk, and any foods containing milk solids, such as cream, butter, and margarines containing whey. In addition, all foods or beverages containing components of milk, such as casein, whey, lactoglobulin, and their hydrolysates, must not be consumed. (See Table 7.2 for help in reading food labels.)

Table 7-2
LABEL-READING GUIDELINES FOR A MILK-FREE DIET

Terms Indicating the Presence of Cow's Milk Components

Butter	Acidophilus milk	Hydrolyzed casein
Butter fat	Lactaid® milk	Ammonium caseinate
Butter-flavored oil	Lacteeze® milk	Calcium caseinate
Butter solids	Condensed milk	Potassium caseinate
Whipped butter	Evaporated milk	Sodium caseinate
Artificial butter flavor	Cultured milk	Rennet casein
Natural butter flavor	Milk solids	Whey
Buttermilk	Malted milk	Whey protein
Buttermilk solids	Milk powder	Whey powder
Cheese	Cream	Sweet dairy whey
Cottage cheese	Whipped cream	Whey hydrolysate
Processed cheese	Half-and-half	Hydrolyzed whey
Cream cheese	Light cream	Delactosed whey
Feta	Ice cream	Demineralized whey
Ricotta	Ice milk	Lactose
Quark	Sherbet	Lactulose
Curd	Yogurt	Lactoglobulin
Homogenized;	Casein	Lactalbumin
1%; 2%; skim;	Casein hydrolysate	
whole; lowfat;		
nonfat milk		

Ingredients That May Contain Milk Proteins

Brown sugar flavoring	Margarine	Natural flavor
Caramel flavor	Chocolate	Simplesse®
High protein flour		

Note: Lactic acid, lactate, and lactylate do not contain milk and need not be avoided.

Alternate Sources of Nutrients

Milk is an important source of protein in the diet of most children. Fortunately, adequate protein is also readily available from meat, poultry, eggs, fish, shellfish, soybeans and other legumes, nuts, and seeds. It is not usually a problem to provide adequate protein for your child unless he or she is allergic to these foods. However, because milk is the most important source of these micronutrients in a child's diet, you will need to find a supplemental source of calcium and vitamin D.

Calcium

Milk is the most abundant and readily available source of calcium in the normal diet. One cup of milk contains about 0.001 oz (290 mg) of calcium.

Good alternative calcium sources include the following (see Table 7.4 for more details).

- Canned fish with bones, such as sardines and salmon, provide calcium. The calcium is in the bones; the canning process softens them, making them more easily digested.

- Green leafy vegetables, such as arugula (rocket kale), kale, beet and turnip greens, collards, mustard greens, and broccoli, also contain calcium. However, the calcium in vegetables is not so readily available to the body as that from animal sources.

- Some nuts and legumes contain calcium.

Calcium Absorption

There is a difference between the amount of calcium consumed and the amount that is actually taken in by a person's body. This is an important consideration in any diet.

- The percentage of the calcium contained in foods that is actually absorbed, used, and retained by the body is variable, depending on age, level of calcium intake, type of food eaten, and other nutrients eaten at the same time.

Table 7-3
DIETARY REFERENCE INTAKE (DRI) VALUES
FOR CALCIUM AND VITAMIN D[5]

Life Stage Group Male and Female	Calcium AI (mg/day)	Vitamin D[b] AI (mcg/day)[c]
0 to 6 months*	210	5
7 to 12 months	270	5
1 through 3 years	500	5
4 through 8 years	800	5
9 through 13 years	1300	5
14 through 18 years	1300	5
19 through 30 years	1000	5
31 through 50 years	1000	5
51 through 70 years	1200	10
> 70 years	1200	15
Pregnancy[a]:		
</= 18 years	1300	5
19 through 50 years	1000	5
Lactation[a]:		
</= 18 years	1300	5
19 through 50 years	1000	5

[a] Female only for pregnancy and lactation values
[b] As cholecalciferol (1 microgram [mcg] = 40 IU vitamin D)
[c] In the absence of adequate exposure to sunlight
*Source of calcium is mother's milk

Table 7-4
NONDAIRY SOURCES OF CALCIUM

NOTE: DO NOT EAT ANY FOOD WHICH CAUSES YOU TO HAVE AN ALLERGIC REACTION.

Listed according to calcium **content**. Ca = calcium

FOOD	PORTION	
	Metric	US/Imperial
More than 300 mg Ca		
Sardines, with bones, canned	85 g	3 oz
Rhubarb*, frozen cooked	270 g	1 cup
Wheat flour, artificially enriched	125 g	1 cup
Collards*, frozen, cooked	170 g	1 cup
Arugula (rocket kale)	170 g	1 cup
250– 300 mg Ca		
Sockeye salmon, with bones, canned (213g/can) (7.5-oz can)	100 g	½ can
Rhubarb*, fresh, cooked	270 g	1 cup
Spinach*, cooked	190 g	1 cup
200–250 mg Ca		
Almonds	125 mL	½ cup
Pink salmon, with bones, canned (213g/can) (7.5-oz can)	100 g	½ can
Oysters, raw, meat only	250 g	1 cup
Sugar, brown, packed down	220 g	1 cup
Turnip greens*, cooked	165 g	1 cup

* Contains oxalic acid, which impairs calcium absorption. Although the calcium is present in the food at the given level, the actual amount absorbed is significantly less.

Table 7-4 (continued) NONDAIRY SOURCES OF CALCIUM		
FOOD	**PORTION**	
	Metric	**US/Imperial**
150–200 mg Ca		
Beet greens*, leaves and stems, cooked	145 g	1 cup
Kale, frozen, cooked	130 g	1 cup
Amaranth (cooked grain): uncooked weight 100 g (cooked)		1 cup
100–150 mg Ca		
Baked beans, canned	250 mL	1 cup
Brazil nuts	125 mL	½ cup
Scallops		7 medium
Sesame seeds	125 mL	½ cup
Soybeans, cooked	250 mL	1 cup
Tofu (8 x 6 x 2 cm)		1 piece
Shrimp, meat only	113 g	4 oz
Molasses, cane, blackstrap	20 g	1 tbsp
Dandelion greens*, cooked	105 g	1 cup
Mustard greens*	140 g	1 cup
Okra pods, cooked	160 g	1 cup
Brussels sprouts*	156 g	1 cup
Broccoli, cooked	250 mL	1 cup
50–100 mg Ca		
Asparagus, fresh, cooked, drained	240 g	1½ cup
Lima beans, cooked	180 g	1 cup
Green beans, cooked	125 g	1 cup
Yellow or wax beans, cooked	125 g	1 cup
Cabbage*, fresh, cooked	217 g	1½ cup
Chinese cabbage* (Bok choy)	76 g	1 cup

Table 7-4 (continued) NONDAIRY SOURCES OF CALCIUM		
FOOD	**PORTION**	
	Metric	**US/Imperial**
50–100 mg Ca (continued)		
Sauerkraut*	235 g	1 cup
Carrots, cooked	234 g	1½ cups
Parsnips, cooked	155 g	1 cup
50–100 mg Ca		
Onions, cooked	210 g	1 cup
Tomatoes, canned, solids and liquid	241 g	1 cup
Chili con carne with beans	250 mL	1 cup
Red kidney beans, cooked	250 mL	1 cup
White beans cooked	250 mL	1 cup
Beans, dry, cooked, and drained	180 g	1 cup
Lentils, cooked	200 g	1 cup
Garbanzo beans (chickpeas), cooked	250 mL	1 cup
Wheat germ	113 g	1 tbsp
Oats, puffed	50 g	2 oz
Orange, raw		1 medium
Orange sections	180 g	1 cup
Hazelnuts, chopped	28 g	1 oz
Cereal, All-Bran	250 mL	1 cup
Cereal, 100% Bran	250 mL	1 cup
Cereal, Branbuds	250 mL	1 cup
Cereal, Granola	150 mL	⅔ cup
15–50 mg Ca *Cereals:*		
Bran flakes and raisins	250 mL	1 cup
Corn bran	250 mL	1 cup

FOOD	PORTION	
Table 7-4 (continued) **NONDAIRY SOURCES OF CALCIUM**		
	Metric	US/Imperial
15–50 mg Ca (continued)		
Cereals:		
Cheerios	250 mL	1 cup
Oatmeal, cooked	250 mL	1 cup
Shredded wheat (10 mg Ca each biscuit)		2–5 pieces
Shreddies	250 mL	1 cup
Bread:		
Cracked wheat	(22 mg Ca per slice)	1slice
Mixed grain	(27 mg Ca per slice)	1 slice
Rye, light	(19 mg Ca per slice)	1 slice
White	(24 mg Ca per slice)	1 slice
Whole wheat 100%	(25 mg Ca per slice)	1 slice
Whole wheat 60%	(23 mg Ca per slice)	1 slice
White bun, hamburger or hot dog	(37–44 mg Ca)	1
Pita, whole wheat 16.5 cm diam.	(49 mg Ca)	1
Tortilla, corn	(42 mg Ca)	1
Vegetables:		
Cabbage, raw, shredded	250 mL	1 cup
Carrot, raw, medium		1
Cauliflower, raw, cooked	250 mL	1 cup
Celery, diced, raw	250 mL	1 cup

Table 7-4 (continued) NONDAIRY SOURCES OF CALCIUM		
FOOD	**PORTION**	
	Metric	**US/Imperial**
Vegetables: (continued)		
Turnip, cooked	250 mL	1 cup
Spinach, raw, chopped	125 mL	½ cup
Olives, black		5 large
Olives, green		5 medium
Parsley, raw, chopped	25 mL	2 tbsp
Peas, boiled	250 mL	1 cup
15–50 mg Ca		
Fruit:		
Grapefruit, raw		1 medium
Kiwi		1 large
Figs, dried, uncooked		1 medium
Pear, raw		1 medium
Raisins	125 mL	½ cup
Other:		
Chocolate	30 g	1 square
Egg, whole, cooked		1 large
Maple syrup	15 mL	1 tbsp
Peanuts, oil roasted	50 mL	¼ cup
Sunflower seeds, kernel	50 mL	4 tbsp
Soymilk, liquid	250 mL	1 cup

- An average adult will absorb approximately 40 percent of the calcium in his or her diet. This increases during growth, pregnancy, and lactation and is reduced during aging. In general, the lower the intake, the more calcium is retained in the body (i.e., less calcium is excreted when intake is low).

- In order for the body to absorb calcium efficiently, an adequate level of vitamin D is necessary. Vitamin D is obtained from some foods (milk, liver, egg yolk), but the best source is the action of sunlight (UV light) on the skin. A diet high in phosphorus and protein (a traditional, high-protein American diet) tends to reduce the amount of calcium retained in the body.

Calcium Supplements

If all milk and dairy products are removed from a child's diet, it is often difficult to obtain sufficient calcium from these alternative sources on a regular basis. A supplement is then necessary. The most well-absorbed and utilized forms of calcium are calcium gluconate, calcium citrate malate, the Kreb's cycle derivatives (citrate, fumarate, malate, succinate, glutamate), and other acidic derivatives of carbonate. These forms are superior to calcium carbonate as a source of the mineral. The various form names will appear on the label of the supplement, so you should become familiar with them when selecting an appropriate calcium supplement.

Calcium Supplements

- Calcium carbonate provides 0.022 to 0.026 oz (625 to 750 mg) of elemental calcium per half-teaspoon (2.5 mL).

- However, calcium citrate malate or calcium gluconate appear to be more effective supplements than calcium carbonate. In addition, some research studies indicate that they may interfere less with the absorption of iron than calcium carbonate.

- Some authorities find that chelated minerals are absorbed and utilized more efficiently than the unchanged mineral salt. A chelated calcium with magnesium product is available (read labels) that also ensures adequate magnesium intake (which tends to be reduced in diets rich in calcium).

The use of calcium-based antacids as a source of calcium is not recommended. Antacids (such as Tums™ and Rolaids™) are designed to neutralize stomach acid in cases of heartburn and acid reflux or indigestion. However, stomach acid is essential for the first stage of protein digestion (acid hydrolysis) and neutralizing this acid reduces the digestion of proteins in food. In addition, the antacid produces an alkaline environment. This alkalinity may reduce the uptake of a variety of minerals (such as iron, zinc, copper, and calcium itself) that require an acidic medium for efficient absorption.

IMPORTANT MICRONUTRIENTS IN MILK

Milk and milk products are an important source of calcium, phosphorus, vitamin D, vitamin B12 , riboflavin, pantothenic acid, potassium, vitamin A, and vitamin E (vitamins D and A are added as fortification during processing).

These nutrients must be obtained from other foods and supplements when all milk is removed from the diet.

Heating and Processing of Milk

Heating or boiling milk will not make it nonallergenic, although a few of the proteins may be decomposed, reducing their allergenicity to some extent. Only children who are allergic to heat-labile proteins (see prior discussion) will tolerate boiled milk and will also be able to tolerate canned milk (evaporated milk) that has been extensively heated. Milk as an ingredient in cooked products is sometimes tolerated when unheated milk is not. However, some of the allergenic milk proteins will cause allergy in very sensitive individuals, even after cooking. The cow's milk in common infant formulas remains allergenic and will induce an allergic reaction in milk-allergic babies.

Milk from Other Animals

Goat's milk may be tolerated for a time by a small number of children with CMA. However goat's milk allergy frequently develops quite quickly in children who are allergic to cow's milk. In one study, 24 out of 26 children with CMA had an allergic reaction to goat's milk.[6] Also, immunological studies have indicated that the proteins in cow's milk and goat's milk are antigenically very similar. The chances of developing an allergy to goat's milk for a person with CMA is obviously quite high, and authorities agree that "the milk of goat and sheep harbor an allergic potential and is not (*sic*)suitable for the nutrition of milk-allergic patients."[7]

If goat's milk is used as a replacement for cow's milk, it is important to make sure that there are adequate sources of folate in the child's diet. In comparison to cow's milk, goat's milk is deficient in this vitamin.

Substitutes for Milk in Meals and Recipes

The following products can substitute for milk in appearance, flavor, and texture, but they are not nutritionally equivalent to milk. None of these substitutes can be used as a sole source of nutrition.

Some of these products contain potentially allergenic ingredients, such as soya or nuts, so it is also important to make sure that your child is not allergic to these alternatives.

Soy Milk

- Soy milk is an acceptable substitute for milk on breakfast cereals and in many recipes. However, some highly allergic children may be or become allergic to soybeans and their products.

- Liquid soy milk can be substituted directly for milk, diluting 1:1 with water (1 cup soy milk added to 1 cup water). Use soy milk undiluted in recipes requiring evaporated milk.

- Many soy beverages are made from uncooked soy beans. Some sensitive people cannot tolerate the raw form of the bean, but tolerate it cooked. If a soy beverage causes digestive tract symptoms, try boiling it for a few minutes and try it again.

- If the taste of soy milk is unpalatable, the addition of lime juice will often make it more acceptable.

- There are several soy-based beverages on the market that are designed as milk substitutes. They are enriched with calcium. These drinks require no dilution.

Rice Milks (e.g., Rice Dream™ [Imagine Foods])

Rice milk is usually made from brown rice and safflower oil. It contains very little protein and therefore, on its own, is not a suitable dietary substitute for milk. Rice milks make an acceptable alternative to milk on cereals and in baking. The calcium-enriched type is recommended for children.

Other Liquids

Meat stock, vegetable bouillon, fruit juice, vegetable oil mixed with water, or just plain water may be added to recipes when only a small amount of milk (less than 1 cup) is needed. When making rice, tapioca, or semolina puddings, use fruit juice instead of milk. Potato water can be used instead of milk in making breads.

Nut Milks

Protein-rich nuts and seeds can be used in place of milk, as long as the child is not also allergic to them. The nuts or seeds can be ground into a fine flour consistency in a blender or coffee grinder, and water is added to make a smooth mixture of the desired consistency. A good mix for most purposes includes 1 cup of nut meal plus 2 cups water. It can be added to recipes in the same quantity as milk.

Whey-Free Margarines

Most margarines are fortified with whey. A few brands, in particular diet spreads, do not contain whey. All of the major ingredients are listed on the product label, so read the labels carefully to determine which margarines are whey-free. Parkay™ Diet Spread, Fleischman's™ low sodium, no salt, and Canoleo™ margarine are examples. Use these in place of butter.

Non-Dairy Creamers and Cream Substitutes

There are several milk-free products on the market designed for use in tea and coffee that are made from oils; an example is Coffee Rich™ (Morningstar Foods).

Nondairy toppings (such as Rich Whip™ [Rich Foods]) can replace whipped cream in desserts.

Read labels carefully. Some products labeled dairy-free contain casein. They are designed for consumption by people with lactose intolerance, but they are not suitable for children or adults with CMA.

Cheese Substitutes

Soybean cake (tofu) can be substituted for cheese in many recipes, and fresh soybean curd may be an acceptable substitute for cottage cheese. Make sure the tofu does not contain milk solids. Some products called tofu cheese do contain milk proteins such as casein. Read labels carefully.

GOAT'S MILK

- Goat's milk proteins closely resemble those in cow's milk.

- Most children who have an established allergy to cow's milk proteins demonstrate, or soon develop, a similar sensitivity to goat's milk proteins.

- Goat's milk is deficient in folate.

- Substituting the milk of animals such as goats and sheep for cow's milk is not recommended.

MARE'S MILK

- Only a few proteins in mare's milk are similar to those in cow's milk.

- In a research study in 2000, only 1 out of 25 children with CMA were allergic to mare's milk.[8]

- Mare's milk may be a good substitute for cow's milk for children with CMA.

Table 7-5
FOODS ALLOWED AND RESTRICTED IN A MILK-FREE DIET

Type of Food	Foods Allowed	Foods Restricted
Milk and Milk Products	• Milk-free substitutes • Soy beverages • Soy-based infant formula • Casein hydrolysate formula • Rice milks • Coconut milk • Nut milks • Seed milks • Non-dairy creamers: e.g., Coffee Rich • Potato starch-based drinks (e.g., Dari-free [Vance's DariFree]) • Clarified butter • Milk-free margarine • Whey-free margarine • Milk-free soybean cake	• All cow's milk (whole; 2%; 1%; skim; Lactaid ™, Lacteeze™, or other lactose-free or lactose-reduced milk; acidophilus milk) • Milk from other animals (goat; sheep; other) • All milk derivatives (cream, half-and-half; whipping cream; light cream; sour cream; ice cream) • All milk products (buttermilk; yogurt; quark; kefir; cheese of all types) • Any manufactured product containing ingredients indicating milk (see section on Label Reading) such as: – Casein – Caseinates – Whey – Lactose – Lactalbumin – Lactoglobulin – Milk solids

Table 7-5 (continued)
FOODS ALLOWED AND RESTRICTED IN A MILK-FREE DIET

Type of Food	Foods Allowed	Foods Restricted
Breads and Cereals	• Breads and baked goods made without milk or milk products • French or Italian bread • Some whole wheat bread • Some rye bread • Soda crackers • Bagels • Pasta without cheese or milk-containing sauce • Plain, cooked, or ready-to-eat cereals • All plain grains, flours, and starches	• Baked products made with milk or milk products, such as breads, crackers, biscuits, muffins, pancakes • Cereals containing milk or milk solids • Commercial baking mixes • Any manufactured food containing ingredients indicating that they were derived from milk

Legumes	• All plain legumes, such as dried beans, dried peas; lentils; dal
	• Milk-free; casein-free tofu
	• Peanut butter
	• Soybeans
	• Any soybean product free of milk components
		• Any prepared with milk ingredients such as:
		  – Milk
		  – Cream
		  – Cheese

Table 7-5 (continued)
FOODS ALLOWED AND RESTRICTED IN A MILK-FREE DIET

Type of Food	Foods Allowed	Foods Restricted
Fruit	• All pure fruits and pure fruit juices	• Any with cream, milk, or butter as additional ingredients, toppings, or sauces
Meat, Poultry, and Fish	• All fresh or frozen meat, poultry, or fish • Kosher-processed meats (may be called "parve" or "pareve") • Processed meats made without milk or milk products • Meat, poultry, and fish canned without milk or milk products	• Commercially produced meat, poultry, or fish that is: – Breaded – Battered – Creamed • Commercially produced meat products containing milk ingredients, such as meat loaf, hot dogs, cold cuts, sausages
Eggs	• Plain, boiled, fried, or poached • Omelette or scrambled made without milk or cheese • Milk-free mayonnaise	• Any egg dish containing milk ingredients such as: – Milk – Cream – Cheese – Commercial mayonnaise
Nuts and Seeds	• All plain nuts and seeds	• Nuts, seeds, and nut and seed mixtures with coatings containing milk or lactose • Any nut or seed candies or confectioneries containing milk ingredients

	Table 7-5 (continued) FOODS ALLOWED AND RESTRICTED IN A MILK-FREE DIET		
Type of Food	**Foods Allowed**	**Foods Restricted**
Spices and Herbs	• All pure spices and herbs	• None
Sweeteners	• All pure sugar, syrup, honey • Sugar Twin®	• Sugar substitutes containing lactose

Fats and Oils	• Clarified butter
	• Pure vegetable oils
	• Milk-free margarines such as:
	  – Fleischmann's® low sodium, no salt
	  – Parkay Diet Spread®
	  – Canoleo® margarine
	• Real mayonnaise
	• Nondairy dessert topping
	• Shortening
	• Lard
	• Meat dripping
	• Gravy made without milk
		• Cream
		• Sour cream
		• Cream cheese
		• Whipped topping
		• Butter
		• Margarine containing whey or milk
		• Salad dressings with milk or milk products

References

1. Crittenden RG, Bennett LE. Cow's milk allergy: A complex disorder. *Journal of the American College of Nutrition* 2005; 24(6):582S–591S.

2. Hill DJ, Hosking CS. The cow milk allergy complex: Overlapping disease profiles in infancy. *European Journal of Clinical Nutrition* 1995;49(Suppl 1):S1–S12.

3. Pumphrey RS. Lessons for management of anaphylaxis from a study of fatal reactions. *Clinical & Experimental Allergy* 2000;30:1144–1150.

4. Hays T, Wood RA. A systematic review of the role of hydrolyzed infant formulas in allergy prevention. *Archives of Pediatrics and Adolescent Medicine* 2005;159:810–816.

5. Dietary Reference Intakes (DRIs): Estimated Average Requirements for Groups. Food and Nutrition Board, Institute of Medicine, the National Academy of Sciences. 1997. Tables may be accessed via www.nap.edu

6. Bellioni-Businco B, Paganelli R, Lucebti P, Giampietro PG, Perborn H, Businco L. Allergenicity of goat's milk in children with cow milk allergy. *Journal of Allergy and Clinical Immunology* 1999;103(6):1191–1194.

7. Bellioni-Businco B, Paganelli R, Lucebti P, Giampietro PG, Perborn H, Businco L. Allergenicity of goat's milk in children with cow milk allergy.

8. Businco L, Giampietro P, Lucenti P, Lucaroni F, Pini C, Di Felice G, Lacovacci P, Curadi C, Orlandi M. Allergenicity of mare's milk in children with cow's milk allergy. *Journal of Allergy and Clinical Immunology* 2000;105(5):1031–1034.

CHAPTER 8

Lactose Intolerance

ABOUT LACTOSE

Lactose is milk sugar.

Lactose intolerance is caused by a lack of the enzyme (called lactase) required to digest it in the digestive tract.

Lactose intolerance is not an allergy.

Milk allergy is caused by an immunological reaction against the proteins in milk.

WHAT IS LACTOSE?

Lactose is a sugar that occurs only in milk. It is found in the milk of all mammals, including humans, cows, goats, sheep, horses, buffalo, and so on. It is the most important source of immediate energy for the immature infant of all species from birth until weaning.

Lactose is actually two sugar molecules joined together; it is known as a disaccharide.[a] The complete lactose molecule is too large to pass through the layer of cells that line the digestive tract (the epithelium), so it must be broken down into smaller pieces in order to reach the circulation and be used as a source of energy for the body. The digestive enzyme that performs this breakdown is called *lactase*. Lactase splits lactose into its two constituent sugars: glucose and galactose. These are single sugars, called monosaccharides.[b] Monosaccharides are small enough to be transported across the cells that line the digestive tract and into circulation, where they are an important source of energy for many body functions.

The normal diet usually contains 10 percent lactose. When this is digested in the small intestine by the lactase enzyme, it produces 5 percent glucose and 5 percent galactose, both of which are carried into circulation by an active transport system across the epithelium.

WHAT IS LACTASE?

Lactase is the enzyme that digests lactose; its chemical name is beta-galactosidase (β-galactosidase). Lactase is made within the epithelial cells lining the digestive tract. If these cells are damaged, they are unable to produce adequate amounts of lactase. As a result, lactose is incompletely broken down into glucose and galactose. The remaining undigested lactose stays in the intestines and eventually finds its way into the large bowel. In the bowel, millions of bacteria use undigested food for their own nourishment, multiplying rapidly, and producing a large number of by-products. Usually, a variety of gases, organic acids, and other irritating chemicals result from the activity of these micro-organisms. The effects are felt as excessive gas or wind (flatus), abdominal bloating, pain, loose stool or diarrhea, and general distress in the lower intestines.

Lactase is produced in quite small amounts compared to the other enzymes that digest disaccharide sugars in the diet, such as sucrose, maltose, and others derived from starches. Lactose is broken down at only half the rate of sucrose, for example. This means that, if a large dose of lactose is consumed,

---

a Disaccharide: double sugar (di = two; saccharide = sugar)
b Monosaccharide: single sugar (mono = one or single; saccharide = sugar)

there may not be enough lactase present to digest it all at once. As a result, some of the undigested lactose finds its way into the colon. In the colon, it causes the imbalance that produces the miserable symptoms of lactose intolerance, even in a baby who is producing a normal quantity of lactase. The consequences of excess lactose in the breast-fed baby are discussed later in this chapter.

ADDITIONAL FACTORS IN THE DEVELOPMENT OF SYMPTOMS IN LACTOSE INTOLERANCE

The severity of the symptoms depends not only on the amount of lactose ingested but also on other factors, especially the following:

- A person's sensitivity to pain in the digestive tract

- The rate at which the contents of the stomach empty into the small intestine

- The speed at which the meal moves along the digestive tract

- The type of microorganisms living in the large intestine

Lactose intolerance does not involve the immune system, and no antibodies are produced. Therefore, lactose intolerance is not an allergy.

INCIDENCE OF LACTASE DEFICIENCY

Normal lactase activity in the human body varies by the individual and age. Deficiencies of lactase can be either an ongoing or a temporary condition.

In Babies and Young Children

Virtually every baby has adequate supplies of lactase to digest the lactose in the mother's milk at birth. Lactase deficiency in infants is uncommon. Lactose is the principal sugar in human milk, and the baby needs lactase in order to digest it and provide the developing body with a crucial source of energy.

There is an extremely rare medical condition known as congenital alactasia, or primary lactase deficiency, in which the baby is born without the ability to produce the enzyme.

A temporary lactase deficiency can develop in babies when the inflammation associated with a bacterial or viral infection in the digestive tract damages the cells that produce the enzyme. This is known as secondary lactase deficiency (as opposed to primary congenital alactasia). Happily, in secondary lactose intolerance, the cells rapidly return to normal when the infection abates, and the usual level of lactase production is quickly re-established.

In Older Children and Adults

The majority of adults lose some degree of lactase activity after puberty. In certain ethnic groups, such as the Asian races, African blacks, people of Middle Eastern origin, aboriginal peoples of North and South America and the Arctic, and Mediterranean people, lactose intolerance may be as high as 80 percent of the population. In contrast, only about 20 percent of people of northern European origin lose the ability to produce lactase. In most cases, complete loss of lactase does not occur. However, the enzyme may be produced at such a low level that consumption of milk and milk products with normal levels of lactose leads to the uncomfortable symptoms of lactose intolerance.

Secondary lactase deficiency can occur in adults as well as children. Bacterial and viral infections and, sometimes, the use of strong drugs and medications such as antibiotics taken by mouth may cause damage to the fragile epithelial cells in the digestive tract. If lactose was tolerated prior to the epithelial damage, regular lactase activity will be resumed as soon as the cells return to normal.

DISTINGUISHING BETWEEN MILK ALLERGY AND LACTOSE INTOLERANCE

It is sometimes difficult to distinguish milk allergy from lactose intolerance on the basis of clinical symptoms alone. This is because some of the symptoms, such as abdominal pain, diarrhea, nausea, vomiting, gas, and bloating, are common to both conditions. However, milk allergy often results in symptoms in other organs, such as the upper respiratory tract (for example, a stuffy, runny nose); pain, itching, fluid drainage from the ears; or skin reactions (such as eczema or hives). Lactose intolerance does not result in these symptoms.

Since secondary lactase deficiency is a consequence of inflammation in the digestive tract, the intestinal inflammation caused by milk allergy can sometimes result in lactase deficiency. Thus, both milk allergy and lactose intolerance can exist together. Because milk is the only source of lactose in the normal diet, eliminating milk from the diet will cure both conditions. But removal of milk will not distinguish the cause of the symptoms. It is important to determine which condition is causing the problem, because milk and milk products are a significant source of nutrients, especially for infants and young children, and should not be eliminated unless it is absolutely necessary. Furthermore, eliminating milk from the diet entirely is not easy, because so many different foods, such as baked goods, soups, salad dressings, gravies, desserts, and so on, contain milk. Avoiding all of these foods can make meal planning very difficult.

LABORATORY TESTS FOR LACTOSE INTOLERANCE

There are a number of laboratory tests that are often used to identify lactose intolerance. They are discussed below.

The **Fecal Reducing Sugar Test** is considered by many clinicians as the most reliable of the currently available tests. After the patient is given a drink containing lactose, the feces are collected and Fehling's solution is added. The presence of lactose is indicated by a change in color, from blue to red. The lactose "reduces" the chemical in the solution. Thus, a change in color indicates that a deficiency of lactase has led to undigested lactose being excreted in the feces.

The **Hydrogen Breath Test** is a more common test for lactose intolerance. In this test, the patient ingests a quantity of lactose, and, after a prescribed interval, a breath sample is analyzed for the presence of hydrogen. If hydrogen is detected, it indicates that bacteria in the digestive tract have acted on undigested lactose and produced hydrogen as one of their metabolic by-products.

Lactose intolerance is defined by a level of breath hydrogen of more than 20 parts per million (ppm) after ingestion of 0.035 ounces per 2.2 pounds (1 gram per kilogram) of body weight or 1.76 ounces (50 grams) of lactose. Unfortunately, this test is not specific for lactase deficiency, because any sugar remaining in the digestive tract will be metabolized by bacteria with the production of hydrogen. Undigested sucrose, maltose, or starch will yield a similar result.

The **Blood Glucose Test** involves measurement of the level of glucose in the blood after the patient has taken a drink containing 1.76 ounces (50 grams) of lactose. An increase in blood glucose concentration indicates that lactose has been broken down to glucose and galactose, the levels of which rise in the blood when the body is producing an adequate amount of lactase. An increase of less than 1.12 millimole (mmol) per liter indicates that lactose has not been digested and, hence, suggests a diagnosis of lactose intolerance. Measuring the level of galactose would be equally informative.

There is also a **Fecal pH Test**. If the feces collected after the lactose drink are acidic, with a pH of 6 or lower[c], it indicates that microorganisms in the large bowel have fermented the undigested lactose. The microbial activity results in the production of acids, which lower the pH of the stool. Thus, the diagnosis of lactose intolerance is further reinforced.

MANAGEMENT OF LACTOSE INTOLERANCE

Lactase deficiency is easier to manage than cow's milk protein allergy (CMA), because any milk or milk product free from lactose can be consumed with impunity. Lactose-free milk is available as products such as Lacteeze™ or Lactaid™. Alternatively, a commercial form of lactase (sold as Lactaid liquid) can be added to the milk before consumption. After 24 hours in a refrigerator, the lactose is split into its two component sugars, glucose and galactose, which the body can absorb and use without harm. All of the nutrients and proteins in milk are thus available to the body, and the risk of nutritional deficiency as a result of long-time avoidance of milk is averted.

---

[c] pH measures acidity and alkalinity. pH 7.0 is neutral. A value above 7 is alkaline; a value below 7 is acidic.

It is more difficult to avoid lactose in prepared foods; anything containing milk or milk solids is likely to contain lactose also. Some people find that they can consume lactose-containing foods with impunity if they take Lactaid in the form of a tablet before eating.

Lactose intolerance is dose-related. Usually, the cells are producing a limited amount of the enzyme lactase, and small doses of foods containing lactose can be processed. Problems occur when the amount of lactose in the food exceeds the capacity of the enzyme to digest it. The important thing is to determine tolerance levels. If lactose-intolerant individuals remain within personal limits, symptoms should not occur. Most people who are lactose intolerant can drink a 6-ounce glass of milk without symptoms, but they may experience abdominal discomfort if they exceed this amount.

When lactose intolerance has been diagnosed, the degree of lactase deficiency can be assessed by taking increasing quantities of lactose in a variety of dairy products (Table 8-1). Most lactase-deficient individuals can process the lactose in one glass of milk, which is about 0.39 ounces (11 grams) of lactose. But taking several types of milk and dairy products in a 24-hour period would exceed their enzyme's capacity to break down lactose, and digestive tract symptoms would result.

Not all foods derived from milk contain the same amount of lactose. In the process of making hard cheeses, whole milk is curdled, resulting in two distinct fractions: the familiar curds and whey. The curd is made up of solidified proteins known as caseins. The whey is the liquid from which the curds separate and consists of a number of soluble proteins that differ from the caseins. This liquid fraction also contains the lactose part of milk. The curds are used to make hard cheeses and are separated from the whey in the cheese-making process. This separation also removes the lactose from the curds. Therefore, the hard cheeses made from the curds are virtually free from lactose. Most lactose-intolerant people can eat almost all hard cheese without any discomfort.

Butter contains virtually undetectable amounts of lactose. In making butter, the fat is removed from the rest of the milk and is churned in a process that results in a solid product. By separating the fat from the rest of the milk constituents, lactose is also excluded, and hence the butterfat is free from lactose.

Table 8-1

LEVELS OF LACTOSE IN NORMAL SERVING SIZES OF COMMON FOODS AND BEVERAGES

Product	Serving Size	Lactose ounces (grams)
Sweetened condensed milk	½ cup (125 milliliters [mL])	0.5 (15)
Evaporated milk	½ cup (125 mL)	0.4 (12)
Whole milk	1 cup (250 mL)	0.39 (11)
2% milk	1 cup (250 mL)	0.39 (11)
1% milk	1 cup (250 mL)	0.39 (11)
Skim milk	1 cup (250 mL)	0.39 (11)
Buttermilk	1 cup (250 mL)	0.35 (10)
Ice milk	½ cup (125 mL)	0.32 (9)
Ice cream	½ cup (125 mL)	0.21 (6)
Half-and-half light cream	½ cup (125 mL)	0.17 (5)
Yogurt, low fat	1 cup (250 mL)	0.17 (5)
Sour cream	½ cup (125 mL)	0.14 (4)
Cottage cheese, creamed	½ cup (125 mL)	0.1 (3)
Whipping cream	½ cup (125 mL)	0.1 (3)
Cottage cheese, uncreamed	½ cup (125 mL)	0.07 (2)
Sherbet, orange	½ cup (125 mL)	0.07 (2)
American (Jack) cheese	1 ounce (30 grams)	0.07 (2)
Swiss cheese	1 ounce (30 grams)	0.035 (1)
Blue cheese	1 ounce (30 grams)	0.035 (1)
Cheddar cheese	1 ounce (30 grams)	0.035 (1)
Parmesan cheese	1 ounce (30 grams)	0.035 (1)
Cream cheese (e.g., Philadelphia™)	1 ounce (30 grams)	0.035 (1)
Lactaid™ milk	½ cup (125 mL)	0.0008 (0.025)
Butter	1 teaspoon (5 mL)	trace

MICROORGANISMS AND LACTOSE INTOLERANCE

Fermented milk products such as yogurt can improve lactose digestion. They are usually well tolerated by most lactose-intolerant people. Studies have shown that, after eating unheated yogurt containing live bacteria, people with lactose intolerance have improved lactose digestion and consequently fewer and less severe symptoms than when they consume milk or pasteurized yogurt. These beneficial effects are due to the production of the enzyme that digests lactose (β-galactosidase) by bacteria in the fermented milk product. This microbial enzyme performs exactly the same function as human lactase and therefore augments the lactase produced in the small intestine.

Another important effect of the intact microorganisms in a live culture is that the cell walls of the bacteria act as mechanical protection for the lactase inside the cells during the movement of the food through the stomach. Thus, this process allows the release of the enzyme into the small intestine, where it has the most effect on lactose breakdown.

In addition, the more solid consistency of the yogurt or other fermented milk product causes a delay in the rate that the food passes through the digestive tract (called gastrointestinal transit time). This allows the digestive enzymes to act on the food for a longer time than if it were in a liquid form, such as milk. Thus, it can digest more lactose than when the food passes through quickly.

Other positive effects of fermented milk with live cultures include an improvement in intestinal functions. This improvement is possibly associated with interactions with the immune cells of the mucous membranes of the digestive tract and a reduced sensitivity to symptoms in the region.

Furthermore, the bacteria in fermented products compete with those established in the colon and may even replace them. This leads to a more "friendly" microflora that has beneficial effects on health and digestion. The bacterial culture that acts in this manner is known as probiotic, a subject discussed in more detail in Chapter 25.

CAN CONTINUING TO DRINK MILK IMPROVE OR DELAY THE ONSET OF LACTASE DEFICIENCY?

Lactase activity in humans and other mammals is not inducible. This means that it is not possible to increase the amount of lactase produced in the epithelial cell of the small intestine. Therefore, lactose digestion is not increased by continuing lactose consumption. However, the ability for lactose-intolerant people to tolerate a higher level of lactose-containing foods can be enhanced by providing lactose to the bacteria that live in the colon. The continued presence of lactose in the colon contributes to the establishment and multiplication of bacteria capable of synthesizing the beta-galactosidase enzyme over time. The undigested lactose enhances the fermentation capacity of bifidobacteria and other lactic acid bacteria, such as lactobacilli and certain strains of streptococci. These are bacteria that metabolize lactose without the production of hydrogen gas. This process reduces the osmotic imbalance within the colon that is the cause of much of the distress of lactose intolerance.

FEEDING THE LACTOSE-INTOLERANT BABY

Providing the lactose-intolerant baby with a nutritionally complete diet will require some care and thought, but it can be done by being careful about diet. Following is the information the parent of a lactose-intolerant baby will need.

The Breast-Fed Baby

A breast-fed baby will ingest significant quantities of lactose in mother's milk. The lactose composition of her milk will remain constant, regardless of whether or not the mother consumes milk and dairy products. The total amount of fat, protein, and lactose in breast milk are relatively unaffected by the mother's diet and nutritional status. This is in contrast to the fatty acid profile and the concentrations of several micronutrients, particularly water-soluble vitamins, which are dependent to some extent on the composition of the maternal diet.

The symptoms of lactose intolerance in a young baby are liquid, frothy stools, frequent passage of gas (wind), and irritability. The usual tests for lactose intolerance, especially the hydrogen breath test and tests for reducing sugars in the stools, are not good indicators in the young baby. These tests are positive in most normal babies under 3 months, so their use in diagnosis of lactose intolerance in this age group is not very useful.

- The lactose intolerance may be secondary to a gastrointestinal tract infection or other condition that is expected to be transient. In that case, some authorities advise continuing breast-feeding. The diarrhea should gradually diminish as the underlying inflammation disappears.

- Some authorities recommend placing a few drops of Lactaid directly into the baby's mouth before each feeding. This may provide enough of the enzyme to break down the lactose in the mother's milk and so reduce or eliminate the baby's digestive tract symptoms.

- Alternatively, the mother can pump her breast milk, treat the milk with Lactaid drops (4 drops per cup [250 ml] of milk), and allow the enzyme to act for 24 hours in a refrigerator. The baby is fed the lactose-free milk the next day. This is continued until the diarrhea abates, when the baby can be gradually put back to the breast.

Lactose Overload

Lactose overload can mimic lactose intolerance and is frequently mistaken for it. An overload is commonly seen in babies consuming large amounts of breast milk in mothers with an oversupply of milk. The baby is producing a normal amount of lactase, but the quantity of lactose entering the small intestine overwhelms the enzyme's capacity to break it down fast enough. This results in excess, undigested lactose passing out of the small intestine and into the colon. In the colon, the lactose causes osmotic imbalance with an increase in the amount of water in the bowel. Then the resident microorganisms ferment the sugar with the production of gas, abdominal bloating, pain, and possibly diarrhea.

Signs of this condition include the following:

- An unsettled, or frankly distressed baby who shows signs of tummy pain (drawing up of the legs) with screaming or crying

- Adequate to large weight gains

- More than ten wet and many dirty diapers in 24 hours

- Sometimes frothy, yellowish stool

- Baby needing to nurse frequently

Typically, these symptoms occur in babies less than 3 months old.

Because of the baby's frequent need to nurse, a mother may mistakenly conclude that she has a low milk supply because her baby always seems to be hungry. However, the diaper count can be the biggest clue to what is actually happening. The large amount of milk the baby is consuming leads to a large production of urine and feces.

The real problem is that a large-volume, lowfat feed goes through the baby so quickly that not all of the lactose is digested. The first milk produced in a feed is lower in fat than the hind milk, which comes later as the baby continues to suckle. A higher fat content would slow the speed at which the milk moves through the digestive tract. The lactose reaching the lower bowel draws extra water into the bowel. Then it is fermented by the bacteria there, resulting in gas and acid stools. Acid stool can cause diaper rash because the acid burns the baby's skin around the anus. Gas and fluid buildup in the bowel causes tummy pain and the baby appears to be hungry. Sucking is the best comfort that the baby knows, and the milk helps move the gas along the bowel. This tends to ease the pain temporarily, and it may result in gas and stool being passed. Since the baby indicates that he or she wants to suck at the breast, the mother, logically, complies. Sometimes it is the only way to provide comfort. Unfortunately, this provides another large feed on top of the previous one. The amount of lactose consumed overwhelms the lactase available to digest it. Then more lactose enters the colon, resulting in more gas and fluid accumulation. This creates a vicious cycle in which the milk seems to, almost literally, go in one end and out the other.

A solution to the problem may be found by a strategy that increases the fat content of the mother's milk and thereby slows the speed at which the milk passes along the baby's digestive tract. This method consists of mothers using the same breast for each feeding during a certain period.[1] For example, set aside a 3-hour period, and every time baby wants to feed during this period, use the same breast. Then use the other breast for the next 3 hours. In this way, each time baby returns to the already used breast, there is a lower-volume, higher-fat feed that helps slow the system down. If there is still an oversupply of milk (as indicated by a continuation of the abdominal symptoms), increase the one-breast feeding to 4 hours. When the baby's symptoms are relieved, go back to a normal breast-feeding routine according to the baby's needs.

Some Important Facts about Lactose Intolerance and Breast-feeding:

Contrary to some popular beliefs,

- Lactose in the breast milk will not be reduced if the mother stops eating dairy products. The nutritional composition of breast milk, especially with regard to lactose, is entirely unaffected by the mother's diet. (Cows never consume milk; they only eat grass and other plant material, and their milk contains about 0.169 oz [4.8 grams] of lactose per ½ cup [100 milliliters] of milk.) The typical lactose content of human colostrum (produced during days 1 to 5 after birth) is 0.183 ounces (5.2 grams) per ½ cup (100 milliliters). Mature milk (produced from day 15 onward) contains 0.246 ounces (7.0 grams) of lactose per ½ cup (100 milliliters) and remains at that level throughout lactation. Table 8-2 provides an idea of the amount of lactose, protein, and fat consumed by the breast-fed baby from birth to 3 months.

- Lactose intolerance in other family members, including the mother, does not mean that the baby is more likely to be lactose intolerant. Lactase deficiency may be inherited, but this defect is not usually apparent until after infancy. Different ethnic groups tend to lose the ability to produce a normal amount of lactase at different ages (see Table 8-3). Almost all babies, regardless of inheritance, produce adequate amounts of lactase in the first few years of life. The very rare exception is a condition known as congenital alactasia, which is present and apparent from birth.

- Breast-feeding should not be discontinued if a baby develops lactose intolerance. Usually, the condition is temporary, often associated with a gastrointestinal infection. Normal lactase production resumes once the tissues of the digestive tract have returned to normal. Then the baby will be able to tolerate lactose without any difficulty.

Table 8-2[2]
TYPICAL DAILY INTAKES (IN GRAMS[d]) OF SELECTED BREASTMILK CONSTITUENTS

Age	Protein	Fat	Lactose
Day 1	5.0	<1	1
Day 3	12.0	5	12
Day 8	9.0	22	40
3 mo	7.5	29	52

Calculated intakes assume the following daily milk volumes:
> Day 1 (0–24 h): 40 milliliters[e] (0.17 cup)
> Day 3 (48–72 h): 200 milliliters (0.85 cup)
> Day 8: 600 milliliters (2.5 cups)
> 3 months: 750 milliliters (3.17 cups)

Table 8-3
AGE OF ONSET OF PRIMARY ADULT ONSET LACTASE DEFICIENCY IN POPULATIONS[3,4]

Ethnic Group	Onset at 2–3 years	Onset at 6 years	Onset at 9–10 years
White American	0%	0%	6%
Americans of Mexican descent	18%	30%	47%
Black South Africans	25%	45%	60%
Chinese and Japanese	30%	80%	85%
Mestizos of Peru	30–55%	90%	>90%

---

[d] 1 gram equals approximately 0.04 ounces; 10 grams equals 0.35 ounces.

[e] 1 milliliter (1 mL) equals 0.03 US fluid ounces or 0.02 teaspoons; 100 milliliters (100 mL) equals 3.38 US fluid ounces or 20.29 teaspoons or 6.67 tablespoons or 0.42 cups.

- Lactose intolerance is quite different from CMA. CMA involves a complex series of events in the immune system, whereas lactose intolerance is merely a deficiency in the enzyme that digests the milk sugar. The symptoms and management of the two conditions are quite distinct.

The Formula-Fed Baby

Infant formulas that are lactose-free can be given to a lactose-intolerant infant.

If the baby is not allergic to milk, suitable formulas are the milk-based formula Enfalac™ Lactose-Free (Mead Johnson) or Similac™ Advance LF (Abbott Nutrition) (LF means lactose-free).

If the infant is allergic to cow's milk proteins, but tolerates soy, soy-based formulas such as Enfamil™ Soy (Mead Johnson), Alsoy™ with omega-3 and omega-6 (Nestlé), or Isomil™ (Abbott Nutrition) may be suitable. None of the soy-based formulas contain lactose.

If the infant is allergic to both cow's milk and soy proteins, a casein hydrolysate formula, such as Similac™ Alimentum (Abbott Nutrition), Nutramigen® (Mead Johnson), or Enfamil® Pregestimil (Mead Johnson), may be tolerated. All are free from lactose.

THE LACTOSE-RESTRICTED DIET

LACTOSE RESTRICTIONS

There are three general guidelines that are helpful for people who need a lactose-restricted diet. These are:

- Foods, medications, and beverages containing milk and milk solids should be assumed to contain lactose unless labeled lactose-free.

- Products should be avoided if they are labeled as containing lactose, milk, milk solids, milk powder, cheese and cheese flavor, curd, whey, cream, butter, or margarine containing milk solids.

- Products containing lactic acid, lactalbumin, lactate, and casein do not contain lactose and can be consumed.

Acidophilus milk is milk to which a bacterium called *Lactobacillus acidophilus* has been added. These bacteria do not break down lactose to any great extent, so the milk would not be tolerated by people with lactose intolerance.

Milk and Milk Products Suitable for a Lactose-Restricted Diet

There are a number of strategies that individuals on a lactose-restricted diet can use to include milk and milk products in their diet. Following are the most important:

- Adding the enzyme lactase (commercially available as Lactaid®) to liquid milk and allowing the enzyme to act for a minimum of 24 hours in the refrigerator will make the milk digestible. No substitutes are then necessary. The amount of the enzyme that needs to be added will depend on the degree of lactase deficiency. Instructions are provided with the product.

   5 drops in 1 liter (approximately 4 cups or 33.814 liquid ounces) of milk will render it 99 percent lactose-free.

   The addition of 10 drops reduces the lactose to 90 percent.

   The addition of 5 drops will provide a milk that is 70 percent

   lactose-free.

- Lactaid® tablets may be taken before eating or drinking lactose-containing products and may be sufficient to break down the amount of lactose consumed in the following meal.

- Lactaid milk® or Lacteeze milk® that are 99 percent lactose-free are available in the dairy section of grocery stores. These are tolerated by lactose-deficient individuals. They are more expensive than regular milk.

- Hard, fermented cheeses may be tolerated since most of the lactose is removed with the whey during their manufacture.

- Although butter and regular margarines contain a small amount of lactose (in whey), they are usually tolerated because the level of lactose is so low and they are only eaten in small quantities.

- Fermented milks such as yogurt and buttermilk may be tolerated because the level of lactose in these products is reduced (but not completely eliminated) by bacterial enzymes. Lactaid® drops may be mixed in the yogurt in the doses as previously indicated. The product should then be refrigerated for 24 hours. This process may render it acceptable for the severely lactose-intolerant individual.

The Diet

There are two phases for creating a diet for lactose intolerant individuals. Restriction of all lactose will be required initially.

Phase I—Should be followed until the digestive tract symptoms improve.

Phase II—Subsequent liberalization of these restrictions, by the gradual re-introduction of increasing amounts of lactose-containing foods, will determine each individual's limit of tolerance for lactose.

Lactose tolerance is determined by introducing milk and milk products in a dose-defined sequence.

Table 8-4
FOODS ALLOWED AND RESTRICTED IN A MILK-FREE DIET

PHASE ONE: AVOIDANCE OF LACTOSE

Type of Food	Foods Allowed	Foods Restricted
Milk and Milk Products	• Milk treated with Lactaid™ drops according to manufacturer's instructions • Lactaid™ milk • Lacteeze™ milk • Other lactose-free milks • Milk-free substitutes: Soy beverages such as SoGood™ SoNice™ EdenSoy™ Rice Dream™ Darifree™ Coffee-Rich™	• Avoid all except those on the FOODS ALLOWED list
Breads and Cereals	• Breads and baked goods without milk derivatives. Read labels carefully to ensure that no milk is included in the list of ingredients; occasionally some of the following manufactured products may contain milk:	• Baked goods made with milk or derivatives of milk • Any labelled as containing milk, milk solids, or other terms indicating the presence of milk (see Chapter 7)

Table 8-4 (continued)
FOODS ALLOWED AND RESTRICTED IN A MILK-FREE DIET

PHASE ONE: AVOIDANCE OF LACTOSE

Type of Food	Foods Allowed	Foods Restricted
Breads and Cereals (continued)	– French bread – Italian bread – Whole wheat bread – Rye bread – Soda crackers – Bagels – Pasta – Plain cooked cereals – Some ready-to-eat cereals – Plain grains	
Vegetables	• All pure fresh or frozen vegetables and their juices, without added ingredients	• Prepared as: creamed, scalloped, mashed with milk, breaded or battered, instant potatoes and similar manufactured foods

Table 8-4 (continued)
FOODS ALLOWED AND RESTRICTED IN A MILK-FREE DIET

PHASE ONE: AVOIDANCE OF LACTOSE

Type of Food	Foods Allowed	Foods Restricted
Fruit	• All pure or frozen fruits and their juices, without added ingredients	• Fruit dishes with milk-containing ingredients or toppings, such as: – Custard – Cream – Ice cream – Any manufactured, packaged, or frozen fruit dishes with added milk solids
Meat, Poultry, Fish	• All fresh or frozen without added ingredients • Any processed meats without milk ingredients • Meat, poultry, or fish canned without milk ingredients	• Any with added ingredients containing milk, such as: – Sauces – Creamed – Breaded – Battered
Eggs	• Plain, without added milk or milk products: – Boiled – Fried – Scrambled – Poached – Omelette	• Prepared with: – Milk – Cheese – Butter – Margarine – Any other milk derivative

Table 8-4 (continued)
FOODS ALLOWED AND RESTRICTED IN A MILK-FREE DIET

PHASE ONE: AVOIDANCE OF LACTOSE		
Type of Food	**Foods Allowed**	**Foods Restricted**

Legumes	• All plain legumes, such as
	  – Beans
	  – Peas
	  – Dried peas and beans
	  – Lentils
	• Peanuts and peanut butter
		• Any prepared with milk or milk derivatives, such as:
		  – Butter
		  – Margarine
		  – Milk or cheese sauces

Nuts and Seeds	• All plain nuts and seeds	• Any with added milk-derived ingredients

Fats and Oils	• Pure vegetable oils
	• Milk-free margarines such as:
	  – Fleischmann's™ low-sodium no salt
	  – Parkay™ diet spread
	  – Canoleo™ margarine
	  – Some other diet spreads (read labels carefully)
	• Real mayonnaise
	• Shortening
	• Lard
	• Meat drippings
	• Gravy made with allowed ingredients
		• Salad dressings with milk or milk derivatives
		• Butter
		• Margarines containing whey (read labels)

Table 8-4 (continued)
FOODS ALLOWED AND RESTRICTED IN A MILK-FREE DIET

PHASE ONE: AVOIDANCE OF LACTOSE

Type of Food	Foods Allowed	Foods Restricted
Spices and Herbs	• All fresh, or dried	• None
Sweeteners	• All except those with added lactose or other milk-derived ingredients • Sugar • Pure syrups • Honey	• Sugar substitutes containing lactose (read labels carefully)

Phase II: Determining Lactose Tolerance Levels

Lactose intolerance is dose related. Usually, a certain amount of the lactase enzyme is being produced, and some lactose can be processed. It is important to establish how much lactose can be broken down at one time (Step 1) and how much lactose can be processed over the day (Step 2). Please refer to Table 8-1 on page 160 to see how much lactose is contained in the various milk products that are consumed in this process.

Step 1:

Day 1: Morning (Breakfast)
      Eat a portion of food containing 1 gram (g) of lactose, for example:
      1 oz or 2 tbsp of cream cheese.

If there are no symptoms of intolerance, double the amount of lactose the next day.

Day 2: Morning (Breakfast)
      Eat a portion of food containing 2 g of lactose, for example:
      2 oz or ¼ cup cream cheese or
      ½ cup of uncreamed cottage cheese.

If there are no symptoms of intolerance, increase the amount of lactose on Day 3.

Day 3: Morning (Breakfast)
      Eat a portion of food containing 5 g of lactose, for example:
      1 cup of yogurt (regular or low fat).

If there are no symptoms of intolerance, increase the amount of lactose on Day 4.

Day 4: Morning (Breakfast)
      Eat a portion of food containing 10 g of lactose, for example:
      1 cup (250 mL) of milk (homogenized; fat-reduced 2 percent, 1 percent, or skim).

Step 2:

To establish how much lactose may be tolerated over the day, go back to the amount last tolerated. (For example, on Day 2, 2 g of lactose were tolerated, but on Day 3, there was bloating, cramping, and diarrhea following 1 cup of yogurt.)

Day 1: Morning (Breakfast)
    Eat a portion of food containing the amount of lactose tolerated in Step 1 (for example, 2 g of lactose).

    Evening (Dinner)
    Repeat the morning procedure.

If there are no symptoms of intolerance, increase the number of servings on Day 2.

Day 2: Morning (Breakfast)
    Eat a portion of food containing the amount of lactose tolerated in Step 1.

Repeat the process at lunch and dinner.

References

1. Anderson J. Lactose intolerance and the breastfed baby. *Essence Magazine.* Australian Breast-feeding Association. August 2006. Retrieved from http://www.breastfeeding.asn.au/bfinfo/lactose.html

2. Prentice A. Constituents of human milk. *Food and Nutrition Bulletin.* The United Nations University Press 1996;17(4). Retrieved from http://www.unu.edu/unupress/food/8F174e/8F174E04.htm

3. De Vrese M, Stegelmann A, Richter B, Fenselau S, Laue C, Schrezenmeir J. Probiotics —compensation for lactase insufficiency. *American Journal of Clinical Nutrition* 2001;73(Suppl 1):421S–429S.

4. Sahi T. Genetics and epidemiology of adult-type hypolactasia. *Scandinavian Journal of Gastroenterology - Supplement* 1994;202:7–20.

CHAPTER 9

Egg Allergy

Egg is a frequent cause of food allergy in children.[1] Allergy to eggs and milk account for the majority of reactions to foods in children under the age of 2 years. Egg allergy typically develops before the child is 2 years old, and, in 55 percent of cases, it disappears during the first 6 years.[2]

Detection of egg-specific IgE antibodies is considered to be the earliest indicator that a baby is atopic.[3] However, several studies indicate that more babies and young children are skin-test positive to egg or have egg-specific antibodies in their blood than actually develop the symptoms of allergy when they consume eggs. As discussed previously, it is not unusual to see evidence of IgE sensitization to a food protein without actual development of symptoms. On the other hand, a negative skin test for egg is generally considered to be an accurate indicator of the absence of egg allergy because negative skin tests for egg have been proven to be very accurate.

ALLERGENS IN EGGS

Eggs contain many different proteins that can lead to allergy. Each individual is likely to be sensitized to more than one such protein. A person who has been proven to be allergic to eggs is usually advised to avoid egg in any form. This is particularly important in children under the age of 7 years because there is a higher risk of a severe or anaphylactic reaction to eggs in this age group. In general, egg-allergic children react principally to the ingestion of egg white. Although egg yolk contains several proteins, egg white contains the greatest number of allergens. Up to 24 different antigenic protein fractions have been isolated, although the ability to trigger an immunological reaction (the antigenicity) of most of these is unknown. The main allergens are ovalbumin, ovomucoid, ovotransferrin, and lysozyme.

Since there is a great deal of difference between the proteins in egg yolk and egg white (the latter tend to be more highly allergenic), it is sometimes useful to find out which of these egg components is the cause of the allergy so that the diet need not be so restricted. In addition, some egg proteins are destroyed by heat, which means that a person sensitized to heat-labile proteins can consume eggs that are well-cooked, especially in small quantities in baked goods, without any harmful effects. However, a person allergic to heat-stable proteins, which are unaffected by heat, must avoid eggs in any form. So, a discussion of egg allergy should start with a brief description of the different proteins in eggs.

Egg Proteins

The white of an egg contains about 10 percent protein and 80 percent water. The yolk is composed of 50 percent water, 34 percent fat, and 16 percent protein. Egg white is considered to be the source of the major egg allergens, which include ovalbumin, conalbumin (ovotransferrin), and ovomucoid (see Table 9-1).

Some egg yolk proteins, especially α-livetin, may also induce the production of IgE antibodies, and there may be some degree of antigenic cross-reactivity between egg yolk and egg albumin proteins.

In most cases of egg allergy, IgE antibodies are produced only in response to the specific proteins associated with the egg. Egg proteins differ from the proteins in chicken flesh. However, some livetins are derived from the blood of the hen. IgE antibodies to these proteins might result in allergy to both egg and chicken. In egg-white allergic individuals, skin tests frequently reveal sensitivity to chicken meat. However, eating chicken does not lead to symptoms in most individuals. An allergic reaction with development of symptoms after eating chicken meat occurs in less than 5 percent of egg-allergic subjects. Children who are skin-test positive to egg need not avoid chicken unless they develop symptoms when they eat it.

Table 9-1 ANTIGENIC EGG PROTEIN	
Antigenic Egg White Proteins:	**Antigenic Egg Yolk Proteins:**
Major Proteins:	**Major Proteins:**
Ovalbumin	Lipovitellin
Conalbumin (ovotransferrin)	Phosvitin
Ovomucoid	Low-density lipoproteins
Ovomucin	Livetins
Lysozyme	
Trace Amounts of:	
Catalase	
Ovoflavoprotein	
Ficin inhibitor	
Ovoglycoprotein	
G2 and G3 Globulins	
Ovomacroglobulin	
Ribonuclease	
Ovoinhibitor	
Avidin	

Cooking may decompose many of the egg proteins. Thus, in some cases, cooked eggs may be tolerated while raw egg causes an allergic reaction. However, some egg proteins, especially ovomucoid, are heat stable, and persons allergic to this component will react to cooked as well as raw eggs. In most children, however, the small amount of cooked eggs in baked goods is usually tolerated.

In some people, contact with eggs can cause hives (urticaria) although they have no symptoms when they eat eggs. These individuals have IgE antibodies that recognize particular egg white molecules that are destroyed by the action of digestive enzymes.[4]

Egg Proteins from Other Birds

Proteins in eggs from different bird species sometimes cross-react antigenically. However, evidence from a single study indicates that people allergic to duck and goose eggs were not allergic to hen's eggs.[5] The subject of cross-reactivity between eggs from different bird species needs to be investigated further.

Based on current knowledge, a person who is allergic to eggs should treat eggs from different birds as if they were an entirely separate food, taking a small quantity at first and monitoring their reaction to it before consuming a whole egg. If the egg has been eaten without incident in the past, there is no reason to avoid eating it in the future.

Children under the age of 7 years who have a known allergy to hen's eggs should not eat eggs from other birds unless it is known that they are tolerated. In this age group, egg allergy can lead to anaphylaxis in severe cases. In the interests of safety, it is therefore advisable for the egg-allergic child to avoid all species of eggs.

SYMPTOMS OF EGG ALLERGY

The only known sensitivity reaction to eggs is an IgE-mediated allergy. Therefore, the symptoms induced by an allergic reaction to eggs are characteristic of any IgE-mediated response[6] and may include the following:

- Symptoms in the skin, such as
  - Reddening (erythema)
  - Hives (urticaria)
  - Tissue swelling, especially of the face (angioedema)

- Gastrointestinal reactions
  - Abdominal pain
  - Nausea
  - Vomiting
  - Diarrhea

- Respiratory reactions
  - Hay fever (rhino-conjunctivitis)
  - Throat tightening (laryngeal edema)
  - Asthma

- Generalized reactions
  - Anaphylaxis

PROGRESS OF EGG ALLERGY WITH AGE

Children frequently outgrow their early food allergies, and allergy to eggs is no exception. There are no tests or signs to predict which child will outgrow egg allergy or at what age eggs will be tolerated. Authorities suggest that children with more severe allergy will be less likely to outgrow their early allergy to eggs than those who experience only mild symptoms. Egg allergy may persist into adulthood, especially when egg causes an anaphylactic reaction.

In many cases, loss of clinical reactivity (no symptoms) precedes loss of IgE antibodies, so skin tests and blood tests may often be positive even though eating the egg causes no problem.

Recent research indicates that, once tolerance develops, it is important for a child to continue to eat the tolerated food in order to maintain their tolerance to that food. It is therefore advisable for the child to undergo a food challenge (eating a small quantity under close supervision) periodically to determine whether he or she continues to be allergic to the food. After the age of 2 years, the child should undergo yearly challenge of foods to which he or she is allergic and which have been avoided in the interim. In the case of egg allergy, it is important that such a challenge be undertaken under medical supervision because of the risk of anaphylaxis.

A safe method of food challenge is described in Chapter 4 "Elimination and Challenge."

COMPOSITION OF THE AVERAGE CHICKEN EGG

Egg white:	56–61%
Yolk:	27–32%
Shell:	8–11%

VACCINES THAT MAY CONTAIN EGG PROTEINS

Viruses need living cells to grow in, so viruses used for vaccines are frequently grown in the chick embryo in an egg. Consequently, such vaccines may contain small quantities of the egg protein when the viruses are harvested. Vaccines that could potentially contain egg proteins include but are not limited to the following:

- The triple virus vaccine of measles, mumps, and rubella (MMR)

- Influenza virus

- Yellow fever virus

Small amounts of egg might also be found in the anti-typhus and anti-rabies vaccines, depending on the way they are prepared.

Anaphylactic reactions to vaccine components are extremely rare. It is often difficult to determine whether a reaction has been caused by the vaccine antigens or by any of the vaccine components (neomycin, sorbitol, and gelatin) or whether the reaction is due to the egg protein the vaccine may contain.

Triple Virus Vaccine

The triple virus vaccine (measles, rubella, mumps) does not contain significant amounts of egg proteins. Egg-allergic children, even those who are highly sensitive, are at very low risk for developing anaphylactic reactions to these vaccines,[7] although such reactions have occasionally been reported.[8] Skin tests with diluted vaccine preparations do not appear to help predict possible allergic reactions after triple vaccine administration. In 1997, The the Committee of Infectious Diseases of the American Academy of Pediatrics proposed routine administration of the vaccine without prior skin tests.[9] They recommend that vaccinated patients should be observed for 90 minutes after vaccination by a team experienced in treating anaphylaxis.

Influenza Vaccine

The influenza vaccine has been reported to contain small quantities (1 to 7 milligrams per milliliter) of egg proteins. The Committee of Infections Diseases of the American Academy of Pediatrics recommends that patients with anaphylactic reactions or very severe reactions after egg ingestion should not be given this vaccine without prior skin testing with a diluted preparation of the vaccine.[9] Vaccine should not be given to anyone who is skin-test positive to the vaccine. The Committee states that children who react positively to the vaccine skin test should not undergo influenza vaccination because of the risk of a reaction and because yearly vaccination might be required.

If the egg-allergic child's clinical situation indicates that the protection of the influenza vaccine is essential and he or she has a negative skin test to the vaccine, the Committee recommends that the vaccine be administered under medical supervision in a facility equipped for anaphylactic emergencies.

Yellow Fever Vaccine

The yellow fever vaccine is also prepared in chicken embryo. Authorities recommend that skin tests with the vaccine should be carried out before yellow fever vaccination only in patients with a history of systemic anaphylaxis after egg ingestion.[10] If immunization is required, the vaccine should be carefully administered in multiple small separate doses at a medical center.

PREVENTION OF EGG ALLERGY

As discussed in Chapter 3, maternal avoidance of eggs, as with any other allergenic food, during pregnancy and lactation does not seem to be effective in preventing sensitization of the fetus to eggs before birth. Nor does maternal consumption of eggs prevent sensitization of the baby during breast-feeding. Of course, if the mother is allergic to eggs, she should be careful to avoid eating them. If the baby is diagnosed with egg allergy, the mother should avoid eggs in her diet while breast-feeding because egg proteins will pass into her breast milk and trigger symptoms in the allergic baby.

MANAGEMENT OF EGG ALLERGY

Avoidance of all forms of egg is important for the child who has an egg allergy and for the mother who is breast-feeding an egg-allergic baby.

Avoidance of egg as an individual ingredient in a meal (such as omelette, scrambled, boiled, fried, etc.) is relatively easy. However, eggs are frequently included as an ingredient in prepared foods. As such, they may not be so easily recognized unless care is taken in reading food labels. Become familiar with the terms that indicate the presence of egg protein and be aware of the foods that are traditionally made with eggs (see Table 9-2).

THE EGG-FREE DIET

The egg-free diet omits eggs and products containing eggs. Because it is almost impossible to separate the white and yolk of the egg, a person with an

---

Table 9-2
TERMS ON LABELS THAT INDICATE THE PRESENCE OF EGGS

Albumin	Eggs of all bird species
Ovalbumin	chicken
Globulin	duck
Ovoglobulin	goose
Ovomucin	turkey
Ovomucoid	ostrich
Ovovitellin	quail
Livetin	plover
Lysozyme	other
Mayonnaise	Frozen egg
Simplesse™	Dried egg solids
Egg powder	Powdered egg
Egg white	Pasteurized egg
Egg yolk	Egg Beaters™
Egg protein	

Table 9-3 NONFOOD ITEMS THAT MAY CONTAIN EGGS	
Photographic film Printed natural fabrics Some fur garments Pet foods	Some vaccines are produced from viruses grown in eggs. The risk of injecting such a vaccine in a highly egg-allergic individual should be discussed with the physician involved.

egg white or egg yolk allergy, especially if it results in anaphylaxis, should avoid all egg proteins until it has been clearly demonstrated that only one part of the egg is responsible for the allergic reaction. If there is any risk of a severe anaphylactic reaction, all forms of egg should be carefully avoided, even if it is known that only the white or the yolk is responsible: both can be contaminated with proteins from the other.

There is evidence that eggs from a variety of different bird species have common allergens, so a person allergic to eggs from one should be advised to avoid eggs from all birds unless it is certain that allergy to specific species does not exist.

Important Nutrients in Eggs

Eggs contribute vitamin D, vitamin B_{12}, pantothenic acid, selenium, folacin, riboflavin, biotin, and iron and, in smaller amounts, vitamin A, vitamin E, vitamin B_6, and zinc. These nutrients can easily be supplied in meat, fish, and poultry products, legumes, whole grains, and vegetables. Therefore, an egg-free diet should not pose any risk of deficiency of any of these nutrients.

General Guidelines for the Egg-Free Diet

Common sense and care go a long way toward helping an egg-sensitive individual consume a healthy diet. The following pointers are general guidelines that you can apply for an egg-free diet.

- Avoid all obvious sources of eggs (omelette, scrambled, poached, boiled, fried) and foods made principally with eggs, such as eggnog, custard, soufflé, meringue, pavlova, quiche, timbale, egg noodles, and angel food cake.

- Avoid packaged foods containing eggs, even as a minor ingredient. Foods with egg, egg powder, egg white, egg yolk, or egg protein obviously should be avoided. Become familiar with the terms on food labels indicating the presence of eggs (see Table 9-2).

- In a restaurant, or when eating a meal with unknown ingredients, avoid foods traditionally made with eggs, including mayonnaise; Caesar salad; some salad dressings; sauces such as Hollandaise, Béarnaise, Newburg, Foyot; meat, fish, or vegetables coated with a batter (such as fritters and tempura); pancakes; waffles. In Chinese restaurants, egg drop soup, wonton soup, and any dish with noodles traditionally contain eggs.

- Some soft drinks (such as root beer), wine, and beer may contain eggs used as "clarifiers."

- Many baked goods contain eggs, and eggs may be present in baking powder. Read labels on these products carefully.

- Some candies, such as nougat and divinity, are made with eggs. Check labels carefully.

- Ice cream usually contains eggs. Children should avoid it unless it is known that the product is made without eggs.

- Eggs may be included as an ingredient in many desserts, especially those containing custard, cream fillings, dessert mixes, and the traditional egg-based desserts such as meringue, pavlova, and angel food cake.

- Eggs may be present as garnish on some dishes and as glaze, especially on pies and other baked products.

- Eggs are often used as a binding agent in meat loaf, dumplings, and similar dishes.

This chapter concludes with a table of foods allowed and restricted on an egg-free diet and with some helpful recipes for substitutes for important cooking ingredients (such as baking powder) that you can create at home.

Table 9-4
THE EGG-FREE DIET: FOODS ALLOWED AND RESTRICTED

Type of Food	Foods Allowed	Foods Restricted
Milk and Milk Products	• Milk (whole, 2%, 1%, skim) • Cream • Sour cream • Yogurt • Buttermilk • Ice cream **without eggs** • Frozen yogurt **without eggs** • Cheese	• Eggnog • Any milk drinks made with eggs • Desserts containing eggs such as custard, cream pies, puddings, some gelatin desserts • Commercial ice creams containing eggs • Any cheese food that may contain eggs in a glaze or coating such as cheese/nut balls (check labels)
Breads and Cereals	• Bread, buns, and baked goods made without eggs and without egg glaze • French or Italian bread • Soda crackers • Plain cooked grains • Plain oatmeal • Regular Cream of Wheat® • Cream of Rice® and other cooked cereals • Ready to eat cereals made without eggs • Egg-free pasta • Egg-free baking mixes	• Commercial or homemade baked goods made with eggs, such as cakes, muffins, pancakes, waffles, fritters, doughnuts, toaster pastries • Quick breads • Cakes, breads, and other baked products with egg glaze • All baking mixes containing eggs • Instant oatmeal and flavored oatmeal • Instant Cream of Wheat® • Commercial pasta (spaghetti, macaroni, egg noodles, etc.)

	Table 9-4 (continued) THE EGG-FREE DIET: FOODS ALLOWED AND RESTRICTED	
Type of Food	**Foods Allowed**	**Foods Restricted**
Breads and Cereals (continued)		• Confectioneries containing eggs, such as divinity, fondants, marshmallows, nougat, meringue, pavlova, mousse, soufflé
Vegetables	• All pure vegetables and their juices	• Vegetable dishes made with eggs • Salads containing eggs • Salad dressings containing eggs, such as traditional Caesar salad • Mayonnaise • Sandwich spreads containing eggs
Fruit	• All pure fruits and fruit juices	• Any fruit dish containing eggs, such as meringue, mousse, soufflé, fruit whips
Meat, Poultry, and Fish	• All pure fresh, frozen, or canned meat, poultry, and fish	• Meat, poultry, and fish dishes made with eggs as a binder or glaze, such as meat loaf, meatballs • Sausages, loaves, or croquettes made with eggs • Some processed meats (check labels) • Soups such as egg drop soup • Consommé cleared with egg white

	Table 9-4 (continued) THE EGG-FREE DIET: FOODS ALLOWED AND RESTRICTED	
Type of Food	**Foods Allowed**	**Foods Restricted**

Eggs	• None	• Eggs from all bird species including
		    Chicken
		    Duck
		    Ostrich
		    Turkey
		    Quail
		    Goose
		    Plover
		    Other
		• Manufactured foods with ingredients indicating the presence of eggs, such as
		    Albumin
		    Globulin
		    Livetin
		    Ovalbumin
		    Ovomucin
		    Ovomucoid
		    Ovovitellin
		• Ingredients made from derivatives of eggs, eg.,
		    Lysozyme
		    Simplesse™

Legumes	• All pure legumes, such as dried peas, beans, lentils, dal • Plain tofu • Plain peanut butter	• Legume dishes containing eggs or derivatives of eggs

Table 9-4 (continued)
THE EGG-FREE DIET: FOODS ALLOWED AND RESTRICTED

Type of Food	Foods Allowed	Foods Restricted
Nuts and Seeds	• All plain nuts and seeds	• Glazed or coated nuts (read label) • Nuts or seeds in baked goods made or glazed with eggs
Fats and Oils	• Butter, cream, sour cream • Margarine • Vegetable shortening • Pure vegetable oils • Lard • Meat drippings • Gravy	• Salad dressings that list eggs in any form as an ingredient • Caesar salad dressing • Real mayonnaise • Sauces made with eggs, such as Hollandaise, Béarnaise, Newburg
Spices and Herbs	• All	• None
Sweeteners	• All	• None

EGG SUBSTITUTES YOU CAN MAKE AT HOME

Eggs serve three purposes in recipes:

1. Act as a leavening agent

2. Act as a binder

3. Provide a source of liquid

There are substitutes you can make at home for these purposes. These substitutes are designed to perform these functions as far as possible, but the finished product may not be exactly the same as when eggs are used.

Substitutes for Eggs as a Leavening Agent

1 tbsp **egg-free baking powder** plus 2 tbsp **liquid** = 1 egg

2 tbsp **flour** plus ½ tbsp **shortening**
plus ½ tsp **egg-free baking powder**   } = 1 egg
plus 2 tbsp **liquid**

(The "liquid" can be water, vinegar, fruit juice, broth, or any liquid that would be appropriate for the recipe.)

Some recipes call for only 1 egg and quite a large proportion of baking powder (2 tsp) or baking soda (1½ tsp). Try these recipes without eggs and add 1 tbsp of **vinegar** instead of the egg with the baking powder or baking soda.

Substitutes for Eggs as a Binder

Recipe 1

Combine ⅓ cup **water** and 3–4 tsp **brown flax seeds**. Bring to a boil on high heat, and then

simmer on low heat for 5–7 minutes until a slightly thickened gel begins to form.

Strain the flax seed out of the liquid and use the gel in the recipes.

This recipe makes enough substitute for 1 egg. Increase the amounts as needed to substitute for 2, 3, or more eggs.

Some people prefer to leave the flax seeds in the mixture after thickening or blend them into the gel before using. This may alter the recipe's taste a little.

Recipe 2

⅓ cup **ground flax seed** plus 1 cup **water**.

Bring mixture to a boil. Simmer 3 minutes. Refrigerate.

One tablespoon of the mixture replaces 1 egg.

Recipe 3

⅓ cup **water** plus 1 tbsp **arrowroot powder** plus 2 tsp **guar gum** (also called guaran) = 1 egg

Recipe 4

2 ounces **tofu** = 1 egg

Substitutes for Eggs as a Liquid

⅓ cup **apple juice** = 1 egg

OR: 4 tbsp pureed **apricot** = 1 egg

OR: 1 tbsp **vinegar** = 1 egg

Commercial egg substitutes that are guaranteed to be free from eggs can be used (for example, Jolly Joan® Egg replacer, or Egg Replacer® marketed by Ener-G-Foods).

DO NOT use Egg Beaters®, which is made from egg whites.

If egg **yolk** is tolerated, but egg **white** causes an adverse reaction, egg yolks separated from the whites can be used as long as the egg white does not cause an anaphylactic reaction.

If the egg white has caused anaphylaxis in the past, do not use egg yolk, because the small amount of albumin that will adhere to the yolk might be sufficient to cause a reaction.

EGG-FREE BAKING POWDER RECIPES

Here are three egg-free baking powder recipes that you can use at home.

Gluten-Free Baking Powder

Baking soda 1 part (⅓ cup)
Cream of tartar 2 parts (⅔ cup)
Cornstarch 1 part (⅓ cup)

Mix and sift all ingredients together. Use in same quantities as baking powder in recipes.

Corn-Free: Arrowroot Baking Powder

Baking soda 1 part (⅓ cup)
Cream of tartar 2 parts (⅔ cup)
Arrowroot starch 2 parts (⅔ cup)

Mix well and store in an airtight container.
1 tsp regular baking powder = 1½ tsp arrowroot baking powder

Hypoallergenic Baking Powder

Baking soda 1 part (⅓ cup)
Cream of tartar 2 parts (⅔ cup)
Ground rice (or brown rice flour) 1 part (⅓ cup)

Sift all ingredients together thoroughly. Use in same quantities as baking powder in recipes.

References

1. Rancé F, Kanny G, Dutau G, Moneret-Vautrin D. Food hypersensitivity in children: Clinical aspects and distribution of allergens. *Pediatric Allergy Immunology* 1999;10:33–38.

2. Position paper. Martorell Aragonés A, Boné Calvo J, García Ara MC, Nevot Falcó S, Plaza Martín AM. Allergy to egg proteins. *Allergology Immunopathology* 2001; 29:72–83.

3. Kulig M, Bergmann R, Klettke U, Wahn V, Tacke U, Wahn U. Natural course of sensitization to food and inhalant allergens during the first 6 years of life. *Journal of Allergy and Clinical Immunology* 1999;103:1173–1179.

4. Yamada K, Urisu A, Kakami H, Koyama R, Tokuda R, Wada E, Kondo Y, Ando H, Morita Y, Torii S. IgE-binding activity to enzyme-digested ovomucoid distinguishes between patients with contact urticaria to egg with and without overt symptoms on ingestion. *Allergy* 2000; 55:565–569

5. Langeland T. A clinical and immunological study of allergy to hen's egg white, VI: Occurrence of proteins cross-reacting with allergens in hen's egg white as studied in egg white from turkey, duck, goose, seagull and in hen egg yolk, and hen and chicken sera and flesh. *Allergy* 1983;38:399–412.

6. Sampson HA. Immediate reactions to foods in infants and children. In: Metcalfe DD, Sampson HA, Simon RA (eds) *Food Allergy: Adverse Reactions to Foods and Food Additives.* Cambridge: Blackwell Science, 1997;169–182.

7. James JM, Burks AW, Roberson PK, Sampson HA. Safe administration of the measles vaccine to children allergic to eggs. *New England Journal of Medicine* 1995;332:1262–1266.

8. Baxter DN. Measles immunization in children with history of egg allergy. *Vaccine* 1996;14:131–134.

9. Peters G (ed). *1997 Red Book: Report of the Committee on Infectious Diseases.* 24th ed. Elk Grove Village, IL: American Academy of Pediatrics Publications, 1997;32–33.

10. Kelso JM, Mootrey GT, Tsai TF. Anaphylaxis from yellow fever vaccine. *Journal of Allergy and Clinical Immunology* 1999;103:698–701.

CHAPTER 10

Peanut Allergy

Peanuts are one of the most frequently cited causes of life-threatening anaphylactic reactions in children and young adults in North America. If an individual has been diagnosed as anaphylactic to peanuts, extreme caution must be exercised in avoiding all sources of peanuts.

SYMPTOMS ASSOCIATED WITH PEANUT ALLERGY

A 2003 review[1] indicates that a child's first allergic reaction to peanuts usually appears between 14 and 24 months of age and commonly occurs at home.

As with any food allergy, the organ systems that may be affected include the following:

- Skin (hives, reddening, tissue swelling, especially of the face)

- Respiratory tract (wheezing, noisy breathing, cough, breathing difficulty, throat tightening, nasal congestion, asthma in asthmatics)

- Gastrointestinal tract (vomiting, diarrhea, abdominal pain)

- Cardiovascular system (drop in blood pressure, irregular heart rate, anaphylaxis)

In addition, eczema (atopic dermatitis) is often reported as a symptom of peanut allergy.

Not all peanut-allergic children have all of these symptoms. As with all food allergies, the symptoms experienced are idiosyncratic; some children develop symptoms in one organ system, but others might experience the peanut allergy in quite a different way.

Peanut Allergy by Contact

Contact dermatitis and hives from direct contact with peanuts, without ingestion of peanuts, have also been reported in the medical literature. I clearly remember an incident that occurred when my son, who was anaphylactic to peanuts from a very young age, was about 2 years old. We were visiting friends and had not noticed a bowl of peanuts that was partially hidden by flowers on a low table. My son thrust his hand into the bowl and then rubbed his eyes. Within minutes, his whole face swelled to an enormous size, and we could barely see his eyes as little slits within the swollen tissue. A similar case of contact angioedema—in a 9-year-old child who had been allergic to peanuts since the age of 1 year—was recently reported in an allergy journal. The child developed angioedema after playing with his "Play Station." The game device had been used previously by his uncle, who had eaten peanuts at a family get-together. The authors suggest that this sequence of events illustrates a new way of transmitting food allergies by proxy.[2]

PRIMARY SENSITIZATION TO PEANUTS

In more than 70 percent of children with peanut allergy, symptoms develop at the first known exposure to peanuts. However, IgE-mediated allergic reactions require an initial exposure to an allergen to induce sensitization. Therefore, this primary exposure is characteristically symptom-free. So it seems logical to assume that children who develop symptoms on the first observed contact with the allergen must have been exposed by an earlier, unknown event.

There is evidence for the presence of peanut protein and blood cells (T cell lymphocytes) that can respond to antigens in amniotic fluid. However, there is no strong evidence to suggest that peanuts in the maternal diet during pregnancy can sensitize the fetus in utero.[3] Nevertheless, authorities recommend that, during pregnancy, the mother refrain from consuming large quantities of any potentially allergenic food. Small quantities of all foods as part of a balanced diet should promote tolerance rather than sensitization to potential allergens.

Evidence for the passage of peanut protein from mother's diet into her breast milk during lactation was provided by a study using a very sensitive assay for peanut allergens in breast milk. Samples of breast milk were tested for the presence of peanut protein at various times after consumption of dry, roasted peanuts by a group of volunteers. The two major peanut allergens associated with anaphylaxis were detected in breast milk within 1 to 3 hours after ingestion in approximately 50 percent of the volunteers.[4]

The authors suggest that exposure to peanut protein during breast-feeding might be a route for sensitization to peanuts for at-risk infants.

However, there is a difference of opinion among clinicians and researchers regarding the response of the infant's immune system to potentially allergenic proteins, both in utero and in breast milk. Exposure to low doses of food proteins has been shown to tolerize the baby to allergens by educating the immune system to recognize the proteins as safe. It is this process of immunological tolerization that allows consumption of foods without the immune systems mounting a defense against the animals and plants consumed—all of which are distinct from and foreign to the human body. Exposure to peanuts and other food allergens during pregnancy, lactation, and early childhood may be important in the development of immunological tolerance and may prevent allergic sensitization to these foods.

Consequently, the concentration of peanut protein, the timing of the child's exposure to it, and the frequency with which the child encounters it may lead either to allergic sensitization or to tolerization. In some cases, exposure to peanut protein in breast milk may actually protect the child against later development of peanut allergy. Therefore, at this stage in our knowledge, it would not be prudent to suggest that all lactating women avoid peanut products during breast-feeding. Although this may protect some babies from peanut sensitization, it may predispose others to acquiring peanut allergy by preventing the process of tolerization.[5]

Given the present state of knowledge, authorities suggest that lactating mothers should avoid peanuts and peanut products while breast-feeding high-risk infants. These are babies with a strong family history of allergies or those who have a first degree relative with peanut allergy.[3]

Before proceeding to the practical aspects of managing peanut allergy, consider what we actually mean by the terms "peanut allergens" and "peanut protein."

PEANUT ALLERGENS

Peanuts contain many different proteins, each with its own distinct structure. Several of these proteins are allergenic and can trigger IgE antibodies; each antibody molecule is specific to its inciting allergen. Peanut protein may include some or all of the known peanut allergens.

The major peanut protein allergens have been characterized and named. The "Ara h" in the name of each of the proteins is derived from the Latin name for peanut, *Arachis hypogaea*. These are the most important of the antigenic peanut proteins:

1. Ara h1
2. Ara h2 (5 subtypes)
3. Ara h3
4. Ara h4
5. Ara h5
6. Ara h6
7. Ara h7
8. Ara h8
9. Ara h Agglutinin
10. Ara h LTP
11. Ara h Oleosin
12. Ara h TI

The relative quantity of each specific allergen affects individuals differently if they are sensitized to one allergen more than another. The assumption that all of the known allergens in a specific food are of equal importance may not hold true.

Some of these allergens are more frequently detected than others as triggers of peanut-specific IgE in peanut-allergic individuals. For example, in a recent study, Ara h2 was recognized most frequently as the causative allergen in all tests for triggering symptoms. It induced a reaction at relatively low concentrations. On the other hand, Ara h1 and Ara h3 were recognized less frequently and reacted only at 100-fold higher concentrations than Ara h2. The authors conclude that, for their patient group, Ara h2 was the most important peanut allergen. The study's authors found that a few of the other proteins may be important allergens, but were important allergens less frequently and at higher concentrations.[6]

In another study, the authors calculated the prevalence of sensitization to every single allergen in a population of 40 individuals sensitized to peanuts. Their results indicated that, in addition to Ara h1 (prevalence 65%) and Ara h2 (prevalence 85%), Ara h4 (53%) was also a major allergen, whereas Ara h5 (13%), Ara h6 (38%), and Ara h7 (43%) were minor allergens. Interestingly, although Ara h6 was considered a minor allergen, the authors also found that sensitization to Ara h6 was associated with more severe clinical symptoms than most of the other allergens.[7]

Future research will reveal which of the allergenic proteins in peanuts are most important to a specific population and which are affected by various processing methods in the manufacture of foods that include peanuts. This information may then explain why certain populations are at risk for peanut allergy and why others are relatively safe.

Furthermore, improved understanding of the molecular structure of the major peanut allergens and the peanut-specific immune response will eventually lead to effective methods for diagnosis, therapy, and, possibly, prevention strategies for peanut allergy.[8]

HOW MUCH PEANUT WILL PROVOKE ALLERGY?

Several studies have attempted to determine the smallest amount of peanut protein that is likely to trigger an allergic reaction in a peanut-allergic person. However, because there are so many variables associated with peanut allergy, it is very difficult to specify a dose of peanut that would elicit symptoms in all peanut-allergic people. It is also difficult to define a dose that would be safe for all peanut-sensitive individuals.

Sometimes contact or inhalation of peanut protein may be sufficient to elicit a potentially life-threatening anaphylactic reaction in a very sensitive individual. As a result, it is usually wise for peanut-allergic people to avoid even the smallest quantity of peanuts in foods or in their environment.[9]

ALLERGENICITY OF PEANUT OIL

Most of the oils available for consumption are highly refined. Oil is subjected to physical and chemical methods of purification, such as degumming, refining, bleaching, and deodorization. It is then referred to as refined oil, and ingredients other than oil from the plant source are usually undetectable. This is the case with refined peanut oil. Until recently, it was thought that refined peanut oil was completely free from peanut protein. Since an allergic reaction requires the presence of the allergenic protein, pure oil was considered to be incapable of eliciting an allergic response.

However, extremely sensitive modern techniques allow detection of much smaller quantities of protein. So, it is now recognized that refined oil does indeed contain sufficient peanut allergen to elicit a reaction in highly sensitive individuals.[10] Nevertheless, all but the most highly sensitive peanut-allergic individuals can consume refined oil with impunity. However, if an oil is used to cook peanuts, peanut protein will be detectable in the previously pure oil, which would then be a great hazard to people with peanut allergy. The reuse of oil is common in some homes. Reuse is especially a problem in fast food outlets, so these sources of contamination with allergenic protein must constantly be avoided by individuals at risk for anaphylaxis.

Not all exposure to peanut allergens is through food. Exposure to peanuts may be through topically applied skin creams containing peanut oil. These creams are frequently used to treat diaper rash and rashes in skin creases in young babies. This has been suggested as the first exposure by a number of studies.[4] It is recommended that any skin creams containing peanut oil should not be used on babies because of the risk for sensitization to peanut allergens through the skin.

SKIN TESTING FOR PEANUT ALLERGY

Because it is possible for sensitization to peanuts to occur through the skin, some authorities are questioning the advisability of skin-testing for peanut allergy at any stage. The pricking of the skin with the peanut allergen provides a route for the allergen to encounter immune cells below the skin surface. The skin test may thus have the potential to cause sensitization of the child who is at risk for allergy.

Most practitioners will not do skin-testing on children who are known to have reacted adversely to peanuts. This is because of the danger of triggering an anaphylactic reaction when the allergen encounters already primed immune cells without the protective moderating effect of the gut-associated lymphoid tissue (GALT) that lines the intestines. (For more information on the immune system of the digestive tract, see Chapter 1.)

PEANUT ALLERGY AND ALLERGY TO TREE NUTS

Peanuts, which are members of the legume family, are botanically unrelated to the nuts that grow on trees. Tree nuts belong to a variety of different botanical families. Most peanut-allergic people are able to eat tree nuts (such as walnuts, pecans, Brazil nuts, almonds, cashew nuts, hazelnuts, macadamia nuts, pine nuts, coconuts, chestnuts, etc.) without difficulty. However, because tree nuts are also highly allergenic foods, they are also frequent causes of strong allergic reactions and anaphylaxis.

Children who are allergic to peanuts should, in the interests of safety, avoid all nuts. Most children are unable to distinguish between peanuts and other types of nuts; in general, they are all small and brown. Besides, in a nut mixture, it may be impossible to determine whether peanuts are present or not. Furthermore, no differentiation may have been made in the marketing of peanuts and nuts, and so the two are often found together in "nut mixtures." When various tree nuts are sold in bulk, the utensil used to handle the nuts has often been previously used with peanuts without cleaning in between. In the manufacture of candies, confectioneries, and ice cream, there is frequent cross-contamination between nuts of different species and peanuts. As a result, anyone with severe peanut allergy is advised to avoid any product containing nuts because of the danger of inadvertently encountering peanuts.

> **Mandalona nut** is a name given to a manufactured product made from deflavored, decolored peanut meal. It is pressed into molds, reflavored, and colored and then sold as a cheaper substitute for tree nuts such as almonds, pecans, and walnuts. Persons with peanut allergy must be cautious when consuming any food that may contain such a product.

Although it is sensible for a peanut-allergic adult to determine his or her sensitivity to nuts of different types to allow more flexibility in the diet, the same is not true for children. Determination of reactivity to nuts for a peanut-allergic child should be delayed until the child is old enough to distinguish one nut from another and to take responsibility for avoiding his or her allergens without supervision. (Tree nut allergy is discussed in Chapter 12.)

EFFECTS OF COOKING METHODS ON PEANUT ALLERGENICITY

The roasting of peanuts tends to improve their flavor and taste. However, roasting has been demonstrated to increase the allergenicity of peanuts compared to the same variety of peanut processed by other methods.[11] This means that roasted peanuts (the form in which most peanuts and peanut butter is consumed in the United States) are more likely to trigger a severe anaphylactic reaction than boiled peanuts. The boiled form is popular in countries such as China, Africa, and in the southern United States.[12] It is a documented fact that the incidence of peanut allergy in China is virtually non-existent. In the United States, in contrast, about 3 million people report being allergic to peanuts.

Other factors that might affect the allergenicity of peanut proteins are thought to include the type and variety of the peanut (of which there are about 14,000), the conditions under which the peanut has been grown, and the degree of maturation of the peanuts.[13]

CROSS-REACTIVITY BETWEEN PEANUTS AND OTHER LEGUMES

Peanuts are legumes. A common problem faced by peanut-allergic people is whether they should avoid all legumes, including soybeans, chick peas, lentils, beans, peas, licorice, carob, and other members of the *Leguminoceae* family.

Although many members of the legume family can be allergenic and trigger allergic symptoms in those individuals sensitized to them, there is no evidence to support the thinking that peanut-allergic individuals should avoid all legumes. In clinical trials, cross-reactivity between different members of the legume family was quite uncommon. One study reported that only 2 out of 41 peanut-allergic children reacted mildly to other members of the legume family.[14] Furthermore, these reactions may not have been because the foods were related. They could have been due to the child becoming sensitized to the different foods independently, just as they would have been to any other allergenic food.

Allergy to multiple foods is usually due to reactions to botanically unrelated, highly allergenic foods such as peanuts, eggs, milk, shellfish, fish, and tree nuts. Highly allergic individuals are most likely to react to the most highly allergenic foods for their age group. Therefore, allergy to specific foods is usually a result of independent sensitization to each individual food allergen.

Allergy to Peanuts and Soy

Previously, the incidence of soy allergy was reported to be low compared to other highly allergenic foods, but recent studies seem to suggest that the prevalence of soy allergy is increasing.[15] It has been suggested that the increase in the incidence of soy allergy in children could be the result of exposure to the allergenic protein (in the form of soy-based infant formulas) in early infancy when the child is at highest risk for allergic sensitization. In addition, recent research suggests that an association between peanut and soy allergy could arise from cross-sensitization from soy-based infant formulas. Both soy and peanuts contain a similar allergen, and it is thought that exposure to the soy allergen in infant formula could prime the child's immune system to respond to the peanut allergen. This may be the case even when the child shows no signs of allergy to soy.[15] As a result, the child could exhibit allergic symptoms on an apparent first exposure to peanuts. (Soy allergy is discussed in Chapter 11.)

PROGNOSIS AND MANAGEMENT OF PEANUT ALLERGY

In spite of the high incidence of peanut allergy in some Western countries and the potential for severe anaphylactic reactions to the food, peanut allergy, like many early food allergies, can be outgrown. In 2001, pediatric allergists in the United States reported that about 21.5 percent of peanut-allergic children will eventually outgrow their peanut allergy.[16] Those with a mild peanut allergy, as determined by the level of peanut-specific IgE in their blood, have a 50 percent chance of outgrowing the allergy.[17] In contrast, only about 9 percent of patients are reported to outgrow their allergy to tree nuts.[18]

Maintaining Tolerance to Peanuts

Recent studies indicate that—when a child has outgrown an early peanut allergy and there is no longer any evidence of symptoms developing after the child has consumed peanuts—it is preferable for that child to eat peanuts regularly. The child should eat peanuts rather than avoid them in order to maintain tolerance to the peanuts. Children who outgrow peanut allergy are at risk for recurrence, but the risk has been shown to be significantly higher for those who avoid peanuts after resolution of their symptoms.[19]

THE PEANUT-SAFE ENVIRONMENT

Currently, there is strong pressure for public places such as schools, hospitals, and airplanes to be peanut-free in an attempt to protect vulnerable individuals, especially children and young adults, from accidental exposure to peanuts. However, declaring an environment peanut-free could, in itself, be a mistake. When people assume that the area is free from contamination, they may relax their guard and thus be at risk for inadvertent exposure to the allergen. A peanut-safe designation indicates that, although people using the facility are requested to avoid bringing peanuts into the area and special precautions are in place to reduce the possibility of exposure of the at-risk population, there must be constant vigilance on the part of everyone to maintain the environment in a peanut-safe condition.

Important measures for a peanut-safe environment should include all of the following:

- Ensuring that all personnel in a peanut-safe facility are well informed about the dangers of accidental contamination to the peanut-allergic person

- Providing clear strategies for maintaining the facility in a peanut-safe condition, including strict rules about cleaning

- Informing everyone entering the facility to avoid introducing peanuts into the area and giving the reasons for the restrictions

- Educating the peanut-allergic persons concerning avoidance of their own exposure to peanuts, including the following:
  - Avoiding foods likely to contain or be contaminated by peanuts
  - Being aware of all terms on food labels that would indicate the possible presence of peanuts (see Table 10-1.)
  - Carrying an EpiPen® or similar device, containing injectable epinephrine (adrenalin) and being familiar with its use in case of accidental exposure and an allergic reaction
  - Wearing a MedicAlert or identification tag or bracelet in case of loss of consciousness in an allergic reaction

- Informing all staff in the facility about emergency procedures should anyone in the area develop symptoms and require medical treatment. Such information should include:
  - Familiarity with the use of the injectable epinephrine (adrenalin) where appropriate
  - Contact with key caregivers, such as parents or guardians of children, and the child's doctor or other health provider according to prior instructions provided to the facility by the parents or guardians
  - Instructions for transporting the child to the nearest hospital in the quickest way possible

THE PEANUT-SAFE LIFESTYLE

The child or adult who is allergic to peanuts must avoid peanuts in any and every form as long as he or she develops symptoms after consuming the food.

It is important that all sources of peanuts should be carefully avoided if there is even a moderate risk of an anaphylactic reaction. However, there is no evidence that even a severe allergy to peanuts requires avoidance of all other legumes. Avoidance of legumes such as soy, lentils, dried peas, and beans is only necessary when allergy to the individual foods has been identified. It is also unnecessary to avoid tree nuts, which are botanically unrelated to peanuts, unless the individual has an allergy to them. However, because of the risk of peanut contamination of tree nuts, especially in nut mixtures, a person who has a demonstrated allergy to peanuts is usually advised to avoid nuts of all types in the interest of safety.

Peanuts are widely used in the food industry because of their nutritive value and their taste. Many manufactured foods contain peanuts, resulting in an increased risk for inadvertent ingestion of peanuts by allergic individuals. Additionally, contamination with traces of peanuts during the manufacturing process of products intended to be peanut-free has sometimes resulted in fatal and near-fatal allergic reactions. It is essential for the peanut-allergic individual and for parents or guardians of peanut-allergic children to be familiar with all of the terms on a product label that could indicate the presence of peanuts (see Table 10-1).

Notes on Peanut Oil

Highly refined peanut oil contains only barely detectable amounts of peanut protein. Although it should therefore be safe for consumption by most peanut-allergic individuals there is no guarantee that any peanut oil is completely free from peanut protein. A child who is potentially anaphylactic to peanuts should avoid entirely all types of peanut oil. In particular, cold-pressed oils (also labeled pure-pressed, expeller-pressed, or unrefined) should be avoided.

Important Nutrients in Peanuts

Peanuts supply niacin, magnesium, vitamin E, manganese, pantothenic acid, chromium, and, in smaller amounts, vitamin B_6, folacin, copper, and biotin.

Table 10-1
TERMS ON FOOD LABELS THAT INDICATE
THE PRESENCE OF PEANUT PROTEIN

Ingredients Indicating the Presence of Peanuts

Peanut protein	Artificial nuts
Hydrolyzed peanut protein	Nu-Nuts® flavored nuts
Peanut oil	Beer nuts
Cold-pressed peanut oil	Mixed nuts
Peanut butter	Goober nuts
Peanut flour	Goober peas
Mandalona nuts	

Products That May Contain Peanuts

Marzipan (almond paste)	Cookies
Prepared soups	Candies
Dried soup mixes	Chocolate bars
Chili	Prepared and frozen desserts
Egg rolls	Ice cream with nuts
Thai dishes	Chocolate ice cream
Chinese dishes	Vegetable oil
Satay sauces	Hydrogenated vegetable oil
Baked goods	Vegetable shortening

These nutrients are easily replaced by including meat, whole grains, legumes, and vegetable oils in the diet. Therefore, a diet completely free from peanuts should not pose any nutritional risk to the average child. However, strict vegans may need to eat tree nuts and seeds in order to obtain adequate quantities of high-grade proteins. So they are strongly advised to undergo a careful investigation of their allergic reactivity to tree nuts and seeds, so that they can be assured that these nutritious foods can be consumed in safety.

The Peanut-Free Diet

The following directives (Table 10-2) should be carefully followed when providing meals for the peanut-allergic child and for the mother who is breast-feeding a baby who has been diagnosed with peanut allergy.

Table 10-2
FOODS ALLOWED AND FOODS RESTRICTED FOR A PEANUT-FREE DIET

Type of Food	Foods Allowed	Foods Restricted
Milk and Milk Products	• Milk • Cream • Plain yogurt • Ice cream made with allowed ingredients • Plain cheese • Sour cream • Quark® • Dips made with allowed ingredients	• Milk-based desserts and confectioneries (e.g., ice cream) containing peanuts or nuts • Chocolate ice cream or other milk-based confectioneries unless labeled peanut-free • Cheese foods (e.g., slices, dips, spreads, cheese balls) containing nuts or undisclosed ingredients
Breads and Cereals	• Any breads, buns, or baked goods that are known to be free from peanut and peanut oil • Plain cooked grains • Plain oatmeal • Regular Cream of Wheat® • Ready-to-eat cereals without added oil or nuts • Homemade granola without peanuts • Dried pasta	• Commercial or homemade baked goods made with peanut oil or peanuts • Baked goods made with undisclosed sources of nuts, oil, or shortening • Baking mixes • Ready-to-eat cereals with added oils and nuts, such as granola
Vegetables	• All pure vegetables and their juices	• Vegetable dishes with sauces containing peanuts, peanut oil, or unknown nuts or oils

Table 10-2 (continued)
FOODS ALLOWED AND FOODS RESTRICTED FOR A PEANUT-FREE DIET

Type of Food	Foods Allowed	Foods Restricted
Vegetables (continued)		• Salads with dressings containing unknown oils or nuts • Vegetables canned in undisclosed oils
Fruit	• All pure fruit and fruit juices	• Fruit dishes containing peanuts or nuts • Fruit dishes made with oil or shortening of unknown origin
Meat, Poultry, and Fish	• All pure fresh or frozen meat, poultry, or fish • Fish canned in broth, water, or nonpeanut oil	• Meat, poultry, or fish dishes made with peanuts or undisclosed nuts or oils • Fish canned in undisclosed oils • Chinese dishes • Thai dishes • Egg rolls • Commercial chili • Vegetarian burgers, unless labeled peanut-free • Peanut protein
Eggs	• All without restricted ingredients	• Egg dishes prepared with oils or nuts of unknown sources • Egg rolls

Table 10-2 (continued)
FOODS ALLOWED AND FOODS RESTRICTED FOR A PEANUT-FREE DIET

Type of Food	Foods Allowed	Foods Restricted

Legumes	• All pure legumes except peanuts
	• Tofu
		• Peanuts and peanut products, including:
		    Artificial nuts
		    Goober nuts
		    Goober peas
		    Hydrolyzed peanut protein
		    Mandalona nuts
		    Mixed nuts
		    Peanut butter
		    Peanut flour
		    Peanut oil
		    Peanut protein
		• Legume dishes containing peanuts or oils or nuts of undisclosed source

Nuts and Seeds	• All packaged plain pure nuts and seeds
	• All pure nut and seed oils and their butters, such as
	    sesame tahini
	    almond butter
	    almond paste
	    cashew butter
		• Mixed nuts
		• Mandalona nuts
		• Artificial nuts
		• Nuts or oils of undisclosed origin
		• Goober nuts
		• Goober peas

Fats and Oils	• Butter • Cream • Pure vegetble, nut, or seed oils with source specified (except peanuts)	• Peanut oil • Salad dressings that list oil without revealing the source

Table 10-2 (continued)
FOODS ALLOWED AND FOODS RESTRICTED FOR A PEANUT-FREE DIET

Type of Food	Foods Allowed	Foods Restricted
Fats and Oils (continued)	• Lard • Meat drippings • Gravy made with meat drippings	• Margarine, unless the source of all oils is revealed and is peanut-free
Spices and Herbs	• All pure herbs and spices • Blends of herbs and spices, without added oils	• Seasoned packets with undisclosed ingredients • Vegetables such as garlic or sun-dried tomatoes packed in oil, unless the source of oil is disclosed and is peanut-free
Sweets and Sweeteners	• Plain sugar • Honey • Molasses • Maple syrup • Corn syrup • Pure chocolate • Pure cocoa • Artificial sweeteners • Homemade cookies and candies with allowed ingredients	• Chocolates with unknown ingredients • Chocolate bars • Marzipan (almond paste) • Cookies and candies • Any confectiionery containing nuts unless specified peanut-free

References

1. Al-Muhsen S, Clarke AE, Kagan R. Peanut allergy: An overview. *Canadian Medical Association Journal* 2003;168:1279–1285.

2. Pétrus M, Villefranche C, Michaud C, Dutau G. Console de jeu: Mode de transmission de l'allergie à l'arachide / Play station: a means of transmitting peanut allergy. *Revue française d'allergologie* 2006;46(4):419–420.

3. Hayday K, Shannon S. Are early exposures linked with childhood peanut allergy? *The Journal of Family Practice* 2003;52(7) [online journal] Retrieved from http://www.jfponline.com/Pages.asp?AID=1503

4. Vadas P, Wai Y, Burks W, Perelman B. Detection of peanut allergens in breast milk of lactating women. *Journal of the American Medical Association* 2001;285(13):1746–1748.

5. Lack G, Fox D, Northstone K, Golding J. Factors associated with the development of peanut allergy in childhood. *New England Journal of Medicine* 2003;348(11):977–985.

6. Koppelman SJ, Wensing M, Ertmann M, Knulst AC, Knol EF. Relevance of Ara h1, Ara h2 and Ara h3 in peanut-allergic patients, as determined by immunoglobulin E Western blotting, basophil-histamine release and intracutaneous testing: Ara h2 is the most important peanut allergen. *Clinical and Experimental Allergy* 2004;34(4):583–590.

7. Becker W-M, Kleber-Janke T, Lepp U. Four novel recombinant peanut allergens: More information, more problems. *International Archives of Allergy and Immunology* 2001;124:100–102.

8. Scurlock AM, Burks AW. Peanut allergenicity. *Annals of Allergy and Asthma Immunology* 2004;93(5 Suppl 3):S12–18.

9. Sicherer SH, Furlong TJ, DeSimone J, Sampson HA. Self-reported allergic reactions to peanut on commercial airliners. *Journal of Allergy and Clinical Immunology* 1999;104(1):25–27.

10. Olszewski A, Pons L, Moutete F, Aimone-Gastin I, Kanny G, Moneret-Vautrin DA, Gueant JL. Isolation and characterization of proteic allergens in refined peanut oil. *Clinical and Experimental Allergy* 1998;28(7):850–859.

11. Maleki SJ, Hurlburt BK. Structural and functional alterations in major peanut allergens caused by thermal processing. *The Journal of AOAC International* 2004;87(6):1475–1479.

12. Beyer K, Morrow E, Li X-M, Bardina L, Bannon GA, Burks AW, Sampson HA. Effects of cooking methods on peanut allergenicity. *Journal of Allergy and Clinical Immunology* 2001;107(6):1077–1081.

13. Chung SY, Butts CL, Maleki SJ, Champagne ET. Linking peanut allergenicity to the process of maturation, curing and roasting. *Journal of Agricultural and Food Chemistry* 2003;51(15):4273–4277.

14. Bernhisel-Broadbent J, Taylor S, Sampson HA. Cross-allergenicity in the legume botanical family in children with food hypersensitivity. II. Laboratory correlates. *Journal of Allergy and Clinical Immunology* 1989;84(5 Pt 1):701–709.

15. Sicherer SH, Sampson HA, Burks AW. Peanut and soy allergy: A clinical and therapeutic dilemma. *Allergy* 2000;55:515–521.

16. Skolnick HS, Conover-Walker MK, Koerner CB, Sampson HA, Burks W, Wood RA. The natural history of peanut allergy. *Journal of Allergy and Clinical Immunology* 2001;107(2):367–374.

17. Fleischer DM, Conover-Walker MK, Christie L, Burks AW, Wood RA. The natural progression of peanut allergy: Resolution and the possibility of recurrence. *Journal of Allergy and Clinical Immunology* 2003;112(1):183–189.

18. Fleischer DM, Conover-Walker MK, Matsui EC, Wood RA. The natural history of tree nut allergy. *Journal of Allergy and Clinical Immunology* 2005;116(5):1087–1093.

19. Fleischer DM, Conover-Walker MK, Christie L, Burks AW, Wood RA. Peanut allergy: Recurrence and its management. *Journal of Allergy and Clinical Immunology* 2004;114(5):1195–1201.

CHAPTER 11

Soy Protein Allergy

Soybeans are legumes. Both soybeans and peanuts (which belong in the same botanic family as soybeans) are the most allergenic of the *Leguminosae* family. There are over 30 species of legumes, including fresh and dried peas, fresh and dried beans, all types of lentils, carob, and licorice. Symptomatic reactivity to more than one member of the legume family is rare. Individuals who are allergic to peanuts or soy or both are not necessarily allergic to other members of the legume family. Each type of legume must be investigated individually to determine the individual's sensitivity to it. Avoiding all legumes when only one causes the allergy would place unnecessary restrictions on a child's diet. This can be especially detrimental to the child's nutritional health if the child and family are vegetarians and even more so if they are vegans.

The first report of soy allergy appeared in 1934. At the present time, the Food and Agriculture Organization of the United Nations includes soy in its list of the eight most significant food allergens. In the United States, the U.S. Food and Drug Administration, Department of Health and Human Services, includes soy as one of the eight major foods or food groups that are responsible for 90 percent of food allergies. (Milk, eggs, fish, crustacean shellfish, tree nuts, peanuts, and wheat are the others.) In an effort to make manufactured foods safe for food-allergic people, the Food Allergen Labeling and Consumer Protection Act (FALCA) took effect on January 1, 2006.[1] It requires that the major food allergens be properly labeled on foods. These actions on the part of the United States government emphasize the fact that allergy to soy, which was previously considered to be a rather unimportant and transient allergy of childhood, has assumed a greater prominence in incidence and severity and is now a significant health concern.

SYMPTOMS OF SOY ALLERGY

It is estimated that up to 43 percent of babies who are allergic to cow's milk develop an allergy to soy when given soy-based infant formulas. Allergy to soy protein has many features similar to those of cow's milk protein allergy (CMA). Like cow's milk, soy is a frequent contributor to eczema (atopic dermatitis) in atopic children. In infants, soy allergy can cause loose stools and diarrhea, vomiting, abdominal discomfort, irritability, crying, intestinal blood loss, anemia, and failure to thrive (slow or no weight gain). Respiratory tract symptoms include coughing, wheezing, asthma, and rhinitis. Symptoms in the skin include hives and angioedema, as well as eczema (atopic dermatitis). Unlike the case of peanuts, anaphylactic reactions to soy are extremely rare and were virtually unknown until a report from Sweden in 1999.[2]

Soy protein has been identified as a cause of a childhood digestive condition known as food-protein-induced enterocolitis syndrome.[3] Symptoms of this condition include vomiting and diarrhea, which may have their onset several hours after the child has consumed soy. In extreme cases, severe dehydration, failure to thrive (little or no weight gain, or weight loss), and shock may occur. The same symptoms may be triggered by cow's milk protein (in which case the condition is known as cow's milk protein-induced enterocolitis). Approximately 50 percent of infants with this condition react to both cow's milk and soy.[3]

SOY-BASED INFANT FORMULAS AND ALLERGY

Soy-based infant formulas were first used to feed babies with CMA in the United States in 1929. Since then, soy protein formulas (SPFs) containing purified soy proteins, a mixture of vegetable oils, and purified carbohydrate have been developed. SPFs have been used for managing various conditions in babies and children, including CMA, lactose and galactose intolerance, and severe gastroenteritis.

PROGRESS OF SOY ALLERGY THROUGH THE LIFE CYCLE

Soy allergy is usually considered to be a transient allergy of infancy and childhood, which is frequently outgrown. In one study,[4] all of the allergic infants became tolerant of soy by the age of 3 years. In another study, two-thirds of the infants lost their soy allergy 2 years after a positive oral challenge.[5] In a study of Danish children with CMA, 5.1 percent demonstrated soy allergy in infancy, but all of the cases had resolved by the age of 3 years.[6]

SOY PROTEIN ALLERGENS

At least 16 potential soy protein allergens have been identified, but their relative clinical significance is presently unknown.

SOY IN MANUFACTURED FOODS

Soybeans and soy products have become a major component in manufactured foods in recent years. They occur in many processed foods, infant formulas, breakfast cereals, baked goods, crackers, soups, packaged meals, and sauces.

Pure soy oil is not considered to be allergenic, unless contaminated by soy protein in its manufacture. This latter source of soy allergen is difficult to detect in a manufactured product. Therefore, people who are very allergic to soy are advised to avoid soy oil as well, although most will tolerate a small amount of the oil without any difficulty.

Most manufactured foods that contain soy will indicate the presence of soy protein on the label. However, sometimes, the word *soy* may not appear, so persons who are soy allergic are advised to become familiar with terms that indicate the likely presence of soy (see Table 11-1).

On a food label, soy may be indicated by terms such as *texturized vegetable protein* or *hydrolyzed plant protein*. Lecithin is often derived from soy. Asian foods such as tempeh, tofu, miso, and bean curd are made from soy, which may not be obvious to the consumer who is unfamiliar with these ethnic foods.

Table 11-1
TERMS THAT INDICATE THE PRESENCE OF SOY IN FOOD PRODUCTS

Terms That Indicate the Presence of Soy Protein:

Tofu	Soy nuts
Kyodofu (freeze-dried tofu)	Soy sauce
Miso	Soy sprouts
Okara (soy pulp)	Soybean
Shoyu	Soybean paste
Sobee	Soy flour
Supro	Soy grits
Tamari	Soy albumin
Tempeh	Soy protein
Yuba	Soy protein isolate
Soy milk	Soy lecithin
Soy beverage	Texturized vegetable protein (TVP)*

Ingredients That May Contain Soy:

Emulsifiers*	Monosodium glutamate (MSG)*
Stabilizers*	Vegetable broth*
Lecithin*	Vegetable gum*
Sprouts (source unspecified)	Vegetable paste*
Bean sprouts	Vegetable protein*
Hydrolyzed plant protein (HPP)*	Vegetable shortening*
Hydrolyzed vegetable protein (HVP)*	Vegetable starch*

* unless the source is specified and is not soy.

Unlabeled products such as bulk foods, unwrapped breads, and baked goods may contain soy, especially if flour is an ingredient. Persons who are allergic to soy are advised not to purchase these products unless the specific ingredients can be ascertained.

Table 11-1 lists the terms most commonly used to indicate the presence of soy and the ingredients that may contain soy.

SOY-FREE DIET

The soy-free diet omits soybeans and all soy products. Soy is widely used in commercial food preparation. Labels should be examined carefully; certain brands of the foods listed may not be soy-free.

Pure soy oil and soy lecithin usually do not contain detectable soy protein and therefore are not usually allergenic. However, sometimes the refining process does not exclude all of the soy proteins. When a child is highly sensitive to soy, all products containing soy oil, especially when it is listed as the main ingredient (for example, soy oil, soy-based margarines, cooking sprays), should be avoided because of the possibility that soy protein may also be present. Cold-pressed oils (also referred to as pure-pressed, expeller-pressed, or unrefined) are very likely to contain soy proteins and should not be used.

Important Nutrients in Soy Beans

Soybeans contribute thiamin, riboflavin, vitamin B_6, phosphorus, magnesium, iron, folacin, calcium, and zinc to the diet. However, soy is typically used in commercial products in amounts that are too small to be considered a significant source for these nutrients. Therefore, elimination of soy from the diet does not compromise the nutritional quality of most diets.

Table 11-2
FOODS ALLOWED AND RESTRICTED ON A SOY-FREE DIET

Type of Food	Foods Allowed	Foods Restricted
Milk and Milk Products	• All except those on the restricted list	• Cheese substitutes • Soy cheese • Tofu cheese • Ice ceam, frozen desserts, and dessert mixes, unless labeled soy-free • Milk or cream replacers • Soy-based infant formula • Soy milk • Soy beverage • Soy yogurt
Breads and Cereals	• All except those on the restricted list	• Homemade and commercial breads and baked goods containing soy • Pancake mixes • Soy grits • Soy flour • Baking mixes • Cereals containing soy • Mixed grain cereals • Multigrain breads • Granola and granola bars • Infant cereals containing soy • High protein flour and bread • English muffins • Stuffings
Vegetables	• All pure, fresh, frozen, or canned vegetables and their juices	• All vegetable dishes made with soy or unknown ingredients

	Table 11-2 (continued)	
	FOODS ALLOWED AND RESTRICTED ON A SOY-FREE DIET	
Type of Food	**Foods Allowed**	**Foods Restricted**
Vegetables (continued)		• Soy sprouts • Mixed sprouts • Salads with sprouts • Imitation bacon bits • Salad dressings containing soy • Some frozen French fries • Commercial vegetable products • Some commercial soups • Commercial dry soup mixes • Some bouillon cubes
Fruit	• All pure fresh, frozen, or canned fruits and their juices	• Fruit dishes made with soy products • Some commercial canned fruit products
Meat, Poultry, and Fish	• All fresh or frozen meat, poultry, or fish • Fish canned in water	• Meat, poultry, or fish dishes with soy • Tuna and other fish canned in oil • Tofu (soybean curd) • Miso • Meat extenders • Textured vegetable protein • Vegetarian meat replacers (analogs) • Veggie burgers • Meat products that may contain soy include: Cold cuts

Table 11-2 (continued)
FOODS ALLOWED AND RESTRICTED ON A SOY-FREE DIET

Type of Food	Foods Allowed	Foods Restricted
Meat, Poultry, and Fish (continued)		Luncheon meat Frozen dinners Hamburger patties Meat paste Meat pâté Meat pies Minced beef Sausages
Eggs	• All plain eggs	• Egg dishes prepared with soy products
Legumes	• All plain legumes except soy and tofu • Dried peas and beans • All green beans and peas • Lentils • Split peas • Peanuts	• All legume dishes containing soy or tofu • Any soy products • Mixed beans • Bean mixtures (e.g., 12–bean soup) • Mixed bean salads
Nuts and Seeds	• All packaged, plain, pure nuts and seeds • All pure nut and seed oils and their butters, e.g., tahini, almond butter • Peanuts • Peanut butter	• Soy nuts • Soy butter • Nuts or mixes containing soy derivatives • Any oils or nuts of undisclosed origin

Table 11-2 (continued)
FOODS ALLOWED AND RESTRICTED ON A SOY-FREE DIET

Type of Food	Foods Allowed	Foods Restricted
Fats and Oils	• Butter • Cream • Pure vegetable, nut or seed oil with the source specified • Lard and meat drippings • Gravy made with meat drippings • Pure olive oil spray • Peanut oil	• Salad dressings that list oil without revealing the source • Soy oil • Margarine, unless the sources of all oils are revealed and the margarine is soy-free • Vegetable oil • Vegetable oil sprays • Shortening

Spices, Herbs, and Seasonings	• All pure herbs and spices
	• Blends of herbs and spices, without added oils
		• Seasoning packets with undisclosed ingredients
		• Sauces containing soy such as:
		    Barbecue
		    Asian
		    Soy
		    Tamari
		    Worcestershire
		• Imitation bacon bits
		• Hydrolyzed vegetable protein (HVP)
		• Hydrolyzed plant protein (HPP)
		• Texturized vegetable protein (TVPJ)

Sweets and Sweeteners	• Plain sugar • Honey • Molasses	• Chocolate • Chocolate bars • Marzipan (almond paste)

Table 11-2 (continued) FOODS ALLOWED AND RESTRICTED ON A SOY-FREE DIET		
Type of Food	**Foods Allowed**	**Foods Restricted**
Sweets and Sweeteners (continued)	• Maple syrup • Corn syrup • Pure chocolate • Pure cocoa • Cocoa butter • Artificial sweeteners • Pure jams and jellies • Homemade cookies and candies with allowed ingredients	• Cookies and candies • Cake icing, unless sources are revealed and are soy-free

References

1. US Food and Drug Administration, Department of Health and Human Services. Public Law 108-282 "Food Allergen Labeling and Consumer Protection Act of 2004". Retrieved from http://www.cfsan.fda.gov/~dms/alrgact.html

2. Sicherer SH, Sampson HA, Burks AW. Peanut and soy allergy: A clinical and therapeutic dilemma. *Allergy* 2000;55:515–521.

3. Sicherer SH, Eigenmann PA, Sampson HA. Clinical features of food protein-induced enterocolitis syndrome. *Journal of Pediatrics* 1998;133:214–219.

4. Bock SA . Prospective appraisal of complaints of adverse reactions to foods in children during the first 3 years of life. *Pediatrics* 1987;79:683–688.

5. Sampson HA and McCaskill CC . Food hypersensitivity and atopic dermatitis: Evaluation of 113 patients. *Journal of Pediatrics* 1985;107:669–675.

6. Høst A and Halken S . A prospective study of cow milk allergy in Danish infants during the first 3 years of life. *Allergy* 1990;45:587–596.

CHAPTER 12

Allergy to Tree Nuts and Seeds

TREE NUT ALLERGY

Nuts represent the reproductive part of the plant. In the majority of cases, the most highly allergenic molecules of plants are associated with the storage proteins in the seed. Nuts, grains, and legumes (peas, beans, lentils), as well as the foods we commonly call seeds, all contain similar types of storage albumins. These storage albumins tend to be highly allergenic. They are used by the growing plant during germination. It is possible they have a defensive role against pathogens, since many of these types of albumins have been shown to have antifungal properties. It is also possible that many of the huge number of dicot seeds contain cross-reacting albumins. Cross-reactivity means that a person who is allergic to one nut, seed, grain, or legume may be allergic to another from a different plant species. However, the degree of clinical cross-reactivity has not been determined with any degree of confidence. It appears that each storage albumin is unique to the species of plant that produces it.

Nuts are produced by trees of diverse and unrelated botanical genera. In theory, it is only necessary to avoid the specific species of nut that has been identified as the culprit allergen. However, because allergy to certain tree nuts is frequently associated with anaphylactic reactions, a child who is known to be allergic to one species of nut should, in the interest of safety, avoid all nuts. It is almost impossible to identify individual nuts in nut mixtures. Additionally, the risk of cross-contamination of one type of nut with another is high.

Botanic Families of Nuts

Nuts belong to a wide array of different biological families, for example:

- Walnuts and pecans belong to the *Judanglacea* family, which also includes the hickory nut.

- Almonds are members of the *Drupacea* family, which includes peaches, apricots, plums, nectarines, and cherries.

- Cashews and pistachios belong to the *Anacardiacea* family group, which also includes mangoes.

- Hazelnuts (filberts) are part of the *Betulaceae* family, to which birch trees belong.

- Chestnuts belong to the *Fagaceae* family, which includes beech trees.

- Coconuts belong to the *Arecaceae* family group, which also includes dates and palm trees.

- Brazil nuts belong to the *Lecythidaceae*, a family of tropical trees, which includes the anchovy pear (*Grias cauliflora*, a West Indian species with edible fruit used for pickles) and several timber trees from South America.

- Macadamia nuts belong to a tropical plant family called the *Proteaceae*, which includes the cone flower and pincushion trees.

Some edible seeds are also highly allergenic, and it is important that the specific seed responsible for a child's allergic reaction be correctly identified. However, as in the case of nuts, if an anaphylactic reaction has been experienced in response to the consumption of seeds, it is usually advisable for the allergic child to avoid all seeds in the interest of safety.

Symptoms that have been reported in response to nuts and seeds include the following:

Contact dermatitis, especially of oral tissues

Oral allergy syndrome

Tingling of lips

Itching of the mouth, ears, and eyes

Conjunctivitis (often from transfer of the allergen to the eye by contaminated hands)

Throat tightening

Hives

Angioedema

Asthma (in asthmatics)

Anaphylaxis

Gastrointestinal symptoms such as abdominal pain, diarrhea, or vomiting

The incidence of both peanut and nut allergy in populations tends to vary. In one reported study, cashew nut allergy was more frequently associated with anaphylaxis than peanut allergy.[1]

Previously, it was believed that allergies to tree nuts—including cashews, almonds, walnuts, hazelnuts, macadamia nuts, pecans, pistachios, and pine nuts—lasted a lifetime. However, recent research indicates that at least 9 percent of young children outgrow their nut allergy.[2] Even children who have experienced a severe nut allergy can outgrow their allergy. However, the study indicated that children who are allergic to multiple types of tree nuts are less likely to outgrow their allergy than children who are allergic to only one or, at most, two types of nuts. Based on their results, the authors recommend that children with tree nut allergies be re-evaluated periodically by an allergist or immunologist. They suggest that oral challenges be considered in children 4 years of age and older who have fewer than five thousand International Units (5 kilounits) per liter[a] of tree-nut specific-IgE in their blood.

Diet Free from Tree Nuts

Tree nuts are not a common constituent of foods, but they are included selectively in recipes and in manufactured foods. Therefore, a specific nut-free diet is not required. It is only necessary to recognize the terms that would indicate the presence of nuts on manufacturers' labels or in recipes. Table 12-1 lists the most commonly used terms and the foods that may contain nuts.

---

[a] International Units are used to measure the amount of a biologically active substance in a given sample. Please see Glossary, "International Units," for a complete explanation.

Table 12-1
TERMS INDICATING THE PRESENCE OF NUTS
AND FOODS THAT MAY CONTAIN NUTS

Terms Indicating the Presence of Nuts

Almond	Pistachio
Brazil nut	Walnut
Cashew	Nut butters
Chestnut	Almond butter
Filbert (Hazelnut)	Cashew butter
Hickory nut	Chestnut spread
Macadamia nut	Other
Mashuga nut	Nut paste
Pecan	Almond paste
Pine nut: also known as:	Marzipan
Pinon	Nut oils
Indian nut	Nut meal
Pignoli	

Foods That May Contain Nuts

Artificial nuts
Nougat
Nutella® (Chocolate/hazelnut spread)
Gianduja (mixture of chocolate and chopped nuts)
Candy bars
Chocolate bars
Boxed chocolates
Flavored ice creams such as:
    Maple walnut
    Pecan
    Pistachio
    Other nut flavors
    Chocolate
Dessert toppings
Cheese balls
Gourmet cheese spreads

ALLERGY TO EDIBLE SEEDS

Sesame seed allergy is becoming more common in children. Sesame seed allergy is not very different from other food allergies. In a study of 14 children with reported sesame seed allergy from three allergy clinics in France,[3] the median age at the beginning of the sesame seed allergy was 5 years (range from 5 months to 16 years). All of the selected children reacted immediately after sesame seed consumption. The symptoms observed included swelling (edema [9 cases, 48%]), hives (urticaria [5 cases, 27%]), and one of each of the following symptoms: vomiting, rhinitis, conjunctivitis, asthma, and anaphylactic shock. One child had recurrent anaphylactic shocks, and another had an anaphylactic shock after subsequent sesame seed exposure; both of these children were asthmatic. Three children outgrew their food allergy. Prior to that study, most of the cases of sesame seed allergy had been reported in adolescents or adults.

Some seeds are eaten as is, some are used as seasoning, and some are pressed for their oil. If a person is allergic to a specific seed, all sources of the seed and seed oil should be investigated and avoided.

Table 12-2 is a list of the seeds known to have caused allergy in susceptible individuals. It is not a complete list of all potentially allergenic seeds.

Table 12-2 ALLERGENIC SEEDS		
Usually Consumed as a Distinct Food	**Usually Consumed as a Seasoning**	**Usually Used as Oil**
• Cotton seed (often added to multigrain products such as breads) * Flax * Melon * Pomegranate • Psyllium • Pumpkin • Sunflower • Sesame	• Yellow mustard • White mustard • Black mustard • Celery • Pomegranate (Anardana) • Poppy	• Flax (linseed) • Safflower • Sunflower

References

1. Davoren M and Peake J. Cashew nut allergy is associated with a high risk of anaphylaxis. *Archives of Disease in Childhood* 2005;90:1084–1085.

2. Fleischer DM, Conover-Walker MK, Matsui EC, Wood RA. The natural history of tree nut allergy. Journal of Allergy and Clinical Immunology 2005;116(5): 1087-1093

3. Agne PS, Bidat E, Rance F, Paty E. Sesame seed allergy in children. *Allergie et Immunologie (Paris)* 2004;36(8):300–305.

CHAPTER 13

Wheat Allergy

Wheat is the grain most commonly reported to cause allergic reactions; it is also the most common grain in the Western diet. Allergy to other grains (such as oats, rye, barley, corn, or rice) is experienced less frequently. It is not uncommon for children to react adversely to wheat but to test negatively in wheat-specific IgE evaluations. Clinical allergy to wheat may cause anything from a mild reaction to anaphylaxis.

SYMPTOMS ASSOCIATED WITH WHEAT ALLERGY

Wheat has been reported to be the provoking allergen in a number of different allergic conditions. The most frequently reported manifestations of wheat allergy are symptoms of abdominal pain and loose stools commencing within 12 to 72 hours after eating wheat. In children, this pattern often accompanies an allergy to cow's milk proteins[1] (CMA), especially when the child has food-associated eczema.

Ingested and inhaled wheat flour has been demonstrated to cause asthma in both adults and children and wheat is one of numerous food and environmental allergens implicated in causing eczema. Wheat allergy may also provoke hives and angioedema. Anaphylactic reactions to wheat have been reported in children, but it is a very rare occurrence[2]. Exercise-induced ana-phylaxis after eating wheat is more frequently reported (for a discussion of exercise-induced anaphylaxis, see Chapter 18).

Allergens in Wheat

Although the carbohydrate content of grains is much higher than their pro-tein content, it is the protein that causes the immune system response in an allergic reaction. Protein makes up about 12 percent of the dry wheat kernel. Wheat proteins are roughly divided into the following four classes:

Gliadins

Glutenins

Albumins

Globulins

Gliadins and glutenins form the gluten complex. Gliadins contain as many as 40 to 60 distinct components; glutenins contain at least 15. The molecular size of the protein components in wheat is between 10 and 40 kilodaltons[a], the size considered optimal for triggering an IgE-mediated allergy. Other cereal grains contain similar mixtures of proteins, which theoretically could trigger an allergic reaction.

Allergy to Wheat Proteins

No single protein or class of proteins seems to be responsible for wheat aller-gy. People allergic to wheat tend to react to the albumins and globulins, rather than to the gliadins and glutenins. However, some researchers disagree with this generalization and think there is more evidence for immune responses to gliadins and globulins[3]. Interestingly, in spite of this demonstrable immune

---

[a] Kilodaltons (1,000 daltons) are the units used to measure the size of molecules. Please see Glossary for more information.

reactivity (IgE positivity in RAST in most cases), some people show no clinical evidence of wheat allergy when wheat is consumed. On the other hand, many people with demonstrable symptoms after consuming wheat are RAST negative, especially when the reaction is delayed for 1 hour or more after the wheat is eaten. These findings simply emphasize the importance of elimination and challenge in the identification of a sensitivity to wheat and any other grain before it is excluded from a person's diet for a prolonged period.

ALLERGY TO OTHER CEREAL GRAINS

The incidence of allergy to other cereal grains and the degree of cross-reactivity among cereal grains is unknown. Allergy to oats, rye, or barley is uncommon and, therefore, restricting these grains is rarely necessary except for the treatment of celiac disease. Corn allergy is rarer, but it has been documented in a number of reports, mainly in childhood. Allergy to rice appears to be equally uncommon. If allergy to any grain is suspected, elimination and challenge should be carried out to confirm the suspicion and determine the specific grain causing the adverse reaction.

GRAINS AND CELIAC DISEASE

Individuals with celiac disease (also called sprue or gluten-sensitive enteropathy) react to the alpha-gliadin fraction of gluten. Although a variety of mechanisms involving immune reactions have been proposed as the primary trigger in the development of celiac disease, there is no evidence that it is due to an allergy.

Symptoms of celiac disease include diarrhea, weight loss, malabsorption (especially of fat), signs of iron or folate deficiency, sometimes rickets, and indications of other vitamin and mineral deficiencies. Occasionally, the condition is accompanied by an itchy rash (dermatitis herpetiformis).

Celiac disease is most definitively diagnosed by a jejunal biopsy (taking a tissue sample from the jejunum, a portion of the small intestine). When a laboratory study of the tissue sample reveals villous atrophy (flattened, short, or absent villi) and other abnormal conditions in the lining of the jejunum, celiac disease can be confirmed. A number of blood tests are available for detecting the presence of a variety of specific antibodies whose presence is indicative of celiac disease. A suspicion that celiac disease is the cause of a person's symptoms should always be confirmed by laboratory data so that treatment is not undertaken inappropriately. Treatment is lifelong and consists of the strict avoidance of all grains that contain gluten, namely, wheat, rye, and barley. However, it is important to realize that not all wheat intolerance, grain intolerance, or even gluten intolerance is due to celiac disease. (Celiac disease and the gluten-restricted diet are discussed in Chapter 24 and in Appendix C).

WHEAT-FREE DIET

In Western countries, avoidance of wheat is one of the more difficult diets to manage because wheat is a principal ingredient in many commonly eaten foods. Breads, cereals, crackers, cookies, muffins, pasta, snack foods, luncheon meats, sausages, candies, desserts, cakes, pies, pancakes, waffles, and many other wheat-containing products are the basis of the convenience foods used in the fast-paced Western lifestyle. These products supply the nutrients occurring naturally in wheat, as well as those added in the fortification of wheat flour, namely, thiamin, riboflavin, niacin, and iron.

Hydrolyzed plant protein (HPP), hydrolyzed vegetable protein (HVP), and monosodium glutamate (MSG) may be made from wheat. However, because the hydrolysis process breaks down the protein to a form that is unlikely to be allergenic, avoiding these products is not always considered necessary.

Wheat is likely to be present in foods containing:

Gluten	Whole wheat flour	High gluten flour
High protein flour	Vital gluten	Wheat gluten
Wheat starch	Enriched flour	Wheat germ
Flour	Starch	Vegetable starch
Modified starch	Bran	Vegetable gum
Wheat bran	Gelatinized starch	Durum
Graham flour	Semolina	Cracker crumbs
Couscous	Farina	

If rye, oats, barley, corn, and rice are tolerated, then baked products, cereals, and pastas using these grains can be used in place of those using wheat. In addition, unusual grains and flours (such as millet, quinoa, amaranth, buckwheat, tapioca, sago, arrowroot, soy, lentil, pea, and bean, as well as nuts and seeds) if tolerated, may be used in interesting combinations to make baked products and cereals.

Spelt, Kamut, Triticale, and flours derived from these grains are too closely related to wheat to be considered safe in a wheat-free diet, unless tolerance is specifically demonstrated by elimination and challenge.

Important Nutrients in Wheat

Wheat and wheat products are a significant source of thiamin, riboflavin, niacin, iron, selenium, chromium, and, in smaller amounts, magnesium, folate, phosphorus, and molybdenum.

Many of these micronutrients are added to wheat cereals and flours as fortifiers. Alternative choices of foods to replace these include oats, rice, rye, barley, corn, buckwheat, amaranth, and quinoa, some of which are fortified with micronutrients similar to those in wheat products. Flours suitable as replacements for wheat flour include flours and starches from rice, potato, rye, oats, barley, buckwheat, tapioca, millet, corn, quinoa, and amaranth.

WHEAT-FREE DIET

The wheat-free diet omits wheat and foods containing wheat products. Foods allowed and restricted on a wheat-free diet are listed in Table 13-2. This diet is not suitable for the treatment of celiac disease because it is not gluten-free.

Label-Reading Guidelines for a Wheat-Free Diet

When restricting any food from the diet, it is important to become familiar with terms that may appear on product labels indicating the presence of the food. Wheat may appear in a food product under the terms listed in Table 13-1.

Table 13-1
TERMS ASSOCIATED WITH WHEAT IN FOOD PRODUCTS

Terms Used to Indicate the Presence of Wheat

Bread crumbs	Phosphated flour
Bran	White bread
Bulgur	Sourdough bread
Gluten	Multigrain flour
High-gluten flour	Multigrain bread
Vital gluten	Seitan
Protein flour	Semolina
High protein flour	Spelt
Graham flour	Triticale
Graham crackers	Kamut
Crackers	Couscous
Matzoh	Anything with wheat in the name, e.g.,
Cereal extract	Wheat berries
Cracked wheat	Wheat germ
Cracker meal	Wheat bran
Durum	Sprouted wheat
Durum flour	Wheatena
Enriched flour	Wheat gluten
Self-rising flour	Whole wheat bread
Pastry flour	60% whole wheat bread
Bread flour	
Unbleached flour	
All-purpose flour	

Terms Indicating That Wheat Is Potentially Present
(unless the source is declared to be other than wheat

Gelatinized starch	Vegetable gum
HVP	Vegetable starch
HPP	Soy sauce
Malt	Malt
Starch (unless origin is specified [e.g., corn starch])	Grain coffee substitute
	Postum
Modified starch (unless origin is specified)	Granola
	Granola bar

Table 13-2 FOODS ALLOWED AND RESTRICTED ON A WHEAT-FREE DIET		
Type of Food	**Foods Allowed**	**Foods Restricted**

Milk and Milk Products	• Milk (whole milk, 2%, 1%, skim, Lactose-reduced (Lactaid®, Lacteeze®, Acidophilus)
	 • Cream
	 • Sour cream
	 • Buttermilk
	 • Yogurt
	 • Cheese of all types
	 • Cottage cheese
	 • Ricotta
	 • Feta
	 • Quark
	 • Any other food made from pure milk
		• Any milk product containing wheat (usually as a thickener), such as:
		   Instant cocoa
		   Hot chocolate mixes
		   Malted milk
		   Ovaltine
		   Coffee substitutes
		     (e.g, Postum)
		   Cheese sauces, spreads,
		     and other dairy foods
		     containing wheat

Grains, Cereals, Flours, and Starches	• Grains, cereals, flours, and starches made with or derived from:
	   Amaranth
	   Arrowroot
	   Barley
	   Buckwheat
	   Corn
	   Lentil or pea flour
	   Kasha
	   Nut meal and flour
	     (all types)
	   Oats
	   Quinoa
	   Rice (all types)
	   Rye
		• Grains, cereals, flours, and starches made with or derived from:
		   Bulgur
		   Couscous
		   Cracked wheat
		   Durum
		   Farina
		   Gluten-enriched
		   Graham
		   Kamut
		   Malt*
		   Matzoh
		   Semolina
		   Spelt
		   Starch*
		   Triticale

Table 13-2 (continued)
FOODS ALLOWED AND RESTRICTED ON A WHEAT-FREE DIET

Type of Food	Foods Allowed	Foods Restricted
Grains, Cereals, Flours, and Starches (continued)	Sago Seed meal and flour Soy flour Tapioca	Wheat Wheatena Wheat bran and germ Wheat berries

Breads and Baked goods	• Any food made from allowed flours and starches such as:
	    Rice bread
	    Rice and soy bread
	    Rye bread
	    Cornmeal bread made without wheat flour
	    Breads, muffins, cookies, pancakes, waflles, and cakes made with allowed grains
		• Any food made from restricted flours or starches
		    Any regular white or whole wheat bread, buns, croissants, bagels
		    Cakes, muffins, pancakes, cookies, waffles, etc. made with wheat or white flour
		    Bread crumbs
		    Cracker meal

Crackers and snacks	• Any food made from allowed grains such as:
	    Corn chips
	    Corn nachos
	    Corn taco chips
	    Potato chips
	    Rice cakes, plain, with seeds, or other allowed grains
	    Rice crackers
		• Any food containin wheat, such as:
		    Graham crackers
		    Cheese crackers
		    Ritz™ crackers
		    Saltines™
		    Champagne™ crackers
		    Vegetable Thins™
		    Matzoh

Table 13-2 (continued)
FOODS ALLOWED AND RESTRICTED ON A WHEAT-FREE DIET

Type of Food	Foods Allowed	Foods Restricted
Breakfast Cereals	• Made from any grain on allowed list, e.g., oats, barley, rye, millet, and corn, such as: Oatmeal Corn Flakes Cream of Rice® Rice Krispies® Puffed Rice Puffed Millet Kenmei Rice Brand® Puffed Amaranth	• Any breakfast cereal containing wheat, such as: Shredded wheat Puffed wheat Weetabix Wheaties Wheatena Creamof Wheat Red River Cereal Miniwheats Other wheat cereals (read labels carefully)
Pasta	• Pasta made from any grain on allowed list, such as: Soy pasta Buckwheat pasta Mung bean pasta Bean vermicelli Rice noodles and pasta Brown rice pasta Wild rice pasta Corn pasta Potato pasta Quinoa pasta (Note: Sometimes wheat is included in the pastas labeled as above. Do not assume that the pasta contains only the named grain. Always check the ingredient list.)	• Any pasta made with wheat flour including: Spinach Carrot Egg noodles Vermicelli Other pastas (read labels carefully)

Table 13-2 (continued)
FOODS ALLOWED AND RESTRICTED ON A WHEAT-FREE DIET

Type of Food	Foods Allowed	Foods Restricted
Vegetables	• All prepared with allowed ingredients • All vegetable juices • All pure, fresh, frozen, or canned vegetables	• Vegetables prepared with a dressing or garnish containing wheat • Salad dressings containing wheat (starch) as a thickener • Sprouted wheat
Fruit	• All pure fruits and fruit juices	• Commercial pie fillings • All fruit dishes containing wheat • Fruit pies with a crust made from wheat flour • Fruit pies with Graham cracker crust

Meat, Poultry, and Fish	• All plain, fresh, frozen, or canned meat, poultry, or fish
	• Those prepared without wheat, wheat batters, or bread crumbs
		• Meat dishes that may contain wheat, such as:
		  Battered
		  Breaded
		  Croquettes
		  Luncheon meats
		  Meat loaves
		  Meat balls
		  Patties
		  Pâté
		  Sausages
		  Spreads
		  Stuffing
		  Wieners
		  Processed meats

Table 13-2 (continued)
FOODS ALLOWED AND RESTRICTED ON A WHEAT-FREE DIET

Type of Food	Foods Allowed	Foods Restricted
Eggs	• All eggs and egg dishes prepared without wheat	• Egg dishes containing wheat • Scotch eggs (wheat is often included in the sausage)
Legumes	• All prepared without wheat • Plain tofu • Peanut butter • Tamari sauce	• Legume dishes containing wheat, usually as a thickener • Soy sauce
Nuts and Seeds	• All plain seeds and nuts	• Snack nuts and seeds with HVP, HPP, or MSG
Fats and Oils	• Butter • Cream • Margarine • Shortening • All pure vegetable, nut, and seed oils • Fish oils • Lard • Meat drippings • Peanut and other pure nut and seed butters • Homemade gravy thickened with non-wheat starch (e.g., corn, tapioca, arrowroot)	• Wheat germ oil • Salad dressings containing wheat • Sauces containing wheat (usually as a thickener) • Gravy thickened with wheat flour or starch

Table 13-2 (continued)
FOODS ALLOWED AND RESTRICTED ON A WHEAT-FREE DIET

Type of Food	Foods Allowed	Foods Restricted
Spices and Herbs	• All plain spices and herbs	• Seasoning mixes containing wheat, HVP*, HPP*, or MSG* such as: Packaged soup seasoning mixes Bouillon cubes
Sweets and Sweeteners	• Sugar • Honey • Molasses • Jams • Jellies • Preserves • Baking chocolate and pure cocoa powder	• All sweets containing wheat, such as: Icing sugar* Candy* Marshmallows*

* Avoid these products unless the source is known not to be wheat.

References

1. Jarvinen KM, Turpeinen M, Suomalainen H. Concurrent cereal allergy in children with cow's milk allergy manifested with atopic dermatitis. *Clinical and Experimental Allergy.* 2003 Aug;33(8):1060–106.

2. Daengsuwan T, Palosuo K, Phankingthongkum S, Visitsunthorn N, Jirapongsananuruk O, Alenius H, Vichyanond P, Reunala T. IgE antibodies to omega-5 gliadin in children with wheat-induced anaphylaxis. *Allergy* 2005;60(4):506–509

3. Takizawa T, Arakawa H, Tokuyama K, Morikawa A. Identification of allergen fractions of wheat flour responsible for anaphylactic reactions to wheat products in infants and young children. *International Archives of Allergy and Immunololgy.* 2001 May;125(1):51–6

CHAPTER 14

Corn Allergy

Although corn is often cited as an allergenic food, cases of allergic reactions after ingestion of corn have rarely been published and very few studies have been devoted to the identification of corn allergens. There is very little evidence to suggest that corn is a food that is likely to trigger severe or anaphylactic reactions. Until recently, few food-induced allergic reactions to corn or maize had been reported. In fact, some allergists questioned whether corn allergy existed at all.[1] Since 2000, a number of investigators have been looking more closely at corn allergy, especially in children, and finding evidence that allergy to corn is a valid reaction and may be more prevalent than previously thought. However, most reactions tend to be mild, and not all children sensitized to corn will develop symptoms when they eat it.

In one reported study, only 6 out of 16 children who were skin-test positive to corn and who had corn-specific IgE antibodies in their blood actually developed symptoms when they ate corn.[2] The remainder were not suffering from food allergy to this cereal, as revealed both by their clinical history and the negative challenge results.

A report published in 2006[3] suggests that " . . . maize-related food allergy is more complex than so far anticipated," so it is logical to expect additional information on corn allergy as more clinicians and scientists become interested in the topic.

ALLERGENS IN CORN

There was virtually no information on the allergenic proteins in corn until about 2001 when a research report identified the major corn allergen as a protein, 9 kilodaltons in size, which has the characteristics of a lipid transfer protein (LTP). These same researchers also identified a 16-kilodalton protein that had the potential to induce IgE antibodies.[4] LTPs are proteins that are present in many foods and are often responsible for the most significant allergies. They are generally heat-resistant, and their allergenicity is unaffected by cooking. Furthermore, they can survive stomach acid and digestive enzymes when they are eaten. Therefore, they are able to induce an immunological response when they encounter immune cells in the intestines.

Another group of researchers found a larger (50-kilodalton) protein that was resistant to both heating and peptic or pancreatic digestion and was thought to be a likely candidate as an important allergen in triggering corn allergy.[2]

Interestingly, the researchers who reported the existence of the 9-kilodalton corn allergen found that the corn LTP cross-reacts completely with LTPs in rice and peach, but not with those in wheat or barley.[5] This is further evidence that foods in the same botanical family rarely cross-react, but proteins that are structurally identical in unrelated plants may trigger allergy in a person who is sensitized to only one of them. (Allergenic relatedness is discussed with oral allergy syndrome in Chapter 21.) A 16-kilodalton protein identified in the same study cross-reacted with similar antigens in grass, wheat, barley, and rice, but the significance of the protein as an allergen was unclear.

CORN-FREE DIET

Avoidance of corn is quite simple as long as only non-manufactured foods are eaten. However, when many prepared foods are included in a person's usual diet, it is an entirely different matter. A large number of manufactured foods contain corn in the form of corn meal, corn starch, corn syrup, and their derivatives. Corn products are likely to be present in cereals, baked goods, snack foods, syrups, canned fruits, beverages, jams, jellies, cookies, luncheon meats, candies, other convenience foods, and meal replacers, as well as in infant formulas. Even medications may contain corn starch as a vehicle for the active drug.

Corn oil is not usually allergenic, unless the product is contaminated during its manufacture by protein from the grain. Corn protein is an extremely rare cause of anaphylaxis and the quantity likely to be present is very small. Therefore, it is not usually considered necessary to restrict corn oil as an ingredient in foods.

Elimination of corn does not lead to nutritional deficiencies as long as the usual intake of corn itself is small. However, if the usual diet contains many convenience foods, alternative corn-free products will be needed for adequate nutrition.

Obvious sources of corn must be avoided, including the following:

- Whole corn or maize

- Popcorn

- Corn flour

- Corn starch

- Corn meal

- Corn alcohol

- Corn gluten

- Corn sweetener

- Corn sugar

- Corn syrup

- Corn oil

The following foods frequently contain corn or one of its derivatives:

- Packaged breakfast cereals sweetened with corn syrup

- Spaghetti sauces

- Canned baked beans

- Canned soups

- Gravies

- Some brands of peanut butter
- Luncheon meats
- Processed meats
- Imitation cheeses, cheese foods, and snacks
- Imitation seafood
- Jams
- Jellies
- Candies
- Cookies
- Canned fruit deserts
- Pudding mixes
- Cake mixes
- Pancake mixes
- Commercial baked goods of all types

Derivatives of corn used in manufactured foods include the following:

- Dextrose (also known as glucose or corn sugar)
- Dextrin
- Dextrate
- Maltodextrin
- Caramel
- Malt syrup

Dextrose is used in cookies, ice cream, and sports drinks.

Dextrose may be used to coat foods such as French fries, fish sticks, and potato puffs because heating causes a reaction (called the Maillard reaction) that imparts new aromas and flavors and an attractive golden-brown color to the food.

Dextrin and maltodextrin are used in sauces, dressings, and ice cream as thickening agents.

Corn syrup can be used in place of the traditional cane or beet sugar to make caramel flavoring.

Corn syrup may also be used in maple, nut, and root beer flavorings for ice cream, fruit ices, candy, and baked goods.

Many soft drinks and fruit drinks contain corn syrup.

Corn starch is added to most confectioner's sugar and baking powder to keep them from caking or clumping.

Marshmallows usually contain corn starch.

When *starch* appears on a food label, it is often corn starch that is included. However, wheat starch is also a common ingredient, so not all products that contain starch without identification of the source actually contain corn.

Similarly, modified food starch, vegetable gum, or vegetable starch may or may not be derived from corn.

HPP, HVP, and TVP also may be made from corn. However, as with similar products derived from wheat, the hydrolysis process breaks down the protein to the point where it is unlikely to be allergenic. As a result, it is usually considered unnecessary to exclude these products from a corn-restricted diet.

If you wish to use foods with ingredients that might be derived from corn, it is wise to contact the manufacturer to see if corn is used in its production.

Other Foods That Might Contain Corn

- Distilled white vinegar

- Bleached white flour

- Iodized table salt

Nonfood Products That Might Contain Corn

Corn oil might be used in emollient creams and toothpastes.
Corn syrup is often used as a texturizer and carrying agent in cosmetics.
Corn may be present in adhesives for envelopes, stamps, and stickers.
Plastic wrap, paper cups, and paper plates can be coated with corn oil.

Medications That Might Contain Corn

Many tablets and liquid medications contain corn derivatives, particularly corn starch.

Some of the most commonly encountered corn-containing medications include the following:

- Aspirin
- Throat lozenges
- Ointments
- Suppositories
- Vitamins
- Laxatives
- Bath powders containing corn starch

The Corn-Free Lifestyle

Obviously, it is not possible to list all of the manufactured foods, medications, and other products that contain corn. Anyone who is dealing with a corn allergy, especially the parent of an allergic child, must carefully read all product labels and become familiar with the terms that indicate an ingredient may be derived from corn.

In spite of the multitude of foods and products that contain corn in our modern world, it is very rare to encounter anyone who experiences a severe allergic reaction in contact or after ingestion of most of them. This is because corn protein is not a highly allergenic allergen, and reactions rarely occur in response to the very small amounts of allergen that are present in most foods. That is the reason why corn is used so extensively. It is considered to be a food derivative that is usually safe and very unlikely to cause an adverse reaction in the greatest number of consumers.

Because manufactured foods are a reality in our fast-paced lifestyle and we demand these products to make our lives easier, we have to accept that a very small percentage of the population might react adversely to them. The alternative, of course, is to cook every meal from scratch using only known, pure ingredients. If the corn-allergic individual is not prepared to do that, then the most important advice is to read all product labels carefully and make choices judiciously.

Table 14-1
COMMON FOODS LIKELY TO CONTAIN CORN

Corn is likely to be present in the following foods:

Corn	Corn flour	Corn on the cob
Corn meal	Corn niblets	Corn starch
Popcorn	Polenta	Hominy
Cornflakes	Grits	Corn bread and muffins
Maize	Kernel corn	Corn sugar
Corn syrup	Caramel corn	Corn sweetener
Corn syrup solids	Corn alcohol	Modified starch
Vegetable starch	Vegetable gum	Vegetable protein
Vegetable paste	Starch	*Caramel flavoring
Dextrose	*Sorbitol	Dextrate
Maltodextrose		

The following Mexican foods are traditionally made with corn:

Tamales	Nachos	Tortillas
Tacos	Masa harina	

Corn-Free Cooking

It is not difficult to avoid corn in recipes. There is no need for a corn-free cookbook or special corn-free recipes. Most recipes in cookbooks are quite suitable for a corn-free diet, as long as they do not use prepared and processed ingredients such as canned soups, packaged soup mixes, flavor packages, or other manufactured additions.

The following guidelines will help you in choosing appropriate recipes in cooking for your allergic child:

- Avoid all recipes with corn in the name of the dish.

- Avoid all recipes where corn is the main ingredient, for example corn bread, corn muffins, polenta.

- Avoid all recipes that include prepared or manufactured foods.

- Always choose recipes that start from single foods, as in traditional cooking, for example, wheat flour, any fruit, vegetables, meat, fish, poultry, nuts, and so on.

- If the recipe calls for corn starch, substitute arrowroot or tapioca starch.

- If the recipe uses corn flour, use wheat flour instead.

- When corn syrup is included in the recipe, use pure maple syrup or honey instead.

- Use canola, safflower, or olive oil in place of corn oil.

You should have no difficulty in providing healthy, balanced meals for your corn-allergic child and your family as long as you use traditional recipes and stay away from prepared, processed, and manufactured foods and snacks. I often advise food-allergic adults or those feeding food-allergic children to stay around the periphery rather than the central aisles of a supermarket when grocery shopping. All of the pure foods are in the produce, bakery, meat, fish, and dairy sections. Most foods in the middle sections are manufactured and are likely to contain common additives such as corn and, of course, preservatives and artificial flavorings and colorings that most children are better off without.

References

1. Moneret-Vautrin DA, Kanny G, Beaudouin E. Food allergy to corn—does it exist? *Allergie et Immunologie (Paris)* 1998;30(7):230.

2. Pasisni G, Simonatao B, Curioni A, Vincenzi S, Cristaudo A, Santucci B, Dal Belin Peruffo A, Giannattasio M. IgE-mediated allergy to corn: A 50 kDa protein, belonging to the reduced soluble proteins, is a major allergen. *Allergy* 2002;57:98–106.

3. Weichel M, Vergoossen NJ, Bonomi S, Scibilia J, Ortolani C, Ballmer-Weber BK, Pastorello EA, Crameri R. Screening the allergenic repertoires of wheat and maize with sera from double-blind, placebo-controlled food challenge positive patients. *Allergy* 2006;61(1):128.

4. Pastorello EA, Farioli L, Pravettoni V, Ispano M, Scibola E, Trambaioli C, Giuffrida MG, Ansaloni R, Godovac-Zimmermann J, Conti A, Fortunato D, Ortolani C. The maize major allergen, which is responsible for food-induced allergic reactions, is a lipid transfer protein. *Journal of Allergy and Clinical Immunology* 2000;106(4):744–751.

5. Pastorello EA, Farioli L, Pravettoni V, Ispano M, Scibola E, Trambaioli C, Giuffrida MG, Ansaloni R, Godovac-Zimmermann J, Conti A, Fortunato D, Ortolani C. The maize major allergen, which is responsible for food-induced allergic reactions, is a lipid transfer protein. *Journal of Allergy and Clinical Immunology* 2000;106(4):744–751.

CHAPTER 15

Seafood Allergy

ALLERGY TO FISH

Fish species are abundant and exist in many edible forms in most countries of the world. The allergenic part of the fish is usually in the meat (muscle) of the fish. However, there is evidence that fish gelatin, made from skin and bones, may also be allergenic. Fish gelatin contains a high level of collagens, so there is concern that certain collagens made from fish might be a cause of allergy. This subject needs to be investigated further.

The incidence of fish allergy varies between populations, depending on whether seafood is a large part of the ethnic diet. A 2004 telephone census of households in the United States that surveyed 14,948 individuals[1] reported that fish or shellfish allergy occurred in 5.9 percent of households. Seafood-allergic individuals reported their specific allergy:

2.3 percent reported seafood allergy

2 percent reported shellfish allergy

0.4 percent reported fish allergy

0.2 percent reported allergy to both types of seafood.

Seafood allergy was more common in adults compared with children (2.8% and 0.6%, respectively) and in women compared with men (3.6% and 2%, respectively).

Sensitization to Fish

Fish consumption during infancy has traditionally been regarded as a risk factor for allergic disease. In fact, some authorities recommend not introducing fish to the diet of a child younger than 1 or even 2 years of age. However, recent evidence suggests otherwise. A study of 4089 newborn infants, followed for 4 years, found that regular fish consumption during the first year of life was associated with a reduced risk for allergic disease by the age of 4 years.[2]

Another study[3] found that frequent intake of fish during pregnancy reduced the incidence of skin-test positivity (SPT) to foods in the offspring of mothers who themselves did not have allergies. In the whole study population (including mothers with and without allergies themselves), there was a similar trend between increased consumption of fish (2–3 times per week or more) and decreased prevalence of SPT to foods. In fact, babies of the mothers who consumed fish regularly had over a one-third less food sensitization compared to infants of mothers who did not consume fish.

In light of the conflicting information, it is difficult to make any clear recommendations regarding the best time to introduce fish to a potentially allergic child. It is probably safe to try fish after 12 months of age (as described in the Introducing Solid Foods section of Chapter 3) until further well-conducted research indicates otherwise.

Allergens in Different Fish Species

The question as to whether antigens in different types and species of fish cross-react has not yet been answered satisfactorily. Thus, it is not clear whether or not it is necessary for fish-allergic individuals to avoid all species of fish if they are allergic to one species. In most cases, it is usually only necessary for the allergic person to avoid the specific type of fish to which he or she is allergic. However, there is increasing evidence that certain fish allergens may be common to several species.

Not a great deal is known about individual fish allergens except for the antigen in cod, named gad c 1, which was one of the first food allergens of any type to be studied. The antigen is a protein called a parvalbumin, which can be found in a variety of fish species unrelated to cod (for example, carp, tuna, and salmon). In some studies, individuals allergic to cod were shown to react to other fish species (such as herring, plaice, and mackerel) in a double-blind, placebo-controlled food challenge.[4] It is still unclear whether a person allergic to one of these species should avoid all fish. At the present time, the directive is this: if there is no risk of an anaphylactic reaction, only the fish species that have triggered clinical reactivity when consumed should be avoided. However, when there is the risk of an anaphylactic reaction, all fish and their derivatives should be avoided in the interest of safety.

Fish and shellfish are quite distinct antigenically, so a person who is allergic to shellfish rarely needs to avoid free-swimming fish (ones with fins). To avoid unnecessary dietary restrictions, it is important that the species of fish to which a person reacts adversely should be clearly identified.

It is usually easy to avoid fish because its presence in a recipe is obvious and its inclusion in a manufactured food is almost always indicated on the label. Table 15-1 lists terms that indicate the presence of fish or fish products in manufactured foods and recipes.

Nonallergic Conditions Causing Adverse Reactions to Fish

Food protein-induced enterocolitis syndrome (FPIES) is an uncommon condition that occasionally occurs in infants. Typical symptoms include profuse vomiting, diarrhea, or both several hours after ingestion of a given food. The disorder is a non-IgE-mediated food hypersensitivity. Therefore, skin tests and blood tests that look for food-specific IgE will be negative. The most frequently involved foods are milk and soy, but some cases of FPIES induced by other foods have been described. Recently, the syndrome was reported in response to fish protein in children aged from 9 to 12 months.[5] As in the case of other food allergies, the diagnosis is confirmed by elimination and challenge (see Chapter 6). In many cases, the child outgrows the condition by about 7 years of age, after a usually prolonged period of avoidance of the food.

Important Nutrients in Fish

Fish is a significant source of niacin, vitamin B_6, vitamin B_{12}, vitamin E, phosphorus, selenium, and, in smaller amounts, vitamin A, magnesium, iron, and zinc. These nutrients are also present in meats, grains, legumes, and oils. So foods with equivalent nutrients can be readily obtained when fish and shellfish are removed from the diet.

Fish Oils

Although pure oils are nonallergenic, it is very likely that any fish oil is contaminated with protein of the fish from which it was extracted. Fish-allergic individuals should avoid oil from the species of fish to which they are sensitive. If the fish species is not specified, then all fish oil should be avoided, especially if there is a risk of anaphylaxis.

SHELLFISH ALLERGY

A person who is allergic to shellfish is usually advised to avoid shellfish of all types. Even unrelated species tend to cause an adverse reaction when eaten by a sensitized individual. Therefore, a shellfish-restricted diet eliminates all species of crustaceans such as crab, lobster, shrimp, and prawn as well as mollusks (bivalves) such as clams, mussels, and scallops. However, a person who reacts to shellfish does not need to avoid fish, since there is no evidence to suggest that there is any relationship between the two types of seafood.

Table 15-2 lists names and terms that indicate the presence of shellfish. Kosher food products do not contain shellfish and therefore are safe for a person with shellfish allergy.

Table 15-1
TERMS ON LABELS THAT INDICATE THE PRESENCE OF FISH

Terms Indicating the Presence of Fish Protein

Fish (all species)	Fish oils, such as:
Roe	cod liver oil
Caviar	halibut liver oil
Surimi	salmon oil
	menhaden oil
	Efamol Marine®

Foods That May Contain Fish Protein

Asian dishes, such as:	Caesar salad (with anchovy)	Baked goods
egg rolls		Cookies
sushi	Chili	Candy bars
sashimi		Prepared and frozen desserts
tempura		
Thai recipes		
Chinese recipes		
satay sauces		

Table 15-2
TERMS ON LABELS THAT INDICATE THE PRESENCE OF SHELLFISH

Terms Indicating the Presence of Shellfish

Crab	Mollusk	Octopus
Lobster	Abalone	Squid
Shrimp	Oyster	Calamari
Prawn	Clam	Escargot (snail)
Scampi	Cockle	Quahog
Crawfish (crayfish)	Mussel	
	Scallop	
	Whelk	
	Winkle	

Food That May Contain Shellfish Protein

Asian dishes	Shrimp noodles	Taro cake
Thai dishes	Shrimp balls	Daikon cake
Chinese dishes:	Shrimp chips	Flavoring in products fish products
Congee	Fish balls, soup	
Oyster sauce	Haw Gow	Stuffing
Satay sauce	Sui My	
XO sauce	Sashimi	
	Sushi	

References

1. Sicherer SH, Muñoz-Furlong A, Sampson HA. Prevalence of seafood allergy in the United States determined by a random telephone survey. *Journal of Allergy and Clinical Immunology* 2004;114(1):159–165.

2. Kull I, Bergstrom A, Lilja G, Pershagen G, Wickman M. Fish consumption during the first year of life and development of allergic diseases during childhood. *Allergy* 2006;61(8):1009–1015.

3. Calvani M, Alessandri C, Sopo SM, Panetta V, Pingitore G, Tripodi S, Zappalà D, Zicari AM. Consumption of fish, butter and margarine during pregnancy and development of allergic sensitizations in the offspring: Role of maternal atopy. *Pediatric Allergy and Immunology* 2006;17(2):94–102.

4. Poulsen LK, Hansen TK, Norgaard A, Vetsergaard H, Skov PS, Bindslev-Jensen C. Allergens from egg and fish. *Allergy* 2001;56:39.

5. Zapatero Remon L, Alonso Lebrero E, Martin Fernandez E, Martinez Molero MI. Food-protein-induced enterocolitis syndrome caused by fish. *Allergology and Immunopathology (Madrid)* 2005;33(6):312–316.

CHAPTER 16

The Top Ten Allergens: Avoidance of Milk, Egg, Wheat, Corn, Peanuts, Soy, Tree Nuts, Seeds, Shellfish, and Fish

It is common for a child with food allergies to react to more than one food. Chapters 7 to 15 provide information on individual food allergies, but it is often difficult to combine the directives for two, three, or more allergens when providing healthy balanced meals. The more foods that need to be avoided, the greater is the risk for nutritional deficiency. Milk and milk products, egg, wheat, corn, soy, peanut, tree nuts, seeds, fish, and shellfish are the most frequent causes of food allergy. When all of these foods are removed from the diet at the same time, it is important to find substitutes that will replace the important nutrients that are restricted. The following table provides lists of substitute foods to ensure adequate nutritional intake when the ten most highly allergenic foods are being avoided.

If your child is allergic to only two or three of these foods, it is a fairly easy matter to follow the guidelines and add the foods that he or she tolerates.

A very restricted diet should not be followed for any longer than 4 weeks, after which time each food should be challenged (see Chapter 6) to confirm that it really needs to be avoided. If one (or more) of the excluded foods is not a problem, it can be included in the diet, which will then become more nutritionally complete and easier to manage.

Each of the foods restricted on this diet can be found in many products and has many derivatives. It would require extensive lists of foods and their products to cover all possible dietary sources. Reading of food labels is essential to detect the allergen as an ingredient in processed and prepared foods. Because so many foods are restricted, information is provided only for the foods allowed. Most of the information for individual restrictions has already been included in Chapters 7 to 15.

If all of the foods included in the following table are consumed and the diet is limited to 4 weeks, nutritional deficiency should be avoided. Possibly the only supplements required are calcium and vitamin D. However, if a child needs this diet for longer than 4 weeks, it is strongly advised to check with a physician and enlist the help of a registered dietitian for guidance in choosing appropriate substitutes and supplements.

Table 16-1
AVOIDANCE OF THE TOP TEN ALLERGENS:
DIET FREE FROM MILK, EGG, WHEAT, CORN, SOY, PEANUT, TREE NUTS,
SEEDS, FISH, AND SHELLFISH

Type of Food	Foods Allowed

Milk and Milk Products	• Milk and soy-free products such as:
	  – Rice Dream® (made from brown rice and safflower oil)
	  – Darifree® (made from potato starch)
	• In recipes substitute:
	  – fruit or vegetable juice
	  – homemade soup stock
	  – water used to cook vegetables or potatoes
	• Instead of butter use:
	  – whey-free, soy-free, corn-free margarine (e.g., Canoleo®)

Table 16-1 (continued)
AVOIDANCE OF THE TOP TEN ALLERGENS:
DIET FREE FROM MILK, EGG, WHEAT, CORN, SOY, PEANUT, TREE NUTS,
SEEDS, FISH, AND SHELLFISH

Type of Food	Foods Allowed
Milk and Milk Products (cont'd)	– pure jelly
	– jam
	– honey
	– olive oil
	• Dressings on vegetables and salads:
	– olive oil with herbs
	– homemade salad dressings made with allowed ingredients
Grains, Cereals, and Bakery Products	**Grains and Flours:**
	– Amaranth and amaranth flour
	– Barley and barley flour
	– Buckwheat and buckwheat flour
	– Chickpea or garbanzo bean flour (Besan)
	– Millet and millet flour (Bajri)
	– T'eff
	– Oats and oat flour
	– Potato starch and flour
	– Quinoa and quinoa flour
	– Rice and rice flour
	– Wild rice and wild rice flour

Table 16-1 (continued)
AVOIDANCE OF THE TOP TEN ALLERGENS:
DIET FREE FROM MILK, EGG, WHEAT, CORN, SOY, PEANUT, TREE NUTS,
SEEDS, FISH, AND SHELLFISH

Type of Food	Foods Allowed
Grains, Cereals, and Bakery Products (cont'd)	**Grains and Flours:** – Rye and rye flour – Sago and sago flour – Tapioca and tapioca starch and flour – Cassava flour and starch **Breads and Baked Goods:** • Baked goods and specialty baking mixes containing allowed ingredients such as: – Ener-G® rice, brown rice, or tapioca bread – Celimix® rice or flaxmeal bread • Homemade baked goods made with allowed flours and grains **Crackers and Snacks:** • Potato chips made without corn oil • Pure rye crisp crackers • Rice cakes without corn, sesame seed, or other restricted ingredients • Rice crackers without corn, sesame seed, or other restricted ingredients

Table 16-1 (continued)
AVOIDANCE OF THE TOP TEN ALLERGENS:
DIET FREE FROM MILK, EGG, WHEAT, CORN, SOY, PEANUT, TREE NUTS, SEEDS, FISH, AND SHELLFISH

Type of Food	Foods Allowed

Grains, Cereals, and Bakery Products (cont'd)	**Cereals:**
	
	• Made from any of the allowed grains such as:
	
	  – Cream of Rice®
	  – Kenmei Rice Bran
	  – Puffed rice
	  – Rice flakes
	  – Oatmeal
	  – Rolled oats
	  – Oat bran
	  – Rye flakes
	  – Granola made with allowed ingredients only
	  – Puffed amaranth
	  – Puffed millet
	  – Quinoa flakes
	
	Pasta:
	
	• Made from any allowed grain such as:
	
	  – Brown rice pasta
	  – Wild rice pasta
	  – Mung bean pasta

Table 16-1 (continued)
AVOIDANCE OF THE TOP TEN ALLERGENS:
DIET FREE FROM MILK, EGG, WHEAT, CORN, SOY, PEANUT, TREE NUTS,
SEEDS, FISH, AND SHELLFISH

Type of Food	Foods Allowed
Grains, Cereals, and Bakery Products (cont'd)	Pasta: – Green bean pasta – Buckwheat pasta (soba noodles) – Rice pasta – Rice noodles – Potato pasta – Quinoa pasta
Vegetables	• All plain fresh and frozen vegetables and their juices except: – Corn – Soybeans – Soybean sprouts – Sprouted wheat – Mixed sprouts
Fruit	• All plain fresh and frozen fruits and their juices
Meat and Poultry	• All fresh or frozen pure meat or poultry Avoid any meat mixed with additional ingredients, such as processed meats, sausages, and all delicatessen meats

Table 16-1 (continued)
AVOIDANCE OF THE TOP TEN ALLERGENS:
DIET FREE FROM MILK, EGG, WHEAT, CORN, SOY, PEANUT, TREE NUTS,
SEEDS, FISH, AND SHELLFISH

Type of Food	Foods Allowed
Fish and Shellfish	• None
Eggs	• None • Use egg-free egg replacer products such as Ener-G® Egg Replacer
Legumes	• All plain legumes and legume dishes prepared with allowed foods (avoid soy and peanut)
Nuts	• None
Seeds	• None

Fats and Oils	• Vegetable oils such as:
	  – Olive
	  – Canola
	  – Sunflower
	  – Safflower
	  – Flaxseed
	  – Grape seed
	• Meat drippings
	• Lard
	• Poultry fat
	• Homemade gravy with allowed ingredients

Table 16-1 (continued)
AVOIDANCE OF THE TOP TEN ALLERGENS:
DIET FREE FROM MILK, EGG, WHEAT, CORN, SOY, PEANUT, TREE NUTS,
SEEDS, FISH, AND SHELLFISH

Type of Food	Foods Allowed
Spices and Herbs	• All pure fresh or dried herbs (leaves and flowers of the plant) • Many spices are derived from seeds, but these are usually tolerated. However, if seed allergy is a severe problem, avoid all spices except for the non-seed spices that are derived from the root or bark of the plant; these are allowed: • Cinnamon • Nutmeg (not a nut) • Mace • Ginger • Turmeric • Clove

CHAPTER 17

Fructose Intolerance

Intolerance of fructose, especially in childhood, probably occurs more frequently than diagnostic figures currently suggest. The condition usually presents itself in the form of loose stools or diarrhea after consumption of fruits such as apples and pears or the juice of these fruits. Fructose intolerance is usually caused by impaired absorption of fructose. However, there are rare cases in which intolerance of fructose is due to a deficiency in one of the enzymes responsible for the digestion of fructose.

THE MECHANISM OF FRUCTOSE MALABSORPTION

Intestinal fructose absorption depends on an energy-requiring carrier mechanism that is facilitated by glucose. The process is not entirely understood, but, when there is an excess of fructose, glucose is preferentially absorbed, resulting in inefficient absorption of the fructose. The resultant unabsorbed fructose moves into the large bowel, where it causes an increase in osmotic pressure and a net influx or reduced outflow of water, resulting in loose stool or frank diarrhea.

Sucrose contains both glucose and fructose in a 1:1 ratio. However, some sucrose-containing fruits, such as apples and pears, contain a higher fructose to glucose ratio than most other fruits. Diarrhea after eating apples, pears, or their juices, when no other cause for the loose stool is evident, is a sign that fructose malabsorption may be the problem.

DIAGNOSIS

Diagnosis of fructose intolerance can be confirmed by giving the child a drink made of water containing a known amount of fructose powder dissolved in it. The amount of hydrogen in the child's breath is then measured every 15 minutes for up to 2 hours following the drink. The contents of the child's breath is determined by having the child breathe into a tube attached to a measuring device.

If the fructose is not carried across the digestive tract lining and transported into circulation (which is what happens in children without fructose malabsorption), it moves into the large bowel. In the large bowel, the fructose is fermented by the resident microorganisms. A major product of fermentation is hydrogen. The hydrogen produced by fermentation of the fructose passes from the bowel into circulation, is removed in the lungs, and finally is exhaled in the breath. This method of testing is often used to diagnose lactose intolerance, but malabsorption of any sugar can be tested in the same way.

The problem with this method of testing for fructose intolerance, is that, if an excessive quantity of fructose is consumed, everyone will experience some degree of malabsorption and will develop loose stool and an increase in breath hydrogen.

Usually, the quantity of fructose used in the test is 2 milligrams per kilogram (kilo) of body weight. (That means a child of 33 pounds [15 kilograms] would be tested with a dose of 30 milligrams of fructose in water.) This is an amount of fructose that is usually tolerated by most people who do not have clinical fructose malabsorption.

MANAGEMENT OF FRUCTOSE INTOLERANCE

Management of fructose intolerance involves reducing the child's intake of foods containing fructose. A fructose-restricted diet inevitably means limiting the consumption of fruit, especially those with a high fructose to glucose ratio. Table 17-1 provides information on the levels of natural fructose and glucose in common foods.

It is usually only necessary to avoid the fruits that contain considerably more fructose than glucose. Apple, pear, cherry, blackcurrant, grape, and honey are probably the worst culprits. Fruits with approximately the same levels of glucose and fructose may be tolerated when they are eaten in small to moderate quantities. However, keep in mind that the sugar content of a fruit will change with the degree of ripeness: the riper the fruit is, the more likely it is that the child will react to it.

Fruit juices are even more problematic than the whole fruit. The sugar tends to be concentrated in the juice, which will then have a higher level of fructose than the whole fruit. It is always wise to dilute all fruit juices in a 1:1 ratio (equal amounts of juice and water) for children under the age of 7 years.

Fructose malabsorption is an individual characteristic. Therefore, the level of fruit or juice that each child can tolerate will probably require some experimentation with different fruits and different quantities of each before the amount that the child can tolerate is known.

Since fruit is an important source of vitamin C, supplementary vitamin C should be taken on a low-fruit diet.

Fructose is sweeter than sucrose and much sweeter than glucose. Hence, fructose is sometimes added to reduced calorie foods to increase the sweet taste without the extra calories of sucrose that would be required to give the same amount of sweetness. Fructose is often used in foods recommended for diabetics, to provide sweetness while avoiding the insulin-dependent mechanisms required for metabolism of glucose. These additional sources of fructose need to be avoided by children and adults who have a problem with the absorption of fructose.

INHERITED CONDITIONS CAUSING FRUCTOSE INTOLERANCE

Although many people, especially children, develop loose stool and diarrhea after consuming a high dose of fructose, there are inherited conditions in which the metabolism of fructose is impaired. These conditions require more careful avoidance of all sources of fructose. These quite rare diseases are more accurately described as inborn errors of metabolism. Diagnosis and treatment typically take place in a specialized clinic staffed by specially trained doctors, dietitians, nurses, and other health care practitioners. The most well-known conditions include the following:

Fructose-1,6-Bisphosphatase Deficiency

Inheritance is through an autosomal recessive gene, and the worldwide incidence of the condition is unknown. The enzyme deficiency leads to the accumulation of certain amino acids, lactic acid, and ketoacids. Symptoms include fasting hypoglycemia (low blood glucose), ketosis (an abnormally high level of ketones[a] in body fluids and tissues), and acidosis(accumulation of acids in body fluids and tissues). Special tests to detect these compounds are used in the diagnosis of the condition. Fructose-1,6-bisphosphatase deficiency can be fatal to newborns. Infections and other fever-inducing illnesses can trigger episodes throughout life.

Hereditary Fructose Intolerance

The inheritance of hereditary fructose intolerance is through an autosomal recessive gene. The condition is due to a deficiency in the enzyme aldolase B. The disease was first recognized in Switzerland, where the incidence has been estimated to be 1 in every 20,000.

The condition is first noticed in infancy, usually after the first feeding of fruit juice or fruit. Symptoms include hypoglycemia, sweating, tremor, confusion, nausea, vomiting, abdominal cramping pain, and, in extreme cases, convulsions and coma. Prolonged consumption of fructose can lead to degeneration of renal function, resulting in cirrhosis and mental deterioration. Ingestion of more than a very small amount of fructose or sucrose results in symptoms.

---

[a]   Ketones or ketone bodies are organic chemicals with a specific structure that are formed during the process of metabolism in the body.

Diagnosis can be confirmed by a fall in blood glucose 5 to 40 minutes after giving 250 milligrams per kilogram of body weight of fructose by intravenous delivery. Liver biopsy shows the absence of the enzyme.

Treatment involves the strict avoidance of dietary fructose, sucrose, and sorbitol.

Essential Fructosuria

This condition is characterized by a deficiency in an enzyme called fructokinase. The condition results in excretion of fructose in the urine. It is inherited as an autosomal recessive gene, and the incidence has been estimated to be 1 in 130,000. Since the fructose is excreted in blood and urine, there is no effect of excess fructose in the digestive tract, and the condition is usually asymptomatic. Usually, no treatment is required, but a false diagnosis of diabetes mellitus might occur due to the high level of fructose in the blood.

Table 17-1
FRUCTOSE AND GLUCOSE CONTENT OF FRUITS AND OTHER FOODS[1]

Food Type	Fructose g/100 g edible portion	Glucose g/100 g edible portion
Fruits		
Apple	5.0	1.7
Banana	3.5	4.5
Blackberry	2.9	3.2
Blackcurrant	3.7	2.4
Cherry	7.2	4.7
Date	23.9	24.9
Fig	8.2	9.6

Table 17-1 (continued)
FRUCTOSE AND GLUCOSE CONTENT OF FRUITS AND OTHER FOODS[1]

Food Type	Fructose g/100 g edible portion	Glucose g/100 g edible portion
Fruits (cont'd)		
Gooseberry	4.1	4.4
Grape	7.3	8.2
Grapefruit	1.2	2.0
Greengage	4.0	5.5
Lemon	1.4	1.4
Loganberry	1.3	1.9
Melon	1.5	2.1
Mulberry	3.6	4.4
Orange	1.8	2.5
Peach	1.6	1.5
Pear	6.5	2.6
Pineapple	1.4	2.3
Plum	3.4	5.2
Prune	15.9	30.0
Raspberry	2.4	2.3
Redcurrant	1.9	2.3
Strawberry	2.3	2.6
Tomato	1.2	1.6
White currant	2.6	3.0

Table 17-1 (continued)
FRUCTOSE AND GLUCOSE CONTENT OF FRUITS AND OTHER FOODS[1]

Food Type	Fructose g/100 g edible portion	Glucose g/100 g edible portion
Other Foods		
Potato	0.1	0.1
Honey	40.5	34.2
Royal jelly	11.3	9.8
Molasses	8.0	8.8

Table 17-2

DAILY VITAMIN C REQUIREMENTS FOR BABIES AND CHILDREN DIETARY REFERENCE INTAKES (DRIs)[2]

Life Stage	Age	Vitamin C mg per day
Infants	0–6 months	40[b]
	7–12 months	50[a]
Children	1–3 years	15
	4–8 years	25
Boys	9–13 years	45
	14–18 years	75
Girls	9–13 years	45
	14–18 years	65

[a] Ketones or ketone bodies are organic chemicals with a specific structure that are formed during the process of metabolism in the body.
[b] Based on Vitamin C content of human milk.

References

1. Adapted from David TJ. *Food and Food Additive Intolerance in Childhood.* Blackwell Scientific Publications, 1993; 164.

2. Dietary Reference Intakes (DRIs): Recommended Intakes for Individuals. Vitamins, Food and Nutrition Board, National Institute of Medicine, the National Academy of Sciences, 2004.

CHAPTER 18

Anaphylaxis and Food Allergy

ANAPHYLAXIS AND FOOD IN CHILDREN

Anaphylaxis is an acute life-threatening condition that can occur at all ages, most frequently in individuals with a previous history of IgE-mediated allergy. Food is responsible for anaphylactic reactions in about one-third of the cases of anaphylaxis requiring hospital treatment in the United States, Europe, and Australia. But it is very rare in countries (such as China) in which people do not consume a Westernized diet.[1]

Anaphylaxis is an immediate, severe reaction, characterized by breathing difficulty (dyspnea); swelling, especially of the face (angioedema); and a drop in blood pressure (hypotension), resulting from the release of inflammatory mediators from mast cells and basophils.[2] Food, insect venom, and drugs are the most common antigens that can cause this extreme IgE-mediated reaction. Exercise, radiocontrast media (used in X-rays and other diagnostic tests), and some nonsteroidal antiinflammatory drugs (NSAIDs) also may induce these clinical symptoms via a mechanism that is not yet completely understood.

Anaphylactic reactions to foods are uncommon in early childhood. The peak age for food-induced anaphylaxis is 17 to 27 years, and it occurs far more frequently in individuals with asthma, which is often an important component of the life-threatening aspect of anaphylaxis. The incidence of food-induced anaphylactic reactions decreases after the age of 27.

Symptoms of Anaphylaxis

Anaphylaxis typically involves all of the organ systems in the body. In the most severe cases, it can progress rapidly to cardiovascular collapse and death. This is a very rare occurrence but the possibility of rapid death generates a great deal of anxiety and fear.

An anaphylactic reaction to a food may progress through a series of symptoms as the inflammatory mediators affect each target organ. The usual symptoms include the following:

- Burning, itching, and irritation of the mouth, oral tissues, and throat

- Feeling of throat tightening and choking

- Nausea, vomiting, abdominal pain, diarrhea as the digestive tract becomes involved

- Generalized itching, warm body feeling, and reddened areas

- Hives, swelling, and reddening of facial tissues

- Feeling of malaise, anxiety ("aura of doom"), and faintness

- Nasal irritation and sneezing

- Irritated eyes

- Chest tightness, bronchospasm (especially in asthmatics), hoarseness

- Rapid pulse that is weak, irregular, and difficult to detect

- Loss of consciousness

- Death from suffocation, cardiac arrhythmia, or shock

The symptoms may appear in any order and, often, at the same time. Furthermore, not all symptoms occur in each case. In general, the later the onset of symptoms occurs after the child has eaten the food, the less severe the reaction is likely to be. A rapid onset (within minutes or while the child is still eating) indicates a fast release of inflammatory mediators, which, in turn, leads to a rapid development of symptoms.

Severe reactions occur within minutes to up to 1 hour of ingestion of the allergen, but, in some cases, the onset of the reaction may be delayed for up to 2 hours.

For both adults and children, in the majority of cases of a fatal anaphylactic reaction to food, the patient is asthmatic. When the patient is receiving desensitization shots (for hay fever, for example), the potential for an anaphylactic reaction increases. This is particularly true when the person is also allergic to wasp and bee venom. It is a frequent observation that individuals who suffer an anaphylactic reaction to a food are rarely monosensitized, meaning that they rarely have only a food allergy. In the majority of cases, they also have other allergies. For example, they may also be allergic to airborne allergens (hay fever or asthma), injectable allergens (insect stings), or both.

In children, the symptoms most frequently indicating anaphylaxis start in the digestive tract, with vomiting (sometimes large quantities of stringy mucus), abdominal (colicky) pain, and diarrhea. Cardiovascular symptoms in children tend to be uncommon.[2] In contrast, in adults, skin and respiratory symptoms are more frequent than gastrointestinal and cardiovascular symptoms and generally have an onset earlier in the reaction.

Causes of Anaphylactic Reactions to Foods in Children

About two-thirds of anaphylactic reactions requiring hospital treatment are reactions to agents other than foods. Allergic reactions to drugs, especially antibiotics (such as penicillin and sulfa drugs); insect venom (wasp, hornet, bee stings, etc.); food additives (for example, sulfites); injected radiocontrast dyes used in diagnostic tests; local anesthetics; immunotherapy injections (for example, shots for desensitization to airborne allergens); latex; and vaccines account for most of the cases of nonfood anaphylaxis. In a significant number of cases, however, the specific trigger is not apparent. These cases are typically referred to as idiopathic anaphylaxis (in other words, the cause is unknown).

In cases of food-induced anaphylaxis, the specific food responsible for the reaction seems to vary among individuals. Reports from different countries indicate differences dependent on local dietary practices. Any food has the potential to cause an anaphylactic reaction in a sensitized individual, as in general food allergy. However, some foods cause anaphylactic reactions more frequently than others. In North America, the foods most frequently reported as triggers of anaphylaxis include the following:[1]

- Peanuts

- Tree nuts

- Shellfish

- Fish

- Eggs

- Milk

- Seeds (most often, sesame, mustard, psyllium, and cotton seeds)

- Fruit (most often, kiwi fruit)

In children under 3 years of age, cow's milk, eggs, wheat, and chicken tend to be more frequent culprits. A report from Italy[2] indicates that seafood and milk were the most common foods that triggered anaphylaxis in the 95 children in their study. The Italian study covered children from ages 1 month to 16 years. Nuts, eggs, fresh fruit, cereals, vegetables, and goat's milk accounted for the rest of the cases in the Italian report; peanuts were responsible for only one episode of anaphylaxis.

It should be emphasized that any food has the potential to trigger anaphylaxis when the child is allergic to it. A list of the foods responsible for reactions in the Italian study included, surprisingly, some foods that are rarely considered to be highly allergenic:[2]

- Fish and shellfish in 16 cases: (shellfish in 4; mussels in 2; various kinds of fish in 10)

- Cow's milk in 12 cases

- Nuts in 7 cases (Brazil nuts in 3 episodes, hazelnuts in 1, peanuts in 1, pine nuts in 1, and chestnuts in 1)

- Egg in 6 cases

- Fruit in 6 cases (1 watermelon, 3 kiwi, 1 date, 1 pomegranate)

- Cereals in 3 cases (barley, oats, and wheat in 1 episode each)

- Vegetables in 2 cases (French beans and celery)

- Goat's milk in 2 cases

In other countries, the foods that cause the majority of reactions in children differ. The greatest difference is the case of peanuts, which, in the United States and England, are the most common cause of life-threatening reactions both in children and adults.[3] In a 2001 report of 32 fatal cases of anaphylactic reactions to foods in adolescents or young adults in the United States,[4] peanuts and tree nuts accounted for more than 90 percent of the fatalities; the rest of the cases were triggered by milk (1 case) and fish (1 case).

In the majority of cases of children who suffer anaphylactic reactions to foods, there are coexistent allergic conditions. Asthma, atopic eczema, and allergic rhinitis (hay fever) were common in these patients.[2] Of these conditions, atopic eczema seems to be the most prevalent.[3]

Exercise-Induced Anaphylaxis

In some cases of anaphylactic reactions to foods, symptoms occur only when exercise takes place within 2 to 4 hours of ingesting the food. When the food is eaten without subsequent exercise, it causes no reaction. Furthermore, if the food is not eaten, exercise can be undertaken without any apparent reaction. This condition is often referred to as food-associated exercise-induced anaphylaxis (FAEIA). FAEIA occurs most often in older children (over 12 years) with a history of hives and tissue swelling, usually of the face (urticaria and angioedema). However, the condition is becoming increasingly recognized in younger children. One study reported incidents of FAEIA in children of 8 years and older.[5] The majority of cases overall occur in people under the age of 30 years.

The foods implicated in cases of FAEIA tend to differ from those responsible for the majority of anaphylactic reactions. Foods such as wheat and other cereal grains have been frequently reported, and celery and shellfish appear quite often as culprits in the condition. Foods that are usually considered fairly innocuous, such as pears and chickpeas, have been reported as causative factors in some cases.[2]

Symptoms often start while the person is exercising, with itching, especially of the scalp, that becomes more generalized. Hives and flushing are common, followed by respiratory obstruction and sometimes cardiovascular collapse.

Patients with specific food anaphylaxis associated with exercise usually have positive skin tests to the food that provokes symptoms. Occasionally, they also have a history of reacting to the food in childhood. Frequently, other allergies coexist, such as asthma and hay fever as well as eczema and digestive tract symptoms.

Symptoms of anaphylaxis while exercising usually occur after ingestion of more than one of the allergenic foods before exercise is performed outdoors in the presence of a high concentration of inhalant allergens. Furthermore, other factors are often involved, such as medications (especially NSAIDs), high humidity, and so on. Consequently, it is often very difficult to predict when the reaction is going to occur.

The best directive for the child or young adult who has experienced FAEIA is to avoid the consumption of any food that has ever caused even a mild adverse reaction for 4 hours before any physical exercise.[5]

Management of Food-Induced Anaphylaxis

Almost all of the reports indicate that children who experienced an anaphylactic reaction to food were experiencing anaphylaxis for the first time; hence, prevention was almost impossible. However, in almost all cases, these children had experienced the symptoms of food allergy, often severe, before the anaphylactic episode.

Anaphylactic reactions in the majority of infants, although definitely dangerous, are usually not life-threatening.[2] Food-related anaphylaxis is more frequent in younger children with a previous history of eczema. The symptoms usually affect the gastrointestinal system and only rarely the cardiovascular one. Exercise-induced anaphylaxis occurs more often in older children with a previous history of urticaria and angioedema. Most fatal anaphylactic reactions occur in adolescents and young adults and are virtually unpredictable.

Accurate Identification of the Food Responsible

In all cases of food-related anaphylaxis, the important first step in the prevention of a subsequent reaction is accurate identification of the food responsible. The culprit food must then be very carefully avoided.

Food challenges are usually unnecessary in children who have had a clear-cut anaphylactic reaction after eating a specific food to which they were already known to have IgE antibodies. Usually, the food has caused a reaction previously. Because the symptoms appear immediately, it is fairly easy to identify the food responsible. However, in a number of cases, the child may be allergic to several foods, and, at the time of developing the anaphylaxis, may have eaten all of these foods in a meal. In these cases, it is essential that the responsible food be identified; food challenges in a suitably equipped medical facility are necessary.

Growing Out of Food Allergy

Many young children who experience food anaphylaxis eventually outgrow their clinical reactivity. Therefore, an oral challenge is appropriate after an extended period of food elimination with no history of adverse reactions. In fact, new research is indicating that, after children no longer experience symptoms on eating a food that previously caused symptoms, they should continue to eat the food regularly in order to maintain tolerance to it (see Chapter 1 for details about oral tolerance to foods). There seems to be an increased likelihood of a recurrence of the allergy, if the food allergy was outgrown but the child continued to avoid the food.[6]

Treatment of an Anaphylactic Reaction

Treatment of an anaphylactic reaction involves immediate injection of adrenaline (epinephrine). Most cases of anaphylaxis occur in the home, in restaurants, outdoors, at school, and other places away from medical facilities. It is wise for children at risk for anaphylaxis to have immediate access to injectable epinephrine. If away from home or school, parents or caregivers should carry the epinephrine. If children are old enough, they should carry it themselves in, for example, a back pack or book bag. Self-administered epinephrine is available as a number of products. EpiPen®; Twinject®; Dey®, Napa, CA are widely used epinephrine products. The most appropriate product for the individual will be prescribed by the child's physician. The EpiPen®, for example, contains 0.3 milligrams of premeasured epinephrine and is recommended for individuals who weigh more than 66 pounds; the EpiPen Jr® is appropriate for children weighing 33–66 pounds. For children weighing less than 33 pounds, instructions for measuring and administering smaller doses will be provided by their doctor or pharmacist.

Authorities suggest that injectable epinephrine kits be prescribed for any food-allergic person who also has asthma or who has experienced a previous reaction involving the airway or cardiovascular systems. In addition, many allergists recommend providing an EpiPen® to patients who are allergic to peanuts, tree nuts, fish, or shellfish; patients who have food allergies and have wheezed during a respiratory illness even if they are not considered to have asthma; and food-allergic children from a family in which another family member has experienced a severe or anaphylactic reaction.[1]

However, authorities are not always in agreement about the universal and wide-scale prescribing of self-injectable epinephrine. Very rarely, deaths have occurred as a result of its inappropriate use. A report from the United Kingdom indicated that adrenaline overdose caused at least three deaths in a 10-year period.[7] The author states that kits for self-treatment depend for their success on selection of appropriate medication, correct dosage, ease of use, and good training. It is very important that the child's family members and other care providers be instructed in the administration of epinephrine, other prescribed medications, and emergency procedures.

After epinephrine has been administered, it is absolutely essential that the child be transported immediately to the nearest hospital or medical facility. So many fatal reactions have occurred when a person appears to be recovering from the anaphylaxis after administration of the epinephrine only to succumb to the second phase of the allergic reaction. Second phase reactions can occur as long as 2 hours or more after the first. This second phase is caused by recruitment of additional granulocytes to the reaction site in response to mediators called chemotactic factors that have drawn them into the area. Release of the additional inflammatory mediators that these cells carry may cause the second phase to proceed faster and more severely than the first. It is often this second phase of the reaction that is responsible for fatal cases of asthma. (For details about the allergic reaction, see Chapter 1.) Too often, caregivers assume that the emergency is over and fail to take the child to the hospital. It is also essential that, if epinephrine has been administered, the child is observed by emergency medical personnel because of the risk (albeit slight) of a fatal reaction to the epinephrine itself.

Because the home is the most frequent place in which an anaphylactic event can occur, all family members, especially parents, should be adequately informed about treatment of an anaphylactic reaction. Education is imperative to ensure that the patient and his or her family understand how to avoid all forms of the food allergen and the potential severity of a reaction if the food is inadvertently ingested. Accidental food ingestion is likely despite avoidance measures, so immediate treatment should be available for such emergencies. Treatment protocols should be prescribed by the patient's physician. Caregivers, school staff, or both should have instructions written by the physician and signed by the parents. A sample plan can be downloaded from the Food Allergy and Anaphylaxis Network's Web site: www.foodallergy.org.

Children who are at risk for anaphylaxis should carry with them at all times medical information concerning their condition (such as a Medic Alert tag or bracelet), emergency medications (EpiPen® and liquid antihistamine such as Benadryl® [diphenhydramine]), and their treatment plan.

Precautions for the Anaphylactic Child in School

When children are old enough to be on their own in school, the risks for accidental exposure to their allergenic foods are increased enormously, as are the fears and concerns of the child's parents and caregivers. The only real protection parents can give the children is education and awareness. The education and awareness program should include the children, the teachers, school staff, and other school personnel who have temporary care of the children. If the children are old enough to be in school, they are old enough to understand the risks involved in their food allergy and the measures they must take to ensure their own safety.

However, the watchwords for any allergic child should be the following: "Be careful, not fearful!" As discussed in Chapter 4, fear is a negative, detrimental emotion that can lead to hiding from life and its challenges. On the other hand, care implies a positive attitude that says, "I'm in control" or "I can handle it." This is what we all want to encourage in our children and what, in the end, will keep the children safe.

Education of the people who have temporary care of the food-allergic child is equally important to the child's well-being. More and more schools are becoming aware of the risks faced by the food-allergic child. Many schools have protocols in place to deal with their allergic students in an environment that is safe from food allergens. Talk to your child's teacher and principal, especially if the child is just starting school or is moving to a new school. Make sure that the following guidelines can be implemented.

Important measures for an environment that is safe from food allergens should include the following:

- Education of allergic children about avoiding being exposed to their allergenic foods, including:

    – Being able to recognize the food

    – Knowing how to avoid foods that are likely to contain or be contaminated by the food

    – Wearing a MedicAlert or identification tag or bracelet in case of loss of consciousness in an allergic reaction

    – Ensuring that, if the child is old enough, he or she understands the importance of the following:

        Being aware of all terms on food labels that would indicate the possible presence of the food

        Carrying an Epipen® or similar device containing injectable epinephrine (adrenalin), and being familiar with its use in case of accidental exposure and an allergic reaction

- Ensuring that all personnel in a school facility, including faculty, administrators, clerical workers, and cafeteria and janitorial staff are well-informed about the dangers to your child in the event of accidental contamination by the allergenic food.

- Having clear strategies for maintaining the classroom in a safe condition, with rules about cleaning the area.

- Informing everyone entering the child's classroom to avoid introducing the food into the area, and—most importantly—giving them the reasons for the restrictions. You need to recruit the help of the other children rather than cause annoyance or rebellion against perceived restrictions to their freedom. If other children rebel against the food restrictions, it could be counterproductive in ensuring your child's safety.

- Informing all staff about emergency procedures in case your child develops symptoms and requires medical treatment. Such information should include:

  - Having an Epipen® or similar device, specifically prescribed for your child, in an accessible place where teachers and staff can find it quickly

  - Ensuring that at least one member of staff is familiar with the use of the Epipen® where appropriate

  - Contact information for key caregivers, such as parents and guardians of children, and the child's doctor or other health provider. These instructions should be provided to the facility by the parents or guardians in the child's treatment plan.

  - Providing instructions for transporting the child to the nearest hospital in the quickest way possible. In most cases, this involves dialing 911 (in North America) or 999 (in the United Kingdom), describing the reaction, and asking for a paramedic to be dispatched immediately.

"Be careful, not fearful!"

Use these watchwords for every allergic child, and make them the motto by which they learn to live.

Fear is a negative, harmful emotion that can lead to hiding from life and its challenges. On the other hand, care implies a positive attitude that says, "I'm in control" and "I can handle it." This is what we all want to encourage in our children and what, in the end, will keep them safe.

References

1. Sampson HA. Anaphylaxis and emergency treatment. *Pediatrics* 2003;111:1601–1608.

2. Novembre E, Cianferoni A, Bernardini R, Mugnaini L, Cafferelli C, Cavagni G, Giovane A, Vierucci A. Anaphylaxis in children: Clinical and allergologic features. *Pediatrics* 1998;101:8–15.

3. Ewan PW. Clinical study of peanuts and nuts allergy in 62 consecutive patients. *British Medical Journal* 1996; 312:1074–1078.

4. Bock SA, Munoz-Furlong A, Sampson HA. Fatalities due to anaphylactic reactions to foods. *Journal of Allergy and Clinical Immunology* 2001;107(1):191–193.

5. Romano A, Di Fonso M, Giuffreda F. Diagnostic work-up for food-dependent, exercise-induced anaphylaxis. *Allergy* 1995; 50:817–824.

6. Fleischer DM, Conover-Walker MK, Christie L, Burks AW, Wood RA. Peanut allergy: Recurrence and its management. *Journal of Allergy and Clinical Immunology* 2004;114(5):1195–1201.

7. Pumphrey RS. Lessons for management of anaphylaxis from a study of fatal reactions. *Clinical and Experimental Allergy* 2000;30:1144–1150.

CHAPTER 19

Hyperactivity and Diet

Occasionally, parents and teachers have to cope every day with an unruly, disruptive, sometimes aggressive child in the home and classroom. When every attempt at control has met with failure, the idea that the child's diet is the cause of the problem is often embraced with great enthusiasm, especially if the alternative is behavior-modifying drugs. This chapter examines a number of ways in which food may trigger behavior problems in children. It also discusses what parents and caregivers might be able to do to help their child in this situation.

THE ROLE OF DIET IN BEHAVIORAL DISORDERS

One of the factors that may be important as a cause for behavioral dysfunction is the child's diet. The idea that dietary components might be a cause of aberrant behavior is not new; it has been considered at various times since it was first suggested in the 1920s. Allergic reactions to wheat and corn were suggested in the 1940s as a cause of fatigue, irritability, and behavior problems.[1]

Since then, numerous theories, some backed by well-conducted research studies, have been put forward to explain why food may be involved in triggering disruptive behavior in children. The most convincing of these suggest the following:

- Components of the food, either naturally occurring chemicals or artificial additives, act in a pharmacological manner on body systems and result in behavioral changes.

- Inflammatory mediators released in an allergic response to the food may be the pharmacological agents responsible for behavioral changes.

- Nutritional deficiencies may result in central nervous system dysfunction.

- Stress or anxiety associated with food may release neuropeptides that can themselves trigger the release of inflammatory mediators and cause clinical symptoms.

A great deal of concern arose in the 1970s from the widespread use of stimulant drugs, such as Ritalin®, to control children's hyperactive behavior. Some clinicians moved to the opposite extreme and advanced claims that childhood hyperactivity was a perception created by intolerant teachers and parents. They proposed that this behavior was caused by environmental factors rather than neurological deficit. In response, components of a child's diet became the focus of attention. The diet was viewed as an alternative to drugs. These attitudes resulted in repudiation of the psychological stigma attached to the caregivers of hyperactive children.

The Feingold Hypothesis

In 1975, Dr. Benjamin Feingold published an article and then a book[2] promoting the theory that a toxic reaction to food additives was responsible for hyperactivity in children. He claimed that up to 70 percent of his hyperactive patients improved when food dyes, artificial flavors, and natural salicylates were eliminated from their diet. After the publication of Dr. Feingold's book in 1975, the Feingold diet became very popular as a nondrug treatment for childhood hyperactivity. As sources of information and support for parents, Feingold Associations were formed in most states within the United States.

In response to Feingold's claims, a number of research studies were conducted in an attempt to confirm or refute his theories. All of these studies can be criticized on the basis of differences in methodology, no clear consensus on diagnostic criteria, inadequate controls, and the diversity of the independent variables employed.   However, the consensus reached was that Feingold's claims were exaggerated and that his findings were anecdotal and lacking in objective evidence. Finally, the idea that diet and food additives were the cause of hyperkinesis (hyperactivity) was strongly refuted in a statement from the National Advisory Committee on Hyperkinesis and Food Additives[3] (1980). Nevertheless, all of the studies had actually demonstrated that a few hyperactive children did benefit from an additive-free diet.

Attention-Deficit Hyperactivity Disorder (ADHD) and Allergy

ADHD is the most recent diagnosis for children with problems in attention, impulse control, and overactivity. However, the diagnosis and cause of the symptoms that constitute this disorder have been in dispute since the condition was first recognized.

The disorder is currently considered to be divisible into several subcategories, such as the Inattentive Type, the Hyperactive Impulsive Type, and the Combined Type.[4] But the debate still continues regarding the degree to which the symptoms are due to a neurological deficit and how much of the problem behavior can be attributed to aberrant environmental factors. Furthermore, there is no clear consensus that these are scientifically divisible conditions based on physiological differences.

In the 1990s, the role of food allergy and intolerance to food additives in learning and behavior disorders in children was the subject of a number of well-conducted studies. A comprehensive review of the research in this field appeared in 1992.[5] This review discusses current thought on the link between diet and behavior disorders. An important point made by these reviewers is the following: "It must be recognized that adverse effects of foods on behavior may be either a manifestation of (probably pharmacologically based) food intolerance, or they may be psychologically based (e.g., via suggestion or adverse conditioning)."[6]

The medical and scientific literature abounds with the results of studies on the role of food components in behavioral dysfunction in children. Few of these reports have been widely accepted. The first criticism that is frequently leveled at these experiments is that the criteria used for selecting the research subjects leave room for doubt about the diagnosis of the behavioral condition being studied.[7]

Experimental Design Problems

All of the studies that are designed to demonstrate a role for food components in children's behavior are plagued by two major handicaps:

- The lack of clear diagnostic criteria for the behavioral conditions being studied

- The absence of definite tests that unequivocally demonstrate allergy to food or intolerance of food additives

Allergy tests such as skin prick and RAST (radioallergosorbent test; see Chapter 4 for details) are notoriously unhelpful in the diagnosis of food allergy and intolerance. The only way to demonstrate an adverse reaction to food components is by elimination and challenge. The suspect food or additive is removed from the child's diet for a specified period and then re-introduced to determine the child's reactivity to it. Double-blind, placebo-controlled, crossover food challenge is the standard method used to identify reactive foods and to rule out as many confounding variables as possible.

Sugar and Hyperactivity

Following the decline in the belief that the Feingold diet was an effective management strategy for childhood hyperkinesis, the idea that refined sugar was an important etiological factor in the disorder became very popular.

Reactive hypoglycemia or functional hypoglycemia (FH) due to sugar in the diet has been blamed for many emotional problems, hyperactive behavior, and irritability. However, there have not been reported studies that conclusively demonstrate low blood sugar levels and impaired insulin response in conditions other than diabetes. The scientific view regarding FH is that the condition is quite rare but "has become popular because it is a respectable metabolic illness rather than a symptom of psychological distress."[6]

The adverse effect of sugar in sensitive individuals may be mediated by mechanisms other than defective insulin control. A 1986 study on the response to sugar and aspartame in 39 children diagnosed with ADHD indicated that catecholamine control of sugar regulation may be impaired in children with ADHD.[8] The ADHD children performed significantly worse on behavioral evaluation following a sucrose challenge compared to an aspartame challenge after a breakfast of carbohydrates. However, behavior improved in these children after a sucrose challenge following a protein breakfast. Normal children in the study were unaffected by the challenges after consuming a carbohydrate, a protein, or a fasting breakfast. This means that children with ADHD require protein to offset the potential adverse effects of sugar.

An excess of sugar in the diet has often been blamed for a range of behavioral problems, such as irritability, anxiety, violent behavior, and fatigue. But, in most cases sugar actually has the effect of making a person feel lethargic, because it promotes the production of serotonin, the sleep chemical, in the brain. Many people are exhibiting the effects of a high sugar or starch breakfast, (such as toast or croissants and jam or breakfast cereals containing high levels of sugars and processed starches) when they reach for a cup of high-caffeine coffee at mid-morning to keep them alert. Or they may feel hungry at that time and compound the problem with a snack of a muffin or doughnut for an energy boost. This is inevitably followed by another rapid drop in alertness and energy as a result of the high sugar and free starch content of the snack. A high sugar or starch lunch is often followed by sleepiness in mid-afternoon. Then these same people wonder why they can't sleep well after a supper high in meat or fish proteins, which is going to promote alertness rather than sleep. Children are no different.

Probably, the reason for the idea that sugar causes hyperactivity in children is that the foods that contain large amounts of sugar—such as soft drinks, candies, and other sweet manufactured foods—also contain artificial food colors and preservatives. It is now thought that it is the latter, and not the sugar, that are responsible for the hyperactive behavior. In addition, a diet high in commercial snack foods and drinks with a great deal of sugar and processed starches tends to lead to a lack of whole foods in the diet, often resulting in nutritional deficiency, especially of essential vitamins and minerals.

Phosphates, as well as a variety of other ingredients, have been considered as dietary components that could play a major role in hyperkinesis, based on anecdotal evidence. Again, this idea was refuted by controlled studies.[1] Importantly, however, children on either a restricted sugar diet or a restricted phosphate diet would avoid many potentially allergenic foods and a variety of artificial colors and preservatives, which might be the real reason for the apparent improvement in their behavior.

NUTRITIONAL DEFICIENCIES AS A CAUSE OF UNACCEPTABLE BEHAVIOR

In 1986, the results were published for a 4-year dietary intervention program in 803 schools in New York City affecting 800,000 children. All school meals were virtually free from sucrose, all artificial food flavors, artificial food colors, and two preservatives (butylated hydroxyanisole [BHA] and butylated hydroxytoluene [BHT]). Academic achievement rather than behavior was chosen as a more objective measure of the performance outcome of this intervention. The average percentile rankings of the students in the study on the California Achievement Test (CAT) over the 4-year test period rose 15.7 percent, from 39.2 to 54.9 percent, with no changes in the school curricula or teaching staff.[9] The hypothesis was made that the improvements in academic achievement were due to diet, which treated marginal malnutrition.[10] Elimination of foods high in sucrose, artificial flavors, artificial colors, and preservatives removes much of the junk foods from a child's diet, giving place to more nutritionally dense foods and a more nutritionally adequate, balanced diet.

FOOD ADDITIVES AS A CAUSE OF HYPERACTIVE BEHAVIOR

A study published in 2004 indicated that all children, regardless of whether or not they would be considered abnormally hyperactive, demonstrate some degree of hyperactive behavior when they consume artificial food dyes and benzoate preservatives. On the Isle of Wight in England, 277 3-year-old children were studied for the effects of artificial food colorings and benzoate preservatives on their behavior.[11] The results showed that these food additives triggered some level of hyperactivity in all children, based on the parents' assessment of their child's behavior. Even children who had no history of behavior problems became more active after consuming the additives. The effect on behavior was more striking on those children already diagnosed as hyperactive; their level of activity increased noticeably. Interestingly, the change in behavior was very obvious to the parents, even though they had no idea whether their child had been given the test drink or a placebo. Nevertheless, psychological tests administered by trained psychologists did not show any changes after either the test drink or the placebo.

SO WHAT IS THE MESSAGE HERE?

At the present stage in our knowledge, we can say that the artificial colors and preservatives, specifically benzoates, in manufactured foods seem to have the potential to trigger hyperactive behavior in the greatest number of children, regardless of whether the child has a food allergy or not. Therefore, they should not be part of any child's regular diet.

AVOIDANCE OF ARTIFICIAL COLORS AND BENZOATES

Artificial colors and preservatives are added to most prepared foods. The four colors and benzoates identified as possible triggers for hyperactive behavior in the IOW study are found in the foods listed in Table 19-1 at the end of this chapter.

MANAGEMENT OF BEHAVIOR DYSFUNCTION THAT RESULTS FROM FOOD INGESTION

The many different types of hyperactivity and related behavior problems in children may or may not be attributable to a variety of biochemical or physiological triggers. Therefore, it is difficult to advocate that diet, either as a cause (for example, a food additive or a natural chemical in the food acting like a drug) or as a deficiency (vitamin or mineral deficiencies) could be the major etiological factor in all of these phenomena. However, it is clear that some food components do trigger hyperactive behavior in some children. Of course, the question asked by every parent and guardian of a child with abnormal behavior levels and patterns is "Which child is affected and what are the food components?"

In response to this question, we can say with some degree of confidence that:

- A child suffering an allergic reaction will respond as any child would to an acute or chronic illness. He or she will feel miserable and appear irritable, be restless, have difficulty sleeping, and may be unable to concentrate. The obverse of this will be that the child will experience fatigue and listlessness. The condition may result in prolonged absences from school, which will have a negative effect on scholastic achievement.

- An allergic condition, such as exercise-induced asthma, may prevent a child from taking part in normal childhood activities, resulting in a feeling of being excluded from his or her peers. Severe eczema can provoke revulsion in other children. Overanxious and overprotective parents may exacerbate the isolation felt by the allergic child, and the need for special diets can impede the normal socializing associated with food. All of these factors may promote an antisocial climate for the allergic child.

- Food allergy may be a direct physiological cause of behavior changes. The hypersensitivity reaction releases inflammatory chemicals, which may have a direct effect on central nervous system functions. The decrease in oxygen reaching the brain (hypoxia) associated with even mild asthma has also been suggested as having significant effects on cerebral function. This might affect behavior.

- Additives in foods, such as azo dyes (for example, tartrazine), preservatives (especially benzoates), and artificial flavors (such as glutamates) have a direct physiological effect on central nervous system functions.

However, when you consider food allergy as a possible cause of your child's allergy, it is important to realize that hyperactivity is never the only symptom of allergy. If your child has allergies, he or she will have other signs of allergy, such as skin reactions (eczema or hives), stomach problems (diarrhea, stomach ache), or a runny, stuffy nose and itchy, watery eyes. Accurate identification of a child's food allergies and removal of the culprit foods from the child's diet are of first importance. But, removal of culprit foods is not a complete response. Equally important is that the allergic child should be provided with alternative foods that supply all of his or her nutritional needs.

Reasons for Improvement on a Modified Diet

Several reasons have been proposed for the observation that a surprisingly large number of behaviorally disturbed children improve significantly on a hypoallergenic diet:

- When food allergens are excluded from the diet, an allergic child's symptoms will disappear. They are then able to sleep, have more energy, and generally feel better; their behavior will naturally improve.

- When food additives are excluded from a child's diet, the junk food and simple sugars are often removed. The resulting diet is often nutritionally much more adequate and balanced. The child's behavior is a response to a more nutritious diet.

- If artificial colors and preservatives have a drug-like effect on a child's behavior, removing them from his or her diet will obviously result in a noticeable improvement in behavior.

- When a specifically formulated diet is prescribed, parents will take extra care in food preparation. The child feels special and commands more attention within the family. This change in status and family dynamics has a positive psychological effect on the child, and behavior improves.

Undoubtedly, most of these factors will have some effect on a child, especially an atopic child. Whatever the scientific basis may be, the opportunity to improve the quality of life for the child and family by dietary management is justified. This is the case as long as the diet does not pose any psychological, nutritional, or economic distress on an already stressed family situation. The best candidates for dietary intervention are children with poor eating habits and physical as well as behavioral symptoms.

STEPS IN THE DIETARY MANAGEMENT OF HYPERACTIVITY IN CHILDREN

- With the help of your child's doctor and a registered dietitian, find out exactly which foods are contributing to your child's allergy symptoms, separate and distinct from his or her behavior. These symptoms typically include skin reactions, such as hives or eczema; respiratory symptoms, such as hay fever or asthma; digestive tract problems, such as stomach ache, diarrhea, nausea, and vomiting; and, occasionally, migraine headaches, with nausea and vomiting. The food identification process ideally will include elimination of the suspect foods, with subsequent challenge. This will clearly identify which foods are involved in your child's symptoms. The child loses the symptoms when the food is eliminated, but they recur when he or she eats the food in the challenge part of the trial. (See Chapter 4 for more specific details about the elimination and challenge process.) Carefully remove all of these problem foods from your child's diet and provide complete balanced nutrition from alternative foods.

- Eliminate all artificial food coloring and preservatives, especially benzoates, from your child's diet. Be particularly careful in reading labels on manufactured foods and become familiar with the terms that indicate the presence of these additives (see Table 18-1 in Chapter 18).

- Make sure that every meal and snack that your child eats contains protein as well as carbohydrates. This is especially important at breakfast and lunch. Eggs, bacon, ham, sausage, milk, and nut and seed butters can be included in breakfast, as long as the child is not allergic to them. Tuna and chicken in sandwiches and salads, and meat in soups and stews are good for lunch. It is usually easy to include protein in dinner or supper, which may be the traditional Western meat and two vegetables, pizza with meat and cheese toppings, pasta with a meat sauce, or even hamburger. However, avoid processed and delicatessen meats that contain additives.

- Limit treats and junk foods that are high in sugars, starches, and artificial additives. (Ideally, you would remove them from the diet entirely, but, in the real world of older children in school, this is next to impossible.) Try to encourage your child to select real foods and beverages instead. You may have to negotiate by allowing a few food items that have ingredients other than the colors and benzoates listed in Table 18-1.

- As much as possible, provide an environment in your home in which all family members eat together, without the intrusion of television and other distractions. Keep the atmosphere calm, and provide meals that are, as much as possible, made with pure foods without a lot of manufactured and processed ingredients.

- Make sure that every meal contains a balanced amount of each of these important three components:

  - Protein

  - Grain or Starch

  - Fruit or Vegetable

For examples of these food categories, see Appendix E.

Table 19-1
FOODS USUALLY CONTAINING ARTIFICIAL FOOD COLOR
(E NUMBERS ARE THE EEC DESIGNATIONS OF ADDITIVES
USED ON PRODUCT LABELS IN EUROPE)

Please note that these lists are by no means exhaustive. Many manufactured foods and beverages contain the additives, and manufacturers are constantly changing ingredients in their products. This table is meant as a general guide only. Parents must read food labels carefully, and when in doubt, contact the manufacturer for up-to-date information.

Tartrazine (E102)

Fruit squash, syrups, and cordials

Colored fizzy drinks (soda pop)

Instant puddings

Packet convenience foods: e.g., Macaroni and cheese

Cake mixes

Soups (packets and cans)

Bottled sauces

Pickles

Commercial salad dressings

Ice creams and sherbets

Candies

Chewing gum

Jams and jellies

Smoked fish

Jello

Mustard

Flavored yogurt

Sunset Yellow (E110)

Used especially in fermented foods that need to be heat-treated

Hot chocolate mix

Packet soups

Candies

Yogurts

Commercial breadcrumbs

Cheese sauce mixes

Jams and marmalades

Canned shrimps and prawns

Pickled cucumbers (dill pickles)

Table 19-1 (continued)
FOODS USUALLY CONTAINING ARTIFICIAL FOOD COLOR
(E NUMBERS ARE THE EEC DESIGNATIONS OF ADDITIVES
USED ON PRODUCT LABELS IN EUROPE)

Ponceau (E124)	Carmoisine (E122)
Cake mixes	Especially useful for foods that are heat-treated after fermentation
Packet soups	Packet soup mix
Seafood dressings	Blancmange
Dessert toppings	Packet breadcrumbs
Canned strawberries	Packet jellies
Canned cherry, raspberry, and red currant pie fillings	Candies
Quick-setting gelatin mixes (Jello)	Packet cheesecake mix
Salami	Brown sauce
	Convenience food mixes (Uncle Ben's Rice mixes, Hamburger Helper, etc.)
	Prepackaged cakes
	Almond paste
	Flavored yogurts
	Ice creams
	Jams and preserves

Table 19-1 (continued)
FOODS USUALLY CONTAINING ARTIFICIAL FOOD COLOR
(E NUMBERS ARE THE EEC DESIGNATIONS OF ADDITIVES
USED ON PRODUCT LABELS IN EUROPE)

Foods Usually Containing Benzoates

Benzoic acid (E210)	Sodium benzoate (E211)
Jams	Caviar
Beer	Prawns
Dessert sauces	Candies
Flavored syrups	Margarine
Fruit pulp and purée	Fruit pies
Fruit juice	Soft drinks
Marinated fish (herring and mackerel)	Oyster sauce
Pickles	Salad dressings
Salad dressings	Barbecue sauce
Yogurts	Taco sauce
Flavored coffees	Cheesecake mix
Margarine	Soy sauce
Table olives	Jams and jellies
Concentrated juices	Dill pickles
Soft drinks	Table olives
	Concentrated pineapple juice

Table 19-1 (continued)
FOODS USUALLY CONTAINING ARTIFICIAL FOOD COLOR
(E NUMBERS ARE THE EEC DESIGNATIONS OF ADDITIVES
USED ON PRODUCT LABELS IN EUROPE)

Foods Usually Containing Benzoates (cont'd)

Potassium benzoate (212)	Calcium benzoate (E213)
Margarines	Concentrated pineapple juice
Table olives	
Dill pickles	
Concentrated pineapple juice	

Ethyl 4-hydroxybenzoate (E214)
Propyl 4-hydroxybenzoate (E216)
Methyl 4-hydroxybenzoate (E218)

Beer	Pickles
Cooked, packed beetroot	Salad dressings
Coffee and chicory essence	
Coloring dyes in solution	
Dessert sauces	
Flavored syrups	
Frozen drink concentrates	
Fruit-based pie fillings	
Fruit pulp or purée	
Glucose	
Marinated fish (herring and mackerel)	

References

1. Randolph TG. Allergy as a causative factor of fatigue, irritability, and behavior problems of children. *Journal of Pediatrics* 1947;31:560–572.

2. Feingold BF. *Why Your Child Is Hyperactive*. New York: Random House, 1975.

3. National Institutes of Health consensus development conference statement: Defined diets and childhood hyperactivity. *American Journal of Clinical Nutrition* 1983;37:161–165.

4. Barkley R. *Taking charge of AD/HD: The complete authoritative guide for parents* (rev. ed.). New York: Guilford, 2000.

5. Robinson J, Ferguson A. Food sensitivity and the nervous system: Hyperactivity, addiction and criminal behaviour. *Nutrition Research Reviews* 1992;5:203–223.

6. Robinson J, Ferguson A. Food sensitivity and the nervous system: Hyperactivity, addiction and criminal behaviour. 220.

7. Egger J. Psychoneurological aspects of food allergy. *European Journal of Clinical Nutrition* 1991; 45(Suppl.1):35–45.

8. Connors CK, Caldwell J, Caldwell L, et al. Experimental studies of sugar and aspartame on autonomic, cortical and behavioral responses of children. Proceedings of Interfaces in Psychology. Lubbock, Texas: Texas Tech Press, 1986.

9. Schauss, AG. New York City public school dietary revisions 1979–1983. Positive effects on 800,000 students' academic achievement. *International Journal of Biosocial Research* 1986;8(1):2–5.

10. Schauss, AG. Nutrition, student achievement and behaviour: Insights from new research. *The Intermediate Teacher* 1986;22(1):5–15.

11. Bateman B, Warner JO, Hutchinson E, et al. The effects of a double blind placebo controlled artificial food colourings and benzoate preservative challenge on hyperactivity in a general population sample of preschool children. *Archives of Disease in Childhood* 2004;89:506–511.

CHAPTER 20

Autism and Diet

WHAT IS AUTISM?

Autism is a life-long developmental disorder affecting as many as 1 in 500 children. Children with autism typically have difficulty with language, communication, and socialization. They have problems in learning and display a variety of atypical behaviors. The disorder is accompanied by mental retardation in three out of four cases. Asperger's syndrome (a high-functioning form of autism without retardation) is one among a range of different presentations of autism.

The number of cases of autism has risen noticeably in recent years. It is unclear whether this troubling observation is a result of: (1) an increasing awareness of the full spectrum of autism disorders; (2) a change in the way autism is diagnosed (so that cases not previously recognized as autism are now correctly diagnosed as such); or (3) a real rise in the number of cases.

DIAGNOSIS OF AUTISM

The diagnosis of autism is usually determined when the child is 2 to 3 years old following extensive evaluation according to criteria of the *Diagnostic and Statistical Manual of Mental Disorders* (DSM-IV).[1] Evidence of the condition may present soon after birth when the child fails to meet expected developmental milestones. In other cases the condition may become evident as the child loses newly acquired skills such as language, making eye-to-eye contact, and sociability after a period of apparently normal development. The latter pattern is often referred to as "regressive autism," and occurs in about one-third of children with autism.[2]

CAUSES OF AUTISM

There appear to be several different causes of autism, none of which is completely understood. Most authorities agree there is a strong genetic factor. It is not uncommon to see several children in one family—usually boys—with the condition. For the great majority of autistic individuals, however, the cause of the disorder has not been determined. It is likely that there are different causes and precipitating factors associated with the way autism is experienced by different individuals. The term *autistic syndrome* may be used to describe a pattern of similar behaviors produced by a variety of different triggers.[3]

DIGESTIVE TRACT DISTURBANCES IN AUTISM

Children with autism commonly experience more digestive tract symptoms than normal children. More than 30 years' anecdotal evidence from parents of autistic children describes disturbed gastrointestinal (GI) tract function, with symptoms such as abdominal pain, bloating, constipation, loose stools, and frequent diarrhea.[4] According to a 2001 survey of 500 parents of autistic children, almost half of those surveyed reported that their children had loose stools or frequent diarrhea.[5] Parents frequently reported an apparent intolerance to certain foods, especially wheat and cow's milk.

Several studies have demonstrated abnormal digestive tract function in autistic children. The abnormality known as "leaky gut" (described as increased permeability of the membrane lining the digestive tract so as to allow food molecules that would normally be excluded to pass into circulation) was demonstrated in some studies. (A detailed discussion of leaky gut follows.) Other studies found evidence of low activity of intestinal carbohydrate digestive enzymes.[6] Taken together, the results of these different studies suggest that significant digestive tract pathophysiology may accompany autism, at least within a subpopulation of patients.[7]

However, other studies have refuted these claims. One study conducted by U.K. researchers in 2002 concluded that there was no substantial association between gastrointestinal illness in children and the development of autism.[8] Nevertheless, the researchers acknowledged that some of their pediatric subjects may have had subclinical GI symptoms that had been overlooked, and that severe GI disease may be associated with autism in certain individuals.

Children with Autism May Be Sensitive to Cow's Milk and Gluten

Parents' frequent reports that exposure to cow's milk and wheat seem to increase their children's autistic symptoms prompted several studies that examined the possibility that components of these foods may trigger or exacerbate autistic symptoms in some children. Two separate studies involving a large number of autistic patients reported an improvement in social, cognitive, and communication skills when the children consumed a diet free of gluten and cow's milk, or a diet free of cow's milk alone.[9]

How Milk and Gluten May Affect Autism

The important types of proteins reported to be involved in triggering or exacerbating certain types of autism are (1) casein (in milk) and (2) the gliadin fraction of gluten (in wheat, rye, and barley). Digestion of dietary casein and gluten in the small intestine by the action of pancreatic and intestinal peptidase enzymes leads to the production of short-chain peptides, which are structurally similar to endorphins.[a] These products are called *exorphins,* to reflect their dietary origin. Gliadomorphins are a family of

---

[a] Endorphins are neuropeptides that bind to opioid receptors in the brain and affect pain perception.

exorphins released from the partial digestion of the wheat protein gliadin. Similarly, casomorphins are a family of exorphins released upon partial digestion of the milk protein casein. Casomorphins and gliadomorphins have been shown to affect the brain in experimental animals, and may be psychosis-inducing agents.[10]

Why is it that in autistic children, but not in normal children, the opioid peptides from the diet move through the lining of the digestive tract into the blood, to be carried to the brain as the blood circulates through the body's various organs? One answer to this question was formulated when it was discovered that the epithelium lining the digestive tract in some autistic children was more permeable than the epithelium lining the digestive tract in normal children—leading to the so-called *leaky gut hypothesis*. According to this theory, the digestion products of natural foods such as casein and gluten-containing grains are able to enter the blood through the leaky mucosa, where they (1) induce immunological responses and (2) interfere directly with the central nervous system.

There is no evidence to suggest that casein or gluten or their products *cause* the leaky gut; the cause remains open to debate. However, some researchers equate the process to celiac disease, in which immunological reactions to the gliadin fraction of gluten trigger a response in the intestinal villi that line the digestive tract epithelium and cause damage. (Please refer to Chapter 24 for more information on celiac disease.) The possible causes of leaky gut, and the possible relationship between autism and milk and/or gluten await further well-conducted research before the theories can be put into clinical practice.

Vitamin B$_{12}$-Deficiency and Nervous System Development

A deficiency in an essential nutrient has often been suggested as a possible contributor to some types of autism. Vitamin B$_{12}$ was thought to be a likely candidate because, when undetected and untreated, vitamin-B$_{12}$ deficiency in infants can result in permanent neurological damage. Furthermore, individuals with disorders of the stomach and small intestine may be unable to absorb enough vitamin B$_{12}$ from food to maintain healthy body stores of it.

According to proponents of the theory that vitamin-B deficiency plays a role in certain types of autism, pathology in the lining of the ileal region of the small intestine in autistic children (which has been observed in some studies) could interfere with the process of transporting vitamin B_{12} into circulation.[11] If absorption is severely inhibited, the resulting reduced amount of vitamin B_{12} in the bloodstream could interfere with the formation of myelin, the lipoprotein material that surrounds the axon of certain nerve fibers. Myelin is necessary for normal conduction of the nerve impulse (i.e., the action potential) in myelinated nerve fibers. Therefore, impairment in nerve conduction could result in the neurological deficits observed in autism. However, direct evidence of a connection between vitamin-B_{12} deficiency and impaired myelin formation in autism is lacking at this time.

Nevertheless, authorities urge (1) regular monitoring of the B_{12} levels in the blood of autistic children, and (2) supplementation of the vitamin, usually by injection, if B_{12} levels are found to be abnormally low.

Adhering to a diet that includes adequate levels of B_{12} is an obvious measure to ensure optimal nutrition in any child, but is especially important for the autistic child, whose diet may be somewhat unbalanced because of his or her food preferences. A discussion of Vitamin B_{12} in foods can be found in Appendix G.

Magnesium, Vitamin B_6, and Autism

Megavitamin therapy became very popular as a treatment for various chronic conditions in the 1950s. It was hoped that extremely large doses of vitamins might improve a child's mental processes and some of the symptoms of autism. Vitamin B_6 (Pyroxidine) was discovered to improve speech and language in some children with autistic syndrome. However, vitamin B_6 in high doses can be quite toxic, and has several unacceptable side effects (some of which are considerably reduced when the mineral magnesium [Mg] is given at the same time).

Since 1980 a number of published studies have attempted to assess the effects on autistic patients of combined treatment with vitamin B_6 and Mg. The subjects' verbal and nonverbal communication, interpersonal skills, and physiological function were monitored following treatment with vitamin B_6 and Mg. The studies were subjected to scientific evaluation and review in 2003.[12] The researchers who critiqued the studies concluded there was insufficient evidence on which to base a recommendation for combined use of B_6 with Mg as a treatment for autism.

Some clinicians have been investigating whether Mg given alone as a supplement may improve symptoms in autism. Their hypothesis is based on the observation that children with autism and children with other autistic spectrum disorders have significantly lower plasma concentrations of Mg than normal subjects.[13] Because Mg is an element that is essential to a number of important physiological processes, it has been suggested that a deficiency may lead to impairment in certain brain functions that could contribute to the autistic disorder. However, studies on Mg and its role in autism have neither defined the deficiency nor established whether supplementation with the mineral is effective in treatment.

WHAT'S THE MESSAGE?

Experts are clearly divided on the subject. There is no agreement on whether dietary manipulation can help prevent autism or aid in its treatment. Researchers do agree that dietary manipulation is strongly recommended if the child's behavior improves after a period of dietary restrictions or when given nutritional supplements. However, many practitioners hold the opinion that "the link between autism and a gastrointestinal pathophysiology is not substantiated by research. The dietary approaches employed are cumbersome and not proven to be efficacious, and may further narrow the food choices of the child with autism."[13]

As their parents well know, autistic children tend to have strong preferences in selection of food. Many have a violent dislike of certain foods, while seeming to crave others that they select repeatedly. Children with autism also tend to have very definite ideas about form and texture. For instance, one of my clients would only eat foods shaped in the form of a patty. This proved ideal because it allowed us to incorporate a wide range of chopped foods into his patties—foods that he would reject outright in their uncut state. Using fish-, meat-, or poultry-based patties containing a variety of chopped vegetables and fruit, we succeeded in creating a well-balanced diet for this client in spite of his very limited food preferences. However, in many cases the selectivity insisted on by the autistic child means that his or her diet is already limited, and parents and caregivers will understandably be reluctant to further restrict their child's food intake. Consequently, a gluten- and casein-restricted diet is not an attractive option for many.

Restricting Gluten and Casein in the Diet

If there is even a chance that your autistic child may be among the few who will benefit from a gluten- and casein-restricted diet, it is worth giving the diet a try, even if for a limited time. If there is no obvious improvement in your child's behavior after one month's strict adherence to the guidelines, simply discontinue the restrictions. See Appendix B for detailed instructions for a gluten- and casein-free diet for individuals with autism. By substituting the allowed foods for the foods that are not allowed, this trial diet ensures that your child will have complete balanced nutrition in spite of the restrictions. A list of foods high in vitamin B_{12} is also provided in Appendix B. If your child is lacking in this vitamin, be sure to regularly include these B_{12}-rich foods in his or her diet.

Keep in mind that there is no evidence that very high doses of a single nutrient are beneficial. In fact, in most cases the contrary is true. Excessive quantities of many vitamins and minerals can be toxic. An excess of one vitamin or mineral frequently leads to a deficiency in another, as they compete for absorption factors and metabolites. Each nutrient plays an essential role in keeping the body healthy. The level of each nutrient that is ideal at each stage of each individual's development is scientifically determined.[15] These levels should not be exceeded unless required by specific medical conditions and as determined in individual cases by a medical specialist.

THE LEAKY GUT

References to *leaky gut* arise in discussions of autism and other conditions involving food allergy or food intolerance. The term was coined to describe the situation that results when food molecules pass especially readily through the lining of the digestive tract into circulation in the bloodstream.

In early infancy the digestive tract lining tends to be quite permeable to food molecules, possibly because components of mother's breast milk must be able to pass readily into the infant's circulation. These components are active immune cells, hormones, and maturation factors that must remain intact in order to exert their effects. After infancy, these molecules are not so essential, and the digestive tract lining starts to "close up" to filter out materials that may be detrimental. The lining of the gut thus becomes less and less permeable as the child grows. By adulthood, only nutrients of smallest molecular weight are able to pass through after food has been fully digested in the lumen.

All along its length, the digestive tract is lined by simple column-shaped (i.e., columnar) epithelial cells. The epithelial cells are linked by tight junction complexes. The epithelial cells and the tight junctional complexes are the principal barriers to free movement into the bloodstream of dietary foods and the products released during their breakdown (i.e., digestion) by digestive enzymes in the lumen of the intestine. This is called the *intestinal luminal barrier*.

Certain conditions can compromise the intestinal luminal barrier and cause the digestive lining to become less permeable. Inflammation in the digestive tract may damage the epithelial cells and allow food molecules through the nonintact epithelium. Infection, food allergy, and autoimmune disease are some of the insults that may cause inflammation, cell damage, and separation of the tight junctional complexes. If the tight junctions separate, molecules of food are allowed to move freely into circulation where they can encounter immune cells and cause a variety of problems.

Testing to Identify Leaky Gut

A sugar permeability test can assess the physical integrity of the luminal barrier. This test measures the ability of small sugar molecules (taken by mouth) to gain entry into the bloodstream and eventually be excreted into the urine.[16]

In the sugar permeability test the patient drinks a measured quantity of two sugars—usually mannitol and lactulose—dissolved in water. The patient's urine is collected, and the ratio of mannitol to lactulose in the urine is measured.

- Mannitol is a monosaccharide that is relatively poorly absorbed by the human intestine. Mannitol molecules pass through the luminal membrane by way of aqueous pores in the brush border membrane. The larger and the more numerous the pores, the more mannitol is allowed to pass through into the bloodstream.

•   Lactulose is a larger dissacharide molecule, which is too large to pass through the pores. The lactulose molecules that do manage to reach the bloodstream do so by passing between the epithelial cells (i.e., through the tight junctions). Therefore, if the tight junctions are weakened, lactulose molecules gain access to the blood in circulation.

If these sugars gain access to the bloodstream, they will be carried to the kidneys and eventually be excreted in the subjects' urine. The quantity of each sugar excreted in urine indicates (1) the degree of permeability of the intestinal membranes and (2) whether the tight junctions are weakened.

It is through the weakened tight junctions that peptides such as gliadin are presumed to pass through a damaged intestinal membrane in celiac disease.

References

1. American Psychiatric Association. *Diagnostic and Statistical Manual of Mental Disorders* (DSM-IV), 4th ed. Washington, DC, 1994.

2. Tuchman RF, Rapin I. Regression in pervasive developmental disorders: seizures and epileptiform electroencephalogram correlates. *Pediatrics* 1997;(4):560–566.

3. White JF. Intestinal pathophysiology in autism. *Experimental Biology and Medicine* 2003;228:639-649.

4. White JF. Intestinal pathophysiology in autism.

5. Lightdale JR, Siegel B, Heyman MB. Gastrointestinal symptoms in autistic children. *Clinical Perspectives in Gastroenterology* 2001;1:56–58.

6. Horvath K, Papadimitriou JC, Rabsztyn A, Drachenberg C, Tildon JT. Gastrointestinal abnormalities in children with autistic disorder. *Journal of Pediatrics* 1999;135:559–563.

7. White JF. Intestinal pathophysiology in autism.

8. Black C, Kaye JA, Jick H. Relation of childhood gastrointestinal disorders to autism: nested case-control study using data from the UK General Practice Research Database. *British Medical Journal* 2002;325:419–421.

314 DEALING WITH FOOD ALLERGIES IN BABIES AND CHILDREN

9. Lucarelli S, Frediani T, Zingoni AM, Ferruzzi F, Giardini O, Quintieri F, Barbato M, D'Eufemia P, Cardi E. Food allergy and infantile autism. *Panminerva Medicica* 1995;37:137–141.

10. Knivsberg A, Reichelt KL, Nodland N, Hoien T. Autistic syndromes and diet: A follow-up study. *Scandinavian Journal of Educational Research* 1995;39:223–236.

11. White, JF. Intestinal pathophysiology in autism.

12. Wakefield AJ, Murch SH, Anthony A, Linnell J, Casson DM, Malik M, Berlowitz M, Dillon AP, Thompson MA, Harvey P, Valentine A, Davies SE, Walker-Smith JA. Ileal-lymphoid-nodular hyperplasia, nonspecific colitis, and pervasive developmental disorder in children. *Lancet* 1998;35:637–641.

13. Nye C, Brice A. Combined vitamin B6-magnesium treatment in autism spectrum disorder (Cochrane Review). In: *The Cochrane Library*, Issue 1, Oxford, 2003.

14. Strambi M, Longini M, Hayek J, Berni S, Macucci F, Scalacci E, Vezzosi P. Magnesium profile in autism. *Biological Trace Element Research* 2006;109(2):97–104.

15. Johnson TW. Dietary considerations in autism: Identifying a reasonable approach. *Topics in Clinical Nutrition* 2006;21(3):212–225.

16. Food and Nutrition Board. *Dietary Reference Intakes (DRIs): Recommended Intakes for Individuals, Vitamins.* Washington, DC. Institute of Medicine, National Academy of Sciences, 2004.

17. White, JF. Intestinal pathophysiology in autism.

CHAPTER 21

Oral Allergy Syndrome

Oral allergy syndrome (OAS) is an allergic reaction to food that is confined to the oral cavity (i.e., to the lips, and around the lips, roof of the mouth, tongue, hard and soft palate, and uvula) and adjacent structures. It differs from other food allergy in that its symptoms do not appear in any other location in the body, and always accompany respiratory allergy to inhaled allergens of plants, particularly plant pollens. Of course, symptoms in the mouth, throat, and upper respiratory tract can be part of a generalized reaction to foods, but in this case they are more accurately described as oral allergy symptoms. The term oral allergy syndrome applies specifically to pollen allergy (pollinosis) accompanied by reactions to certain raw foods when they are in direct contact with oral tissues. Individuals with OAS typically have hay fever-type symptoms caused by allergies to trees, grasses, and weeds. They experience irritation in the mouth (lips, tongue, roof of the mouth) and sometimes the throat after eating specific types of raw fruits, vegetables, and sometimes nuts.[1]

Some authorities have suggested using the term pollen-food allergy syndrome (rather than oral allergy syndrome) to avoid confusing OAS with food allergy with oral symptoms in which the primary sensitizing allergen is food, not pollen.

The syndrome has been diagnosed with increasing frequency in recent years as more patients and clinicians have become familiar with it. The majority of cases occur in adults, but wider familiarity with the syndrome has led to

315

its being increasingly recognized in children. A 2004 study on the incidence of food allergy in children from birth to 17 years of age in Berlin[2] reported that most of the reactions were the result of pollen-associated food allergy, and were generally mild.

SYMPTOMS

Children who have OAS experience almost immediate symptoms, usually beginning just a few minutes after eating the offending food. Symptoms include itching, irritation, and sometimes swelling of the lips, tongue, throat, and palate. Occasionally these tissues blister and papules form. These symptoms can be uncomfortable. A swollen lip or tongue may make it difficult for the child to speak normally. In extreme cases, the tongue or throat may swell and block the airways, creating a possibly life-threatening condition that requires immediate medical attention. Most children exhibit symptoms within 5 minutes of contact with the food, and all but a few exhibit symptoms within 30 minutes. On rare occasions, symptoms may appear 2 hours after contact with the food.

Oral allergy syndrome is characterized by three factors:

1. Symptoms are confined to the mucosal surfaces of the oral cavity and adjacent tissues.

2. Symptoms occur immediately after contact with the allergenic food.

3. The syndrome involves a coexisting allergy to inhaled plant materials, usually pollens that contain protein antigens related to those of the food that is responsible for the oral symptoms.

MECHANISMS OF REACTIVITY

Oral allergy symptoms are caused by a rapid response of the mast cell–bound pollen-specific IgE to allergens released from raw fruits and vegetables as they enter the mouth and come into contact with saliva. Unusually high concentrations of mast cells in the oral and pharyngeal tissues result from continual response to pollen allergens in their native form. The tissues of the upper respiratory tract become sensitized to a pollen allergen as both cause and consequence of long-standing hay fever.[3] Foods that contain a protein that is structurally indistinguishable from the allergenic protein in the pollen can cause release of inflammatory mediators from the primed mast cells. For example, the food allergens can attach to the pollen IgE molecules sitting on receptors on the mast cells and act as if they were pollen proteins. (Please see Chapter 1 for a detailed discussion of what happens when inflammatory mediators are released from mast cells.) The released inflammatory mediators then affect tissues adjacent to the upper respiratory tract in the oral cavity and cause inflammation.

Interestingly, the proteins in foods that can mimic pollen proteins come from plants that are botanically unrelated to the plants that produce the pollens. This is further evidence that botanic relatedness has little or nothing to do with antigenic (or allergenic) relationships, and shows that the old idea that allergy to foods in one plant family predicts allergy to other foods in the same plant family is mostly invalid.

FOODS INVOLVED IN ORAL ALLERGY SYNDROME

Oral allergy syndrome has been most often reported in people who have respiratory allergy (such as hay fever) to specific plant pollens. The pollens most often implicated are produced by

- Birch and alder trees

- Ragweed

- Mugwort

- Grasses of various types, especially timothy grass, widely grown for hay in the United Sates

Birch and alder tree allergy seems to be the most frequent accompanying allergy in OAS.

Table 21-1 lists the foods that most frequently trigger OAS in children sensitized to certain inhaled allergens. The inhaled allergens are listed in column 1 and the trigger foods are listed in columns 2 through 5.

Oral contact with the related fruit, vegetable, or nut causes symptoms when the food is eaten raw, but there is usually no problem when the food is eaten in cooked form. Cooking changes the nature of the protein and the immune system does not recognize the cooked form of the protein. Therefore, for example, someone with OAS can eat stewed apples, but not raw chopped apple in a fresh fruit salad. Many of the fruits tend to increase in allergenicity as they ripen, so people with OAS tend to have more severe symptoms, the riper the fruit they eat.

DIETARY MANAGEMENT OF ORAL ALLERGY SYNDROME

It is important that any child with an allergy avoid nutritional deficiencies by consuming the widest possible range of foods from all food groups. It is therefore essential that the foods that do cause symptoms be correctly identified. Only those causing an immediate reaction should be avoided; all other foods not causing symptoms should be included in the diet. The challenge, of course, is to accurately identify the specific foods that are responsible for the symptoms.

Managing OAS in children often presents a puzzle because the symptoms start very mildly, and the child usually reacts to only one or two of the foods listed in Table 21-1. In addition, the foods that trigger OAS rarely result in a positive skin test or radio allergosorbent test (RAST). This is because the antibodies are formed in response to the pollen, not in response to the food. Results of the skin test and RAST are usually positive for the pollen, but these results tell nothing about the child's likely response to the cross-reacting foods.

Over time, OAS symptoms may become more severe, and the child may start to react to other foods that cross-react with his or her pollen allergens. Parents often question whether they should eliminate all the foods listed in Table 21-1 if their pollen-allergic child reacts to one or more of the related foods. The following guidelines will help you answer questions about food elimination:

- Eliminate only the foods to which you child is reacting. Which foods will usually be obvious because the reaction will usually be clearly visible in the child's mouth, and he or she will complain of tingling or irritation.

Table 21-1

FOODS THAT TRIGGER OAS IN CHILDREN SENSITIZED TO INHALED ALLERGENS[4]

TRIGGERING FOODS				
Inhaled Nonfood Allergens	Fruits and Vegetables	Legumes and Grains	Nuts and Seeds	Other Foods
Birch pollen	Apple	Peanut	Hazelnuts	Some spices
Alder pollen	Apricot		Other tree nuts	Echinacea
Mugwort pollen	Carrot		Sunflower seeds	Chamomile tea
Grass pollens	Celery			
Timothy grass	Cherry			
Ragweed	Fennel			
	Kiwi fruit			
	Melon			
	Nectarine			
	Orange			
	Peach			
	Potato			
	Tomato			
	Watermelon			
	Banana			
	Cantaloupe			
	Cucumber			
	Honeydew			
	Melon			
	Watermelon			
	Zucchini			

- If your child wants to continue eating the food, offer it only in well-cooked form. The cooked form will usually cause no problem, but you should remain alert to the remote possibility that a reaction to the cooked food may occur in children who are very sensitive to the food. Avoid the food entirely if your child reacts to it in well-cooked form.

- Do not avoid other foods from the list in Table 21-1 unless and until your child displays allergic symptoms after eating the food.

- Remain alert to the possibility that over time your child may develop a reaction to other foods listed in Table 21-1.

Identification of Foods Responsible for Oral Allergy Syndrome

Some practitioners use the prick-in-prick (or prick + prick) method for testing foods involved in OAS. A sterile needle is inserted into the suspect raw food (such as an apple). The child's arm is then pricked with the same needle. In some cases, transferring the raw allergen to the child may induce a wheal and flare reaction that allergists consider an indication of the child's reaction to the food.

In practice, however, the only truly accurate way to identify the foods your child reacts to is to carefully observe how the child reacts when he or she comes into contact with the foods.

Topical Application of Suspect Food

When the symptoms occur (1) predominantly in the oral tissues, and (2) upon immediate contact with the food, it may serve to apply just a small amount of test food to the outer border of the child's lip. The site of application should be observed for development of overt signs of a reaction—itching, reddening, blistering, or swelling. Half an hour's observation is usually sufficient, but signs of reaction may become apparent at the site for up to 2 hours following application of the test food.

If OAS has ever led to throat tightening or tongue swelling in your child, the topical application of suspect food should always be used as the first method of testing, prior to methods that allow the child to ingest the test food. This is because allergic reactions can increase in severity upon repeated exposure to culprit food. In extreme cases the reactions can be life-threatening.

If topical application does not elicit an adverse response, an open food challenge should confirm whether the food is indeed responsible for the child's symptoms.

In situations where the food could cause a severe reaction, ingestion should take place only under medical supervision in a fully equipped facility.

Open Food Challenge

In most cases, open food challenge with increasing doses of the test food will identify the foods that must be avoided. The sequential incremental dose challenge (SIDC) is a very effective method of challenge. The key components of SIDC are outlined as follows:

- Consult your pediatrician before starting the test.

- With your doctor's OK, begin with topical application of a test food to your child's lip. If topical application causes no reaction, give your child a teaspoon-sized portion of the food and monitor for reactions for 4 hours.

- If the child has not reacted during the 4-hour period of monitoring, give him or her a tablespoon-sized portion of the test food and again monitor for response for 4 hours.

- If no symptoms have appeared during these 8 hours, allow the child to eat as much of the food as he or she wishes while continuing to monitor for reactions for another 4 hours.

- If there is no sign of symptoms after the last dose, the food can be considered safe.

- If a reaction appears at any time during the challenge, remove the food immediately. Your doctor may suggest an antihistamine medication to keep on hand for troublesome allergy symptoms that may arise during the process of open food challenge.

Finalizing the Diet

When the culprit foods have been identified by challenge, they should be strictly eliminated from the diet. Take care to provide your child complete balanced nutrition from alternate sources, especially when the foods eliminated were important sources of essential nutrients.

References

1. Joneja JMV. Oral allergy syndrome, cross-reacting allergens and co-occurring allergies. *Journal of Nutritional and Environmental Medicine* 1999;(9):289–303.

2. Roehr CC, Edenharter G, Reimann S, Ehlers I, Worm M, Zuberbier T, Niggemann B. Food allergy and non-allergic food hypersensitivity in children and adolescents. *Clinical and Experimental Allergy* 2004;34(10):1534–1541.

3. Amlot PL, Kemeny DM, Zachary C, et al. Oral allergy syndrome (OAS): Symptoms of IgE-mediated hypersensitivity to foods. *Clinical Allergy* 1987;17:33–42.

4. Joneja JMV. Oral allergy syndrome, cross-reacting allergens and co-occurring allergies.

CHAPTER 22

Eczema and Diet

Eczema (known in medical terminology as atopic dermatitis) is one of the most troublesome allergic conditions in infants. Eczema is regarded as the most common skin disease of childhood. It may start as early as the first few weeks of life, and may occasionally be present at birth. In most cases, eczema appears within the first 3 months. The baby is obviously distressed by the condition. He or she appears irritable and uncomfortable, rubs or scratches the affected areas (which makes the situation seem worse), and often has restless, disturbed sleep. Parents and caregivers are frequently even more distressed than the baby. Eczema is unsightly. When a baby is obviously uncomfortable, everyone is anxious to relieve the problem in any way possible. Because food allergy frequently plays a key role in the genesis of the condition, food restrictions are often undertaken for baby and breast-feeding mother. These can create nutritional deficiencies in both.

SYMPTOMS OF ECZEMA

Eczema appears in a fairly typical pattern that changes at the different stages of infancy, childhood, and mature life.

Infantile Eczema

Infantile eczema usually starts between the first 2 and 6 months of life, although it often begins earlier if the baby is highly food-allergic. The baby develops a red rash, which may weep. It first appears on the cheeks and may spread to the forehead and the back of the arms and legs. In severe cases, infantile eczema may involve the whole body. Heavy scaling may occur. Infantile eczema is often associated with food allergy. It tends to disappears between ages 3 and 5, as food allergies are outgrown.

Childhood Eczema

Childhood eczema may follow the infantile phase almost immediately, or it may start for the first time between the ages of 2 and 4. The rash in childhood eczema is found in the creases of the elbows, behind the knees, and across the ankles, and may involve the face, ears, and neck as well. This form of eczema is frequently associated with allergy to airborne and contact allergens (such as dust mites, animal dander, mold spores, and plant pollens). It often disappears by age 10, but may continue into adult life.

Adult Eczema

Adult eczema usually appears as large areas of very itchy, reddened, weeping skin. The elbow creases, wrists, neck, and ankles, and the area behind the knees are especially affected. Troublesome adult eczema may also appear on the palms of the hands and between the fingers. The condition tends to improve in mid-life, and occurs only unusually among the elderly.

CAUSES OF ECZEMA

It is important to understand that food does not cause eczema (nor does food cause allergy). The symptoms of allergy are caused when the immune system reacts to food as though it were a threat to the health of the body. In infancy, eczema is one of the earliest signs that a baby may have food allergy. Of course, not all babies with eczema have food allergy. For about one-third of young children with atopic dermatitis, the condition is attributed to food allergy. One typical study found 33.8 percent (25 of 74) of pediatric patients with atopic dermatitis were diagnosed with food allergy.[1] The foods most frequently identified as allergens for this group were eggs, milk, and peanuts.

Eczema can also occur as a response to an allergic reaction to environmental allergens such as dust mites, mold spores, animal dander, and plant pollens, among others. These allergens usually become a greater problem as the baby grows up, and the allergens gain access to the immune cells through the non-intact skin of the patches of eczema that were induced by earlier food allergy.

Eczema as a symptom of food allergy seems to be much more frequent in early childhood than later in life. The first symptoms that a baby may be allergic (sometimes said to be atopic) present in the digestive tract (often exhibited as prolonged colic-like symptoms) and in the skin (exhibited as eczema and hives). In babies younger than 6 months, eliminating the foods that trigger the symptoms often leads to a significant improvement in the eczema—in some cases leading to total remission. The triggering foods may be in the diet of the breast-feeding mother or in the diet of the baby if he or she is formula-fed or has begun to consume solid foods.

FOODS ASSOCIATED WITH FOOD ALLERGY IN BABIES AND CHILDREN WITH ECZEMA

The food allergens that most frequently trigger the onset of eczema in babies and children are

- Egg
- Milk and milk products
- Peanut
- Soy
- Shellfish

Occasionally green peas and tomatoes are added to the list of food allergens that trigger eczema in children, usually after the peas or tomatoes have been introduced as solid foods.[2] Researchers in one study found that all of their young subjects who were allergic to sesame seed had atopic dermatitis.[3]

Eczema can be almost completely controlled in food-allergic babies up to about age 6 months by avoiding the foods most frequently associated with infant allergy. For breast-fed babies, this means that mother must avoid these foods (and must include nutritionally equivalent substitutes in her diet to ensure complete balanced nutrition for herself and for baby). For formula-fed babies, this means that an extensively hydrolyzed casein formula (ehf) must be fed, to avoid the milk proteins in conventional milk-based infant formulas.

Of course every baby is an individual. Your baby may have become sensitized to foods other than those listed among the food allergens that commonly trigger eczema. If elimination of the trigger foods does not result in complete resolution of your baby's eczema, proceed to eliminate other foods. Keep careful records of both mother's and baby's diet and of baby's symptoms. (Please refer to Chapter 6 to learn how to complete a food and symptom record for baby and lactating mother.) Reintroducing each separate food into the mother's diet while monitoring baby's response should provide the information needed to formulate a diet that (1) is free from the baby's eczema triggers and (2) provides complete balanced nutrition from alternate sources for both baby and breast-feeding mother. (Details of elimination and challenge in the breast-fed baby are covered in Chapter 6.)

Unfortunately, older children do not improve as markedly as babies when food allergen avoidance is undertaken as a means to control eczema. This is because after age 1, the child is as susceptible or more susceptible to environmental allergens as to food allergens. After a first encounter with the allergens, the baby's immune system is primed to respond with symptoms of allergy. The allergy may be expressed as eczema, or as rhinitis (nasal stuffiness) and wheezing (which can be a symptom of asthma) when the allergens have sensitized tissues of the respiratory tract.

It is not uncommon for eczema in a 2-year-old to increase in severity while rhinitis and wheezing simultaneously and suddenly appear. This sequence would be especially likely to occur among children in an environment where airborne allergens—typically dust mites, molds, pollens, and animal dander—are unusually high. This scenario is typical of the atopic child who starts out with infantile eczema as a symptom of food allergy and becomes sensitized to environmental allergens as he or she grows up. Up to the age of about 5, but more commonly at age 2 or 3, food and inhalant allergy often coexist, making any symptoms worse in the face of what are now a multiplicity of allergens to trigger the release of inflammatory mediators and increase symptom severity and incidence.

MANAGEMENT OF FOOD ALLERGY IN A CHILD WITH ECZEMA

The first step in determining the cause of pediatric eczema is to consult your child's pediatrician. He or she may refer you to a pediatric dermatologist or to an allergist. If allergy is suspected, the specialist will typically carry out an allergy evaluation and order a radio allergosorbent test (RAST), a blood test to demonstrate whether your baby has been sensitized to specific allergens in foods and in the environment. Skin-testing is not advisable for babies or children who have eczema, because their skin is already highly reactive and will frequently produce false positive results. Skin-testing a patient who has eczema may also create a route for sensitization to allergens in the test reagents. Many authorities recommend "diagnostic evaluation of food allergy be performed in all children" with atopic dermatitis.[4]

A short time trial on a diet that excludes the foods most frequently associated with eczema (eggs, milk and milk products, peanuts, soy, tomatoes, shellfish, sesame seed, and green peas) and the foods that test positive in the RAST should result in improvement in the baby's or child's symptoms if foods are playing a significant role in the eczema. Separately reintroducing these foods and monitoring the child's response (for example, by looking for reddening of the skin, itching, and an obvious increase in eczema) will confirm that the food that triggered the response should be avoided. A registered dietitian should assist in the food elimination process. Professional supervision is recommended because it is essential that foods excluded from the child's or lactating mother's diet be replaced by foods of equal nutritional value. We do not want to put mother or child at nutritional risk as a result of removing important food groups.

Table 22-1 lists foods that are allowed on a test diet that excludes the suspect food allergens associated with eczema. Chapters 7 to 16 provide more details about the foods that should be avoided and about their replacements.

The test diet should be followed for 4 weeks. If significant improvement in the child's eczema is achieved on this regimen, individual reintroduction of each of the eliminated foods—either into the child's diet (if he or she is eating solids) or into the mother's diet (if she is breast-feeding the baby)—should determine exactly which foods are contributing to the eczema. These foods must be avoided as long as the child displays symptoms (usually until age 5), at which time retesting of the foods should be undertaken.

RECIPES AND MEAL PREPARATION TIPS

This section provides a few recipes that can be incorporated into the test diet for food allergy associated with eczema outlined in Table 22-1.

Clarified Butter (Ghee in South Asian and Indian Cooking)

- Over low heat, melt 1 lb of butter (4 sticks), cut into pieces, in a heavy saucepan.

- Milk solids will sink to the bottom, and may rise to the top as foam.

- Skim the foam off the top and discard.

- Allow the residue of milk solids to sink to the bottom and pour off the clear oil.

- Discard the bottom solids.

- The remaining clear yellow oil (about one-fourth less than what you started with) is clarified butter.

Light Whipped Butter

Clarified butter is very hard and is difficult to spread when solidified. A light whipped butter, with the addition of a polyunsaturated vegetable oil such as canola, makes a softer spread and reduces the saturated:unsaturated fat ratio, which is beneficial in lowering cholesterol.

Table 22-1

**TEST DIET FOR FOOD ALLERGY ASSOCIATED WITH ECZEMA
DIET FREE OF MILK, EGG, SOY, PEANUT, SESAME SEEDS,
SHELLFISH, TOMATO, AND GREEN PEA**

Food Group	Foods Allowed

Milk and Milk Products	• Milk-free and soy-free products
	   – Rice Dream® (made from brown rice and safflower oil)
	   – Darifree® (made from potato starch)
	• Substitute these in recipes:
	   – Fruit or vegetable juice
	   – Homemade soup stock
	   – Water used to cook vegetables or potatoes
	• Substitute these for butter:
	   – Clarified butter (recipe below)
	   – Whey-free, soy-free, corn-free margarine (e.g., Canoleo®)
	   – Pure jelly
	   – Jam
	   – Honey
	   – Herb-flavored olive oil
	• Salad dressings, vegetable dips
	   – Olive oil with herbs
	   – Homemade salad dressings made with allowed ingredients

Table 22-1 (continued)
TEST DIET FOR FOOD ALLERGY ASSOCIATED WITH ECZEMA
DIET FREE OF MILK, EGG, SOY, PEANUT, SESAME SEEDS,
SHELLFISH, TOMATO, AND GREEN PEA

Food Group	Foods Allowed

Grains, Cereals, Bakery Products	**Grains and Flours**
	• All cereal grains
	• All flours from grains, including
	   – Wheat and wheat flour
	   – Amaranth and amaranth flour
	   – Barley and barley flour
	   – Buckwheat and buckwheat flour
	   – Chickpea (also called garbanzo bean, besan) flour
	   – Corn, corn flour, corn starch
	   – Millet and millet flour (also called bajri, or bajra, flour)
	   – T'eff flour (produced in Ethiopia)
	   – Oats and oat flour
	   – Potato starch and flour
	   – Quinoa and quinoa flour
	   – Rice and rice flour
	   – Wild rice and wild rice flour
	   – Rye and rye flour
	   – Sago and sago flour
	   – Tapioca, tapioca starch, tapioca flour
	   – Cassava flour and starch

Table 22-1 (continued)
TEST DIET FOR FOOD ALLERGY ASSOCIATED WITH ECZEMA
DIET FREE OF MILK, EGG, SOY, PEANUT, SESAME SEEDS,
SHELLFISH, TOMATO, AND GREEN PEA

Food Group	Foods Allowed

Grains, Cereals, Bakery Products (cont'd)	**Breads and Baked Goods**
	
	 • Baked goods and baking mixes containing allowed ingredients
	
	 • *Avoid* any containing[a]
	
	   – *Milk*[b]
	
	   – *Eggs*[c]
	
	   – *Peanut or peanut oil*
	
	   – *Soy or soy oil*
	
	   – *Sesame seed*
	
	 • Homemade baked goods made with allowed ingredients
	
	 Crackers and Snacks
	
	 • Potato chips made *without soy or peanut oil*
	
	 • Any made with allowed grains and flours such as wheat, but *avoid* *snacks containing sesame seeds, peanuts and peanut oil, soy or soy oil, eggs (sometimes added as a glaze)*
	
	 • Pure rye crisp crackers

[a] Italic type indicates a food that must be avoided.
[b] This ingredient must only be avoided by *the child* who is eating the food—not by the lactating mother, unless the item is a major ingredient. (The amount of milk in most baked goods is too small to cause problems for the breast-fed baby.)
[c] See Note b. (The amount of egg in most baked goods is too small to cause problems for the breast-fed baby.)

Table 22-1 (continued)
TEST DIET FOR FOOD ALLERGY ASSOCIATED WITH ECZEMA
DIET FREE OF MILK, EGG, SOY, PEANUT, SESAME SEEDS,
SHELLFISH, TOMATO, AND GREEN PEA

Food Group	Foods Allowed
Grains, Cereals, Bakery Products (cont'd)	**Crackers and Snacks (cont'd)** • Rice cakes but ***avoid*** *rice cakes made with sesame seed or other restricted ingredients* • Rice crackers but ***avoid*** *rice crackers made with sesame seed or other restricted ingredients* **Breakfast Cereals** • Made from any of the allowed grains • ***Avoid*** *cereals containing* – *Soy, soy derivatives, soy oil* – *Peanut, peanut oil* – *Sesame seeds* **Pasta** • Pasta made from any allowed grain, including – Wheat – Rice pasta – Brown rice pasta – Wild rice pasta – Mung bean pasta – Green bean pasta – Buckwheat pasta (soba noodles) – Rice pasta

Table 22-1 (continued)
TEST DIET FOR FOOD ALLERGY ASSOCIATED WITH ECZEMA
DIET FREE OF MILK, EGG, SOY, PEANUT, SESAME SEEDS,
SHELLFISH, TOMATO, AND GREEN PEA

Food Group	Foods Allowed
Grains, Cereals, Bakery Products (cont'd)	**Pasta (cont'd)** – Rice noodles – Potato pasta – Quinoa pasta *Avoid any noodles that contain egg, soy or soy oil, peanut or peanut oil*
Vegetables	• Most plain fresh and frozen vegetables and their juices but *avoid* – *Soy beans* – *Soy bean sprouts* – *Mixed sprouts* – *Tomatoes* – *Green peas* – *Snow peas* – *Split peas*
Fruit	• All plain fresh and frozen fruits and their juices
Meat and Poultry	• All fresh or frozen pure meat or poultry but *avoid any meat mixed with additional ingredients, including processed meats, sausages, and all deli meats that may contain soy, soy oil, or peanut oil.*

Table 22-1 (continued)

TEST DIET FOR FOOD ALLERGY ASSOCIATED WITH ECZEMA
DIET FREE OF MILK, EGG, SOY, PEANUT, SESAME SEEDS,
SHELLFISH, TOMATO, AND GREEN PEA

Food Group	Foods Allowed
Fish	• All are allowed
Shellfish	• *None allowed* ***Avoid*** *all crustaceans (lobster, crab, prawns, shrimp, scampi, crayfish, crawfish, etc.) and mollusks (bivalves such as mussels, scallops, whelks, cockles, winkles, etc.)*
Eggs	• *None allowed* • Use egg-free replacement products such as Ener-G® Egg Replacer
Legumes	• Most plain legumes and legume dishes prepared with allowed foods, but ***avoid*** – *Soy, peanut, green peas, snow peas, split peas (green and yellow)*
Nuts	• Most are allowed, but ***avoid*** – *Peanuts, soy nuts, any nuts roasted in or containing peanut or soy oils*
Seeds	• Most are allowed, but ***avoid*** – *Sesame seed, any seed roasted in or containing peanut or soy oils*
Fats and Oils	• Vegetable oils, including – Olive

Table 22-1 (continued) TEST DIET FOR FOOD ALLERGY ASSOCIATED WITH ECZEMA DIET FREE OF MILK, EGG, SOY, PEANUT, SESAME SEEDS, SHELLFISH, TOMATO, AND GREEN PEA	
Food Group	**Foods Allowed**
Fats and Oils (cont'd)	– Canola
	– Corn
	– Sunflower
	– Safflower
	– Flaxseed
	– Grape seed
	– ***Avoid*** *peanut oil, soy oil*
	• Meat drippings
	• Lard
	• Poultry fat
	• Homemade gravy with allowed ingredients
Spices and Herbs	• All pure fresh or dried herbs (including leaves and flowers of the plant)
	• All pure fresh or dried spices (including root, bark, and seed of the plant)

Following this recipe for whipped butter will ensure that the canola oil is well integrated into the butter oil and won't separate upon standing:

- Pour liquefied clarified butter (the yellow oil) into a blender. Start blending on the lowest setting.

- As slowly as possible, add canola oil to the clarified butter in the blender, using ½ cup canola for the amount of clarified butter derived from 1 lb of butter.

- The two oils blend together best as butter oil begins to cool. Whip mixture to form a light whipped product.

- Pour whipped butter into a plastic container and refrigerate.

Tomato-free Sauces for Spaghetti and Other Pasta

If tomatoes are a food allergen that triggers eczema or another form of dermatitis in your baby or child, you will want to prepare dishes based on tomato substitutes. You may be surprised to know that **mangoes** make a great substitute for tomatoes in recipes for

- Salsa

- Antipasto

- Pasta sauces

- Pizza toppings

If you are cooking for someone who must avoid tomato, you may want to try the three recipes provided below.

Basil Pesto Sauce

Ingredients

Fresh basil leaves (strip leaves from stalks)	2 cups (packed leaves)
Sea salt	¼ teaspoon
Garlic, peeled and crushed	2–3 cloves

| Olive oil | ¼ cup |
| Pine nuts | 1 tablespoon |

Preparation

- Put basil, olive oil, pine nuts, garlic, and salt in a blender or food processor.

- Blend until contents form a smooth purée.

- For thinner sauce, add 2–3 tablespoons of water from cooked pasta.

- Freeze pesto sauce, if required for later use.

- To serve immediately, add pesto sauce (uncooked) to hot, drained pasta, tossing to coat all strands.

Makes enough for 4 servings of pasta.

Garlic and Olive Oil Sauce

Ingredients

Olive oil	¼ cup (90 mL)
Garlic, peeled and finely chopped	2 or more cloves
Black pepper, freshly ground	To taste
Salt	To taste
Parsley, fresh, chopped	2 tablespoons

Preparation

- Cook oil and garlic in a small saucepan over very low heat for 1 to 2 minutes—just until the garlic begins to changes color.

- Add hot oil and garlic sauce to cooked, drained spaghetti or other pasta.

- Toss rapidly, coating all strands of pasta.

- Season with fresh ground black pepper; garnish with parsley.

- Serve immediately.

Makes enough for 4 servings of pasta.

Zucchini and Basil Sauce

Ingredients

Olive oil	¼ cup (90 mL)
Garlic, peeled and sliced	2 cloves
Zucchini	1½ lbs (675 g)
Black pepper, freshly ground	To taste
Salt	To taste
Clarified butter, melted	3 tablespoons (40 g)
Basil, fresh, finely chopped	6 leaves

Preparation

- Cut off and discard both ends of the zucchini.

- Wash, dry well, and slice into thin rounds.

- Heat oil in a large, heavy frying pan.

- Add garlic and fry until golden; remove garlic and discard.

- Add zucchini slices to the pan.

- Fry with pinch of salt and freshly ground black pepper until tender, stirring frequently to prevent burning (for about 8 to 10 minutes)

To complete the dish:

- Drain cooked spaghetti or other pasta and place on warmed serving dish.

- Add melted clarified butter, zucchini and their cooking oil, and the basil.

- Toss until all strands of pasta are thoroughly coated.

- Serve immediately.

Makes enough to serve 4 to 5.

References

1. Eigenmann PA and Calza A-M. Diagnosis of IgE-mediated food allergy among Swiss children with atopic dermatitis. *Pediatric Allergy and Immunology* 2000;11(2):95–100.

2. Eigenmann PA, Sicherer SH, Borkowski TA, Cohen BA, Sampson HA. Prevalence of IgE-mediated food allergy among children with atopic dermatitis. *Pediatrics* 1998;101:e8.

3. Eigenmann et al. Prevalence of IgE-mediated food allergy among children with atopic dermatitis.

4. Fiocchi A, Bouygue GR, Martelli A, Terracciano L, Sarratud T. Dietary treatment of childhood atopic eczema/dermatitis syndrome (AEDS) *Allergy* 2004;59:78.

CHAPTER 23

Asthma and Food Allergy

As discussed earlier, food allergy involves an IgE-mediated response to specific foods, which results in the release of inflammatory mediators. (Please see Chapter 1, What Is Food Allergy?) It is the action of these mediators on the tissues of various organ systems that results in the symptoms of allergy. When the mediators act on tissues in the respiratory tract, for example, we see signs of rhinitis that resemble hay fever, or we see symptoms in the lungs that resemble asthma.

The primary modes by which food allergy can trigger the symptoms of asthma are (1) by inhalation of the allergenic food, and (2) by ingestion of the allergenic food.

ASTHMA AND THE INHALATION OF FOOD PARTICLES

Allergenic foods can impact the lungs when an allergic individual inhales food particles that may have been released when the food was cooked or that were dispersed in aerosol form. An example of the latter is baker's asthma, an occupational hazard for bakery workers who inhale wheat particles in aerosolized flour. Allergy to the allergens in cooked food has been reported by highly allergic patients who were exposed to their allergenic foods (say, fish, shellfish, or eggs) in an enclosed area (for example, a restaurant dining room) or during meal preparation. Most cases of asthma triggered by aerosolized food allergens involve adults engaged in specific occupations that regularly expose them to the allergens. In contrast, most cases of asthma in children are triggered when the allergen is eaten, not inhaled.

ASTHMA AND THE INGESTION OF FOOD ALLERGENS

One of the earliest studies to link asthma and food allergy was published in 1992.[1] In 279 children with asthma, 168 experienced wheezing in double-blind placebo-controlled food challenges. The foods in this study that triggered wheezing were: peanut (19); milk (18); egg (13); tree nuts (10); soy (2); wheat (2); legumes (beans) (2); and turkey (1). In all cases the wheezing occurred within 2 hours of the children's having eaten the test foods. The children in the study were all known to be allergic to the foods, and had other symptoms that indicated their allergic status.

Another study of asthma triggered by foods[2] identified six culprit foods in order of their prevalence in triggering the allergic reaction as follows: (1) egg; (2) milk; (3) peanut; (4) wheat; (5) soy; and (6) fish.

In most cases of food-associated asthma in children, the asthma symptoms rarely occur alone. This is because additional symptoms of allergy are triggered when the offending food is ingested. Food-induced anaphylaxis is the most dramatic example of the involvement of multiple organ systems in responding to food allergy.

The relationship between food allergy and asthma is most obvious in children (as opposed to adults), and is strongest in the youngest of the young subjects. In a group of milk-allergic babies with mean age of 10 months, 29 percent of 27 infants had lung responses typical of asthma on challenge with milk.[3]

Asthma and Food Intolerance

Certain types of food ingredients and food additives that cause a non-immunological reaction in the body (food intolerance[a]) can make asthma worse. Artificial food colors called azo dyes, especially tartrazine (which is yellow); preservatives such as sulfites and benzoates, and forms of these chemicals that occur naturally in some foods; and salicylate (which is the active ingredient in aspirin), are chemicals that may enhance the asthmatic response to allergens in a child who is sensitized to them.

The reaction of asthmatics to these chemical compounds is not an allergy, but is more correctly described as an intolerance because the initial response is not a triggering of the immune system. The process involves an increase in the level of the inflammatory mediators that are responsible for the bronchospasm of asthma. These mediators include histamine and leukotrienes. They are released during the reaction to an allergen, and cause the muscular contractions that result in the difficulty in breathing and wheezing that are typical of asthma. By inhibiting (or turning off) other types of mediators, the chemicals in the food additives cause an increase in the level of histamine and leukotrienes. This results in increased bronchospasm, and a definite worsening of the asthma symptoms[b].

By avoiding the food ingredients and additives that are responsible for this type of enhancement of an allergic reaction, an asthmatic child will not lose his or her asthma. However, an asthmatic child who does have an intolerance to these chemicals will definitely benefit from avoiding them because their asthma symptoms will be less severe than when they are eaten frequently.

For more information about food additive intolerance, and sources of foods in which these additives are found, please see the companion book, *Dealing with Food Allergies*.[4]

---

[a] Please see Chapter 1 for a definition of food intolerance.

[b] For more information on the process, please see Reference 4.

MANAGEMENT OF FOOD-ASSOCIATED ASTHMA

If you suspect that certain foods trigger wheezing or asthma symptoms in your child, your first action should be a consultation with your pediatrician to determine the exact inventory of foods your child is allergic to. The doctor will probably refer you to a pediatric allergist, or may carry out the tests him- or herself to identify your child's reactive foods. (Please see Chapter 5, Diagnosis of Food Allergy.) It is essential that once you know your child's food allergens, you remove all sources of them from his or her diet, and provide alternative foods with equal nutritive value to ensure that your child receives complete and balanced nutrition for optimum growth and development.

Food allergy contributes to asthma only in limited cases. Because there are so many other asthma triggers that contribute to the condition—inhaled dust mites, mold spores, animal dander, pollens, and so on—it is very unlikely that removing the allergenic foods will allow you to completely control your child's asthma. It is most probable that food allergy is making your child's asthma worse rather than being solely responsible for triggering its symptoms. The role of food allergy as aggravator, not the sole cause, of asthma increases as children grow older.

Nevertheless, it is possible to gain some idea of whether and which foods are triggering wheezing and asthma by carrying out a food challenge. Introduce suspect foods individually and monitor the child's symptoms, following a period of having avoided the suspect food. (See Chapter 6, Elimination and Challenge, for details.) Food challenge procedures should be conducted under the supervision of a physician because the symptoms—if and when they are triggered—must be controlled with appropriate medication. Changes in airway response during food challenge can be measured in older children with a peak flow meter (or by using an instrument called a spirometer[c]). The physician will rely on symptoms alone to monitor infants' pulmonary function during food challenge.

The food allergy associated with asthma in childhood is no different from the food allergy that causes other symptoms. The offending foods must be

---

[c] A spirometer is an instrument that measures the air taken into and exhaled from the lungs.

avoided as long as the child presents symptoms after eating the foods. Parents and caregivers must become familiar with terms printed on product labels, and with the entire range of food products in which the allergen may be present as a minor, or even hidden, ingredient.

After long-term avoidance of the offending foods, many children outgrow their food allergies. Subsequent periodic challenge with the offending food should therefore be undertaken to determine whether your child remains allergic to it. The results of skin and blood tests tend to remain positive long after symptoms have resolved, so direct challenge with the offending food is usually necessary. Once a food ceases to cause problems, it should be eaten regularly to maintain tolerance.

An asthmatic child is likely to be sensitive to ingredients in manufactured foods which will tend to make their asthma worse. This type of food intolerance is not usually outgrown. It tends to persist into adulthood and to increase the response to an allergen as long as the asthma continues. Asthmatic children should not consume manufactured foods containing artificial colors and preservatives. Unfortunately, this includes most of the candies and other brightly colored and artificially flavored high-sugar foods and beverages that the average child sees as "treats". The parents of asthmatic children need to put in place an alternative way of rewarding the child, so that the asthma is not perceived as a "punishment" of withholding pleasures in addition to the misery of the condition itself. In dealing with my own asthmatic children, I developed a system of "bartering" in which the undesirable foods had relative values that could be exchanged for a desired object. In my son's case this was a collection of miniature cars, Star Wars figurines, replica football team helmets, and so on, that he still treasures as an adult. This exchange system worked especially well for Halloween. With the exchange system, my son still had the pleasure of dressing up and "trick or treating" but had no desire to eat the chocolates and candies that he collected. They were valuable to him as a means of exchange for more treasured items.

The most frequently reported food additives that exacerbate asthma are artificial food dyes, especially tartrazine, and preservatives such as benzoates and sulfites. Interestingly, food coloring agents and benzoates are the additives that have been most often associated with hyperactivity in children. Details about avoiding these additives can be found in Chapter 19, "Hyperactivity and Food." It is a good idea to start with the food plan described in that chapter, with the additional elimination of sulfites (a list of foods containing sulfites can be found in Appendix H) to determine whether your asthmatic child benefits from such dietary management strategies.

PREVENTION OF ASTHMA IN THE FOOD-ALLERGIC CHILD

Although avoidance or late introduction of highly allergenic foods is thought to prevent food allergy in young infants, the vast majority of studies seem to agree that the early food restriction has no effect on respiratory allergies such as asthma and hay fever after about age 2. By the age of 5 to 7 all benefit of early food avoidance on any allergy except food allergy is lost.[5] The number of children with asthma and hay fever tends to be exactly the same, whether their diet was restricted in infancy or not. This indicates that inhaled allergens predominate in older children with respiratory allergy. Foods probably contribute very little to these conditions, except for their role in aggravating the situation when inflammatory mediators are released in the food-induced allergy, or when food additives enhance the production of inflammatory mediators responsible for the bronchospasm of asthma.

References

1. Bock SA. Respiratory reactions induced by food challenges in children with pulmonary disease. *Pediatric Allergy and Immunology* 1992;3:188–194.

2. Sicherer SH, Sampson HA. The role of food allergy in childhood asthma. *Immunology and Allergy Clinics of North America* 1998;18(1):49–60.

3. Hill DJ, Firer MA, Shelton MJ, et al. Manifestations of milk allergy in infancy: Clinical and immunological findings. *Journal of Pediatrics* 1986;109:270–276.

4. Joneja JMV. *Dealing with Food Allergies.* Boulder CO: Bull Publishing Company, 2003.

5. Zeiger R, Heller S. The development and prediction of atopy in high-risk children: Follow-up at seven years in a prospective randomized study of combined maternal and infant food allergen avoidance. *Journal of Allergy and Clinical Immunology* 1995;95:1179–1190.

CHAPTER 24

Immunologically Mediated Adverse Reactions to Foods in Childhood: Food Allergy, Food Intolerance, or Something Else?

As the definition of food allergy has expanded to encompass any immunological response to food components that results in symptoms when the food is consumed,[1] a number of conditions are now included in the definition of the term *food allergy* that were previously excluded.

EOSINOPHILIC ESOPHAGITIS

A prime example is eosinophilic esophagitis (EE).[2] Before 1995 this condition, which mainly affects children and young adults (rarely babies), was thought to be associated with esophageal reflux disease. More recent research has identified an allergic component of the disease in which immune cells characteristic of allergic conditions such as asthma and hay fever (allergic rhinitis)—called eosinophils—are present in significant numbers. Because most studies suggest that an immunological response to foods can be an important precipitating event, many allergists consider EE to be a distinct type of food allergy.

Eosinophils are white blood cells (also called leukocytes) that are often found in tissues where an inflammatory response is occurring (for example, where the inflammation associated with asthma occurs in the lungs or where the inflammation associated with hay fever occurs in the upper respiratory tract). Eosinophils are also found in abundance in the intestinal canal in such disorders as inflammatory bowel disease and in infections caused by such parasites as helminths and nematode worms, among others.

In EE, a large buildup of eosinophils develops in the esophagus, the muscular canal that connects the mouth to the stomach. Eosinophils are rarely seen in this location in healthy people. Eosinophils are granulocytes. Like other granulocytes (such as mast cells and basophils), they contain inflammatory chemicals (mediators). The inflammatory mediators are released from the eosinophils, act on local tissues in the esophagus, and cause inflammation.

Eosinophilic esophagitis differs from the type of food allergy that typically results in such symptoms as hives and swelling (angioedema), digestive disorders (including vomiting, painful diarrhea, bloating), and in severe cases anaphylaxis. These conditions are triggered by the IgE antibodies that are produced against a specific food and that cause the release of inflammatory mediators from mast cells. We do not see any food-specific IgE in EE. In EE it is eosinophils, not mast cells, that release the inflammatory mediators.

Symptoms of Eosinophilic Esophagitis

Children with EE frequently experience these symptoms typical of the disease:[3]

- Vomiting

- Regurgitation of food

- Difficulty in swallowing (e.g., food said to be "sticking on the way down")

- Choking on food

- Heartburn and chest pain

- Water brash (regurgitation of a sour fluid or nearly tasteless saliva that contains no food material)

- Poor eating

- Failure to thrive (poor or no weight gain, weight loss)

Although the symptoms of EE resemble gastroesophageal reflux disease (GERD), the reflux of EE does not respond to customary antireflux therapy. The medications typically used to suppress the gastric acid and control regurgitation in GERD provide no relief to EE sufferers.

Eosinophilic esophagitis occurs in toddlers, older children, and adults but rarely in babies. In adults EE typically persists for many years—even indefinitely. In infants the symptoms frequently clear up in the first few years, especially when they are triggered by a few specific foods that can be removed from the baby's diet early on. When the symptoms arise in older children and young adults, they usually last for many years. Boys are more frequently affected than girls.

Diagnosis of Eosinophilic Esophagitis

The symptoms of EE are so distinctive, your doctor will suspect the condition when you describe them. He or she will refer you to a gastroenterologist, a specialist in stomach and digestive tract diseases, who will look at the child's esophagus with an endoscope and take a tissue sample (biopsy) for evaluation by a pathologist. The presence of large numbers of eosinophils will confirm the diagnosis. The gastroenterologist may also order the drawing of a blood sample. A higher than normal level of eosinophils in the blood will also suggest the diagnosis of EE.

Other evidence that the disease is indeed EE is the finding that the usual antireflux medications are of no benefit, but that elimination diets are often helpful, suggesting an underlying food allergy or intolerance as a triggering event. Medications to reduce inflammation, typically corticosteroids such as Prednisone, are effective in treating the symptoms of EE. Elimination diets are also helpful.

Potential Causes of Eosinophilic Esophagitis

Although IgE-mediated food allergy does not seem to be involved in EE, there are some foods frequently associated with the condition. In this sense we can

consider EE to be a variant of food allergy. The foods most frequently reported to be triggers of EE are the same ones involved in the majority of cases of
IgE-mediated food allergy:

- Egg
- Cow's milk
- Soy
- Wheat
- Corn
- Peanuts
- Tree nuts
- Shellfish
- Fish

Eosinophilic Esophagitis May Result from Pollen or Food Allergy

Even though EE is not caused by IgE-mediated allergy, as many as 80 percent
of patients with EE report such symptoms of allergy as hay fever or asthma.
Because the immunological response in hay fever and asthma typically leads
to a large number of eosinophils in the respiratory tract, it has been theorized
that the close proximity of the upper-gastrointestinal (GI) tract tissues to the
inflamed tissues of the upper respiratory tract may result in infiltration of the
eosinophils associated with asthma and hayfever into the esophageal tissues,
causing EE. This theory remains to be proven.

Some patients with EE find that their symptoms appear only during the
seasons in which they are exposed to their allergenic pollen. This observation
would seem to reinforce the hypothesis of the respiratory allergy–EE connection, because active allergy to pollen will result in large numbers of
eosinophils in the upper airways and lungs.

Not All Eosinophilic Esophagitis Is Related to Allergy

Close to one quarter of EE sufferers present no evidence of allergy. Some have
underlying conditions that can cause similar inflammation in the digestive

tract. Children in this group will not respond to diet manipulation, but may respond to medication.

It is puzzling to observe that some children do feel better when certain foods are removed from their diet—even in cases when, upon examination, their doctors still find evidence of inflammation in the esophagus. This suggests that although the foods contribute to the symptoms in these cases, in fact the foods are only aggravating the symptoms and are not involved in causing them.

If EE is left untreated, the inflammation may damage the esophagus, resulting in narrowing of the canal (known as stricture) and an increase in the fibrous tissue surrounding it (known as fibrosis). It is therefore essential that any child with the symptoms listed above be immediately seen by their pediatrician for examination, diagnosis, and treatment.

Dietary Management of Eosinophilic Esophagitis

Because IgE-mediated food allergy is not a cause of EE, skin tests and blood tests for allergen-specific IgE will be of no value in identifying foods that may be involved. We do know that certain foods can trigger EE or aggravate EE, making it definitely worthwhile to find out whether your child will benefit from eliminating foods from the diet. The most important questions ask (1) which foods should be avoided, and (2) how to tell which foods are actually associated with the condition.

The foods most frequently associated with EE (listed above in the section on Potential Causes of EE) should be removed from your child's diet for a defined period to see whether his or her symptoms improve. While the foods are being avoided, replace them with foods of nutritional equivalence so that your child is never at risk for nutritional deficiency. Carefully follow the dietary directives in Chapter 16, The Top Ten Allergenic Foods. Ask your child's pediatrician or gastroenterologist to refer you to a registered dietitian for personalized assistance in this process.

At the end of the period of food avoidance, separately reintroduce each food, in increasingly larger quantities, while you monitor the child's symptoms. This should give you a good idea of whether a suspect food is causing a problem. If reintroducing the food makes no difference in your child's wellbeing, it can be continued as part of his or her regular diet. If the reintroduced food triggers symptoms or makes existing symptoms worse, the food should be permanently removed from your child's regular diet.

Your child's symptoms may improve over time, so you will want to try again to reintroduce the suspect foods one at a time, again carefully monitoring your child's reactions. If you find that your child has outgrown some of the earlier reactions to food triggers, he or she will now be able to eat the foods without problems. If the foods continue to provoke an adverse reaction, they will have to be avoided for the long term.

Please read Chapter 6, Elimination and Challenge, for detailed information on this process of removal and reintroduction of suspect foods. It is essential that all the nutrients required for your child's growth and healthy development be provided in his or her diet, in spite of the limitations of a food-restricted diet. Please refer to Appendix E for information regarding alternative sources of the nutrients that will be deficient when important food groups need to be avoided for the long term.

FOOD PROTEIN–INDUCED ENTEROCOLITIS SYNDROME

Food protein–induced enterocolitis syndrome (FPIES) is another condition triggered by foods but not mediated by IgE. The symptoms of FPIES in infants typically include profuse vomiting and diarrhea, which can progress to dehydration and shock in severe cases. Because FPIES is not mediated by IgE, the results of skin tests and blood tests including the radio allergosorbent test (RAST), for IgE-mediated allergy, are typically negative.

Most reports of FPIES indicate that the condition develops in response to food proteins and results from digestive tract and immunological immaturity. Symptoms develop in the young infant after exposure to certain proteins in foods. Early reports indicated that cow's milk and soy proteins, common ingredients in infant formula, were the most frequent causes of the reaction. Milk- and soy-associated FPIES usually starts within the first year of life, most frequently within the first 6 or 7 months as a result of exposure to the proteins in infant formulas. When solids foods are introduced, these other foods may cause the condition.[4] Foods that have been identified in individual cases as triggers of FPIES include cereals (oats, barley, rice); legumes (peas, peanuts, lentils);[5] vegetables (sweet potato, squash); poultry (chicken, turkey); and egg.[6] Removal of the culprit foods leads to immediate recovery from the symptoms. After the child has avoided the offending foods for a period, resuming consumption of them may cause a recurrence of the syndrome in which the symptoms are mild, and with symptom onset occurring after a delay of 2 or more hours, not immediately after ingestion.[7]

Cause of the Syndrome

The immune system reaction in FPIES appears to involve T helper cells that release TNF-α, which is typical of a Th1 response. This is in contrast to allergy, in which a Th2 response releases the cytokines that result in the production of IgE. (For an explanation of Th1 and Th2 responses, please refer to Chapter 1, What Is Food Allergy?) In addition, a low level of TGF-β, the cytokine most frequently involved in developing tolerance to foods, suggests that a lack of immunological tolerance causes the immune system to treat the food as if it were a threat to the body's health and survival.[8] The subsequent release of inflammatory mediators (in response to the entry of the offending food into the body) results in the "defensive" symptoms of copious vomiting and diarrhea.

Breast-feeding and FPIES

Most reports of FPIES indicate that exclusive breast-feeding is protective in potential cases of FPIES.[9] None of the infants who later developed FPIES after the introduction of solids had symptoms while being exclusively breast-fed. Authors of these studies suggest that, while being breast-fed, babies with FPIES were sensitized to the proteins through an infant formula given during a period of immunological susceptibility.

Diagnosis of FPIES

There are no diagnostic tests for FPIES at present. The clinical picture of development of acute symptoms immediately after consumption of the offending foods (often milk- or soy-based infant formula), together with the absence of positive tests for food allergy, will usually alert your child's pediatrician to the possibility that FPIES is the cause of the problem.

Management of FPIES

Like food allergy, FPIES is managed by avoiding the food that triggers the child's symptoms. In most cases, a reaction to milk- and soy-based formula with severe vomiting and diarrhea, without other signs of allergy such as skin reactions, is suggestive of the diagnosis. Elimination and challenge of the suspect foods, under the supervision of your child's pediatrician, will usually confirm the syndrome. In most cases you will be advised to delay introducing solid foods because of the possibility that, until your child's immune system has matured, a similar reaction to proteins in other foods may elicit the same response.

We are far from understanding all the different immunological and physiological mechanisms responsible for FPIES, and how to best manage the condition. Until more well-run research studies have been conducted, the wisest directive is to avoid the foods that clearly trigger FPIES (usually milk- and soy-based formulas) in the early months, and to delay the introduction of solids until after 6 or 7 months of age.[10] Undertake the introduction of solid foods with greatest caution. Follow the protocols in Chapter 3 that prescribe the method and sequence for introducing solid foods. Adhering to these conventions will enable you to detect any adverse response to FPIES triggers upon your child's first exposure to them.

Exclusive breast-feeding is the best prevention against early development of FPIES. If the infant has already developed FPIES, the lactating mother should remove all milk and soy from her own diet. If the baby who has developed the syndrome is formula-fed, an extensively hydrolyzed casein formula (ehf) such as Nutramigen®, Alimentum®, or Pregestimil® may be tolerated. If the baby cannot tolerate an ehf, the pediatrician will probably recommend an elemental formula such as Neocate®.

Most babies outgrow FPIES by age 2 or 3, when their immune and digestive systems have matured. If a child has exhibited symptoms of FPIES and the offending foods have been avoided, the foods can be reintroduced, usually under medical supervision, at about age 2 years or later.

FOOD PROTEIN–INDUCED PROCTITIS, OR PROCTOCOLITIS

It's easy to understand parents' concern over finding flecks of blood, often mixed with mucus, in the stool of their apparently healthy baby. Food protein–induced proctitis, or proctocolitis (FPIP), is often the cause.[11] The condition typically appears in the first few months of life, on average at the age of 2 months. The absence of other symptoms (such as vomiting, diarrhea, failure to thrive) usually rules out food allergy or food protein enteropathy as the cause of blood in the stool. The blood loss is usually very slight, and anemia as a consequence of loss of blood is rare. A diagnosis of FPIP is usually made after other conditions that could account for the blood, (for example, anal fissure, infection) have been ruled out.

Cow's milk proteins and soy proteins are the most common triggers of food-protein proctitis. Many babies develop the symptoms during breast-feeding in response to milk and soy in the mother's diet.[12]

Causes and Management of Food Protein–Induced Proctitis, or Proctocolitis

Although the exact cause of FPIP is unknown, it does not involve IgE, so tests for allergy are usually negative. In most cases, avoidance of the offending food leads to resolution of the problem. When the baby is breast-fed, elimination of milk and soy from the mother's diet is usually enough to resolve the infant's symptoms. Occasionally egg can cause the symptoms, in which case mother must avoid all sources of egg in her diet as well.[13] When the baby is formula-fed, an extensively hydrolyzed infant formula (ehf) such as Nutramigen® will often lead to recovery, although a few babies do develop symptoms on an ehf. In these cases an elemental formula such as Neocate® is usually the answer. Bleeding usually disappears within 72 hours of exclusion of the protein responsible for the reaction.

In most cases, the disorder resolves by the age of 1 or 2 years. After this age, the offending foods may be gradually reintroduced with careful monitoring for reappearance of blood in the baby's stool.

CELIAC DISEASE: GLUTEN-SENSITIVE ENTEROPATHY

Another disease that is caused by an adverse reaction to specific foods, mediated by the immune system but not an IgE-mediated allergy, is celiac disease, or gluten-sensitive enteropathy (previously referred to as celiac sprue).

Celiac disease is a genetically inherited condition that affects the small intestine. Gluten in certain cereal grains (such as wheat, rye, barley) triggers an immune response that results in damage to the cells in the epithelium lining the intestines (called brush border cells). Protruding from these cells are numerous projections, called villi, that serve to increase the total surface area over which food can be absorbed into circulation. In celiac disease, the brush border cells are "attacked" by components of the immune system, causing damage to the villi. Under a microscope, the damaged villus appears flattened and distorted—the clearest diagnostic indicator of celiac disease. Damage to the villi impedes absorption of food across the epithelial lining of the intestine, which prevents the child with celiac disease from absorbing nutrients efficiently and causes weight loss or failure to thrive. In addition, celiac disease allows unabsorbed food materials to pass into the colon where they ferment and result in the gas, bloating, and diarrhea typical of the disorder.

The components of cereal grains that can cause this immunological response are in the gluten fraction of wheat, rye, and barley—more specifically, the alpha-gliadin component of glutens (in wheat), hordeins (in barley), and secalins (in rye).

Although celiac disease can be diagnosed at any age, it appears most commonly in early childhood (between 9 and 24 months) and in the third or fourth decade of life. Close to the same number of girls as boys have the disease, although in adults, twice as many women as men are diagnosed with it.

Recent reports indicate that celiac disease is much more common than previously thought, affecting about 1 in 250 people. The increase in incidence can be explained by doctors' greater awareness of the disease, and by the fact that many more symptoms than previously recognized are now included in the diagnosis. Over the last 20 years, more accurate immunological tests have been developed and biopsy techniques have been used more frequently, resulting in many more individuals being investigated for and diagnosed with celiac disease.[14]

Symptoms of Celiac Disease

The symptoms of celiac disease most commonly begin in children younger than 1 year old, although the condition can manifest at any age, sometimes well into adulthood.

Celiac disease was once thought to be characterized by the "classic" symptoms of the gastrointestinal malabsorption syndrome. These included diarrhea, unabsorbed fat in the stool (steatorrhea), weight loss, fatigue, and anemia. In infants, the symptoms were understood to include chronic diarrhea, weight loss, and failure to thrive. In children, vomiting, poor appetite, short stature for their age, iron deficiency anemia, and a protuberant abdomen were the signs that alerted the clinician to the possibility of celiac disease.

These symptoms are now associated only with severe celiac disease. Most patients today are recognized to have the milder symptoms of abdominal discomfort, bloating, and indigestion, or the nongastrointestinal symptoms of fatigue and anemia. (Some patients present with no symptoms at all.)[15]

How Does Gluten Cause Celiac Disease?

Our understanding of the key steps in intestinal inflammatory response to celiac disease has increased dramatically in recent years.

The first stage in the immunological reaction sequence that ultimately leads to damage of the brush border cells is release of a specific molecule present in certain types of gluten. This molecule is found in wheat, rye, and barley glutens, but not in the gluten from any other grains. The molecule is different from the ones that are responsible for triggering IgE-mediated allergy to these grains. The so-called celiac molecule is freed from the complete protein by an enzyme called transglutaminase that is present in the digestive tract.

Celiac molecules are recognized by the immune system. Together with a specific type of "self-antigen" called HLA-DQ2 that is present in most children who inherit the tendency to develop celiac disease, the celiac molecules interact with the epithelium and cause the cell damage characteristic of the disorder.[16] In addition, research evidence suggests that this interaction weakens the tight junctions between epithelial cells, leading to increased permeability of the digestive tract lining. (For more information on digestive tract permeability and the condition known as leaky gut, please see the section in Chapter 3 titled Permeability, or "Leakiness," in the Digestive Tract.)

Celiac disease is an example of tissue damage that results in malabsorption of nutrients, not in a net increase in permeability of mucosal tissue, although the two mechanisms are not mutually exclusive. Inflammation causes tissue damage. In the case of celiac disease, the absorptive villous cells are damaged, significantly reducing their capacity to transport nutrients. However, access to antigens through the damaged epithelium is increased. This means that food molecules and other material that would normally be excluded can readily pass through the more porous epithelium. This may explain why other immunologically mediated conditions may accompany celiac disease.

Diagnosis of Celiac Disease

Celiac disease is diagnosed with the aid of highly sensitive immunological tests. The tests identify antibodies in blood that are produced against antigens that arise when celiac disease causes damage to tissues. When the tests are positive, the diagnosis is confirmed through microscopic examination of biopsied samples taken from the lining of the intestine.

Testing for celiac-related antibodies in children younger than 5 may be unreliable. However, because celiac disease is hereditary, first-degree relatives—such as the parents, siblings, and offspring—of patients diagnosed with the disease may wish to be tested for it. Between 5 and 15 percent of the first-degree relatives of a person with celiac disease generally also have it. About 3 to 8 percent of people with type 1 diabetes will have biopsy-confirmed celiac disease, and 5 to 10 percent of people with Down syndrome will be diagnosed with celiac disease.

Previously IgA antibodies against gliadin and reticulin (a connective tissue component released when tissue damage occurs), and an antiendomysial antibody formed against transglutaminase in blood were measured in active cases of celiac disease. These antibodies disappear when a gluten-free diet is followed. Today's modern tests, which detect the presence of sIgA antibodies against transglutaminase, have proven to be more reliable than any of the older methods.[17] The presence of these antibodies in blood is an indication that celiac disease may be the cause of a patient's symptoms. However, because of false positive and false negative reactions associated with the tests, a diagnosis of celiac disease cannot be based solely on the presence of these antibodies. False negative reactions can result from an IgA deficiency sometimes associated with the condition, and false positive reactions appear more frequently in communities where other causes of enteropathy are common (for example where intestinal parasites are endemic), and when an inflammatory bowel disease (such as Crohn's disease) is involved.[18]

Positive immunological tests are almost always followed by examination of the cells lining the digestive tract. These are taken by biopsy using a long, thin tube called an endoscope. In the biopsy, the doctor removes a tiny piece of tissue from the small intestine to check for damage to the villi. To obtain the tissue, the doctor eases the endoscope through the mouth and stomach into the small intestine, and takes the sample using instruments passed through the endoscope. Changes in the appearance of the brush border cells' villi tell the pathologist that celiac disease is present.

In a child, symptoms of celiac disease quickly resolve when all sources of the gluten responsible for the disease are removed from his or her diet. Strict avoidance of wheat, rye, and barley lead to recovery of the intestinal villi. They return to their normal shape and the IgA antibodies associated with celiac disease disappear from blood. This means that if the child has been on a gluten-free diet for about 1 month before the test, there will be no evidence of the disease. For the tests to be valid, therefore, the child must consume gluten regularly for at least two to four weeks prior to the test so that evidence of the disease can be detected. Eating gluten may cause temporary digestive tract distress, but is nevertheless necessary if an accurate diagnosis is to be made.

An accurate diagnosis is essential because celiac disease is a lifelong condition. Gluten must be avoided throughout life for the patient to remain symptom-free and avoid the condition's complications. The complications of celiac disease may include the consequences of chronic malabsorption of essential nutrients, such as osteoporosis and iron deficiency anemia, and a troublesome skin condition called dermatitis herpetiformis. In addition, there is evidence that, in extreme cases, certain malignancies in the digestive tract may result from untreated celiac disease. However, if the results of all the tests for celiac disease are negative, there is no reason to subject the child to the often cumbersome and tedious dietary restrictions of a gluten-free diet.

Management of Celiac Disease

All of the acute symptoms in the gastrointestinal (GI) tract resolve when all sources of gluten are removed from the diet. This diet requires complete avoidance of wheat, rye, and barley, and of all foods containing them or their derivatives. For most people, following a gluten-free diet will end the symptoms, heal existing intestinal damage, and prevent further damage. Improvements begin within days of starting the diet. The small intestine usually heals completely in 3 to 6 months in children and younger adults, and within 2 years for older adults.

Lifelong adherence to the dietary restrictions is essential because tissue damage and resulting symptoms recur rapidly when gluten is reintroduced. Within a few hours of eating gluten, damage can be detected in microscope preparations of epithelial tissue. It is important that celiac disease be detected early because of the grave risk of developing more persistent conditions, especially the malignancies, associated with celiac disease.

Oats and Celiac Disease

Oats were once excluded from the diet of persons living with celiac disease. However, studies in 1995[19] demonstrated that after 6 to 12 months, patients with celiac disease who had avoided wheat, rye, and barley but had continued to consume oats presented no signs of the disease. Subsequent studies have confirmed these results in children.[20]

In some cases, concern has continued over children with celiac disease who continue to eat oats. There is evidence that imported oats may be contaminated with the gluten of other gluten-containing grains. In general, however, pediatricians and dietitians have encouraged the consumption of oats to liberalize the gluten-free diet and encourage compliance by children and adults alike. A few patients have been reported to show both clinical and immunological responses to a pure-oat product, so signs and symptoms of the disease should be carefully monitored in children who are consuming oats while on a gluten-free diet.[21]

Guidelines for a gluten-free diet that excludes wheat, rye, barley, and oats is provided in Appendix C. When the child's symptoms resolve, oats and oat products can be reintroduced to the diet in increasingly larger servings. If symptoms remain latent, oats can be eaten regularly—provided the child's symptoms are carefully monitored, and the oats are immediately removed at the earliest sign of digestive tract disturbance.

For more information on celiac disease and its management, consult the very informative U.S. National Institutes of Health Web site on Digestive Diseases at http://digestive.niddk.nih.gov/ddiseases/pubs/celiac/#4

OTHER FOOD-ASSOCIATED INTESTINAL ENTEROPATHIES

A number of other foods, including soy-based products and cow's milk, have been found to cause alterations in children's small intestinal mucosa that are similar to those of celiac disease. Occasionally implicated as the cause of food-associated enteropathy are cereal grains, egg, and seafood.[22] The symptoms of dietary protein enteropathy characteristically include diarrhea and vomiting with resulting malabsorption of nutrients, typically resulting in slow or no weight gain—the condition known as failure to thrive. These enteropathies, like celiac disease, are not IgE-mediated allergies, so all tests for allergy will have negative results. Unlike celiac disease, which is a lifelong condition, these changes in the cells of the small intestine are usually of short duration and improve quickly when the offending food is avoided. Most children outgrow food-associated enteropathies within 1 to 2 years. The immunological mechanism that causes the damage in these cases remains to be determined.

References

1. Johansson SGO, Hourihane JOB, Bousquet J, Bruijnzeel-Koomen C, Dreborg S, Haahtela T, Kowalski ML, Mygind N, Ring J, van Cauwenberge P, van Hage-Hamsten M, Wüthrich B. A revised nomenclature for allergy. An EAACI position statement from the EAACI nomenclature task force. *Allergy* 2001;56:813–824.

2. Liacouras, CA and Ruchelli E. Eosinophilic esophagitis. *Current Opinion in Pediatrics* 2004; 16(5):560–566.

3. Liacouras, CA. Eosinophilic esophagitis in children and adults. *Journal of Pediatric Gastroenterology and Nutrition* 2003; 37 Suppl 1:S23–28.

4. Nowak-Wegrzyn A, Sampson HA, Wood RA, Sicherer SH. Food protein–induced enterocolitis syndrome caused by solid food proteins. *Pediatrics* 2003;111:829–835.

5. Levy Y, Danon YL. Food protein–induced enterocolitis syndrome—Not only to cow's milk and soy. *Pediatric Allergy and Immunology* 2003;14(4):325–329.

6. Nowak-Wegrzyn et al. Food protein–induced enterocolitis syndrome caused by solid food proteins.

7. Nowak-Wegrzyn et al. Food protein–induced enterocolitis syndrome caused by solid food proteins.

8. Chung HL, Hwang JB, Park JJ, Kim SG. Expression of transforming growth factor β1, transforming growth factor type I and II receptors, and TNF-α in the mucosa of the small intestine in infants with food protein–induced enterocolitis syndrome. *Journal of Allergy and Clinical Immunology* 2002;109:15–154.

9. Nowak-Wegrzyn et al. Food protein–induced enterocolitis syndrome caused by solid food proteins.

10. Nowak-Wegrzyn et al. Food protein–induced enterocolitis syndrome caused by solid food proteins.

11. Sicherer SH. Clinical aspects of gastrointestinal food allergy in childhood. *Pediatrics* 2003;111(6):1609–1616.

12. Anveden HL, Finkel Y, Sandstedt B, Karpe B. Proctocolitis in exclusively breast-fed infants. *European Journal of Pediatrics* 1996;155:464–467.

13. Sicherer SH. Clinical aspects of gastrointestinal food allergy in childhood. *Pediatrics* 2003;111(6):1609–1616.

14. Van Heel DA, West J. Recent advances in celiac disease. *Gut* 2006;55:1037–1046.

15. American Gastroenterological Association medical position statement: Celiac sprue. *Gastroenterology* 2001;120:1522–1525.

16. Nowak-Wegrzyn et al. Food protein–induced enterocolitis syndrome caused by solid food proteins.

17. Nowak-Wegrzyn et al. Food protein–induced enterocolitis syndrome caused by solid food proteins.

18. Calabuig M, Torregosa R, Polo P, Tomas C, Alvarez V, Garcia-Vila A, Brines J, Vilar P, Farre C, et al. Serological markers and celiac disease: A new diagnostic approach? *Journal of Pediatric Gastroenterology and Nutrition* 1990;10(4):435–442.

19. Janatuinen EK, Pikkarainen PH, Kemppainen TA, et al. A comparison of diets with and without oats in adults with celiac disease. *New England Journal of Medicine* 1995;333:1033–1037.

20. Hogberg L, Laurin P, Falth-Magnusson K, et al. Oats to children with newly diagnosed coeliac disease: A randomised double-blind study. *Gut* 2004;53:649–654.

21. Lundin KE, Nilsen EM, Scott HG, et al. Oats induced villous atrophy in coeliac disease. *Gut* 2003;52:1649–1652.

22. Sicherer. Clinical aspects of gastrointestinal food allergy in childhood.

CHAPTER 25

Probiotics and Allergy

There are about 10^{12} to 10^{14a} fairly harmless microorganisms in 1 mL (0.20 of a teaspoon) of the contents of the gastrointestinal tract of the healthy human, mostly in the large bowel. More than 500 different species of these microorganisms have been identified. Taken together, they weigh more than one kilo (2.2 pounds) of our body weight. These microorganisms are essential for the health of not only the intestines, but the whole body. Laboratory rats that are born and reared in a completely sterile environment, so that they never have microorganisms in their digestive tract, quickly sicken and die. Like rats and other mammals, we humans are dependent on our digestive tract microorganisms for achieving and maintaining optimal health.

There are several ways the microorganisms in our digestive tract help us:

- They break down undigested food that moves into the bowel from the small intestine (where most of the digestion of food and absorption of nutrients take place). Micronutrients such as vitamin K, biotin, thiamin, vitamin B_{12}, and folate are produced as a result of their metabolic activities. We absorb these vitamins, and they form an essential part of our nutritional resources.

---

[a] To understand these numbers, write down 1 and add the number of 0s in the superscript (10^{12} = 1,000,000,000,000, or one trillion).

- Microorganisms in the large bowel defend the bowel from invasion by nonessential, even harmful, microorganisms by competing with them for space and nutrients.

- Microorganisms in the large bowel also perform a vital role in stimulating the immune system of the digestive tract, which is known as gut-associated lymphoid tissue (GALT). Constant interaction between microorganisms and immune cells maintains a healthy balance that aids in the defense of GALT against invasion by potential pathogens (known as the Th1 response). The constant interaction is also how balance between the Th1 and Th2 response to microorganisms and foods may be maintained in oral tolerance. (For a discussion of oral tolerance and Th1 and Th2 responses in allergy, please refer to Chapter 1, What Is Allergy?)

- Research in the past decade indicates that the risk for allergy in infants may be reduced by using probiotic bacteria to maintain a good bacterial balance in pregnant mothers and to modulate intestinal flora in infants. Research also seems to indicate that some strains of bacteria have the potential to speed recovery from food allergy in babies and children (discussed in more detail later in this chapter).

WHICH MICROORGANISMS LIVE IN THE BOWEL?

The environment of the bowel determines precisely which microorganisms survive there. Factors that determine which species survive in the bowel include the presence or absence of oxygen (measured as eH); the degree of acidity or alkalinity (measured as pH); whether nutrients passing through the bowel are in solid, liquid, or gaseous form; interaction with other microorganisms and their metabolic products; and how well the immune system of the gut tolerates the microorganisms.

Once the microbial flora is established—usually soon after weaning (soon after solid foods are introduced)—it remains more or less unchanged throughout life unless significant modifying events occur within the gut environment. People living in the same household who eat more or less the same diet may have in their bowel vastly different microorganisms (referred to as the indigenous microflora, or microbiota). Even if many species succumb to oral antibiotics used in treating an infection, over time the microorganisms that were present prior to the antibiotic therapy become reestablished in more or less the same proportions.

Many studies have indicated the possible value of modifying the indigenous microflora, especially in situations where existing microbial activity appears to be detrimental. However, this can be quite a challenge. Once the microflora is established, it can be likened to a city in which all the houses are occupied by people of a specific race and culture. Introduction of a new group of residents with different dietary and ethnic practices will require not only displacing the established population, but also providing the nutrients and environment required by the "immigrants" to allow them to survive and flourish. This is where the science of probiotics fits in with the populating of the large bowel.

WHAT ARE PROBIOTICS?

The term probiotic was coined in the early 1990s to describe a culture of living microorganisms within a food designed to provide health benefits beyond its inherent nutritional value.[1] The types of microorganisms used in such foods must have certain characteristics to be of any value: specifically, they must have a beneficial effect within the bowel, and they must be capable of living within the human bowel without causing any harm.

In order to colonize the area, the microorganisms must survive passage through the hostile environment of the stomach (which is very acidic) and upper small intestine; resist the effects of intestinal secretions, including evading the effects of digestive enzymes and bile salts; attach to intestinal cells on reaching the large bowel; and thrive within their physiological and nutritional milieu.[2]

It is thought that probiotic microorganisms alter the gut microflora by competitively interacting with the existing flora through the production of chemicals that are toxic to other microorganisms (called antimicrobial metabolites), or possibly by affecting the local immune response within the digestive tract so that it becomes hostile to the indigenous microorganisms.[3]

The microorganisms most frequently used in probiotics are human strains of lactobacilli, bifidobacteria, and a few enterococci. Given the enormous number of different species resident in the healthy human digestive tract, it is probable that many more types of bacteria will be identified as beneficial in the future. At present, however, research is being directed toward the saccharolytic strains,[b] which use sugar for their nutrition and multiplication. These seem to promise the greatest benefit.

HOW DO PROBIOTICS WORK?

The value of the probiotic microorganism lies in its ability to produce chemicals that are beneficial to the body. Microorganisms act on the substrate (nutrients) available to them, and produce end products that are determined by (1) the enzymes they are able to produce, and (2) the environment in which they are growing. The substrate and environment can be readily manipulated in the laboratory, where most microbiological studies have been conducted. However, within the complex environment of the bowel it is not so easy to achieve the desired end products.

In order to ensure that the desirable microorganisms survive in the colon and generate end products of greatest benefit, current research is focused on not only the appropriate selection of the strains of microorganisms to be incorporated into the probiotic food, but also on the substrate that will yield the desired end products. The term prebiotic has been coined for the substrate; synbiotic refers to the combination of the specific microbial strain (probiotic) with its specifically designed prebiotic. It is hoped that this new research will allow colonic colonization by the beneficial microorganism and will decrease the undesirable strains as a more healthy environment is established under the influence of increasing numbers of probiotic strains.

---

[b] Saccharolytic strains are microorganisms that use a sugar as a source of nutrients, and whose products result from the breakdown, or fermentation, of the sugar.

PREBIOTICS

Much of the research on prebiotics has centered on the oligosaccharides, carbohydrates consisting of chains whose construction ranges from 3 to 10 glucose molecules and which are indigestible by human enzymes. The indigestibility of oligosaccharides means they will pass unchanged into the large bowel, where they will provide a substrate for nutrition and for multiplication of the bacteria that are being introduced. The deposition of undigested oligosaccharides into the large bowel is akin to sending a population into an unknown region, together with food packages to ensure their survival! In the United States and Europe, the fructo-oligosaccharides (FOS, also called fructans) and inulin are the most common oligosaccharides in use as prebiotics because of their economy of manufacture and their proven value in human health.[4] Galacto-oligosaccharides (GOS) are also coming on the market in Europe and the United States, but are not presently as widely used as the fructans. Many more oligosaccharides—including isomalto-oligosaccharides, soybean oligosaccharides (raffinose and stachyose), xylo-oligosaccharides, and gentio-oligosaccharides—are available in Japan. Unfortunately, the precise metabolism of these substrates by specific strains of probiotic bacteria has only recently begun to be studied. Furthermore, if the substrate is not provided continuously, the newly introduced probiotic bacteria will not survive and the original inhabitants of the area will quickly return and reestablish themselves.

HOW ARE PROBIOTICS USED?

Probiotic microorganisms have been utilized in therapy for certain types of dysfunction within the colon in some quite specific ways. For example, it has been known for some time that yogurts containing live bacterial cultures of bacteria such as lactobacilli, bifidobacteria and *Streptococcus thermophilus*, assist in reducing the symptoms of lactose intolerance. The beneficial effects result from (1) the production of the enzyme beta-galactosidase (lactase) by the bacteria in the yogurt, which breaks down lactose, and (2) the thick fermented milk itself, which delays gastrointestinal transit and thus allows a longer period in which both the human and the microbial lactase enzyme can act on the milk lactose. It has been suggested that lactose tolerance in people who are deficient in lactase (see Chapter 8) may be improved by continued ingestion of small quantities of milk. There is no evidence that this will improve or affect the production of lactase in the brush border cells of the small intestine in any way, but it seems that the continued presence of lactose in the colon contributes to the establishment and multiplication of bacteria capable of synthesizing the beta-galactosidase enzyme over time. Thus, when lactose reaches the colon undigested, large numbers of the resident microflora will break down the lactose, preventing the osmotic imbalance within the colon that causes much of the distress of lactose intolerance.[5]

Probiotics may also be of benefit in fighting gastrointestinal infections associated with diarrhea. The probiotic appears to balance the intestinal flora during a period of diarrhea and enhance the immune response to the infective microorganism. After oral antibiotics have killed off some of the regular microflora, probiotics may serve to reduce the risk of diarrhea, shorten the duration of acute diarrhea, and reduce the risk of antibiotic-associated intestinal symptoms.

HOW PROBIOTICS HELP FIGHT ALLERGY

Studies in the past decade indicate that intestinal microflora may be the major source of microbial stimulation that promotes maturation of the immune system in early childhood.[6] The appropriate microbial stimulus soon after birth may be extremely important in balancing the Th1 and Th2 responses of the immune system, which are skewed at birth to the Th2 (allergy) type.[7] (For details about the Th1 and Th2 responses in the fetus and newborn, please read Chapter 1, What Is Allergy?, and Chapter 3, Prevention of Allergy.) Research studies suggest that such harmless probiotic bacteria as lactobacilli may stimulate a Th1 (protective) response in the digestive tract without causing disease. Introducing these bacteria during infancy may help halt the atopic process.

A number of studies suggest that the selection of appropriate probiotic bacterial strains may help in certain allergic conditions. At present, however, we have insufficient evidence to recommend probiotics as therapy for or prevention of allergy in regular clinical practice.[8] The use of probiotic therapy to prevent allergic disease in neonates has been demonstrated in a few studies based on the probiotic strain *Lactobacillus rhamnosus* GG. The therapy seems particularly effective in reducing the incidence and severity of atopic eczema.[9] Unfortunately, these positive results have not been repeated in studies with older patients. Researchers who attempted to achieve the same positive results of earlier studies recently published a paper reporting they found no apparent benefit from supplementation with *Lactobacillus rhamnosus* in their subject children.[10] In a Finnish study, infants with milk allergy and atopic dermatitis had milder symptoms and reduced incidence of intestinal infections when their milk formula was fortified with *lactobacilli*.[11] However, many more large-scale studies must be conducted, and much more must be learned about how microorganisms interact with the immune system in allergy prevention, before we can state with any confidence that probiotics is the answer.

WHICH ORGANISMS AND WHICH FOODS ARE PROBIOTIC?

Current evidence suggests that probiotic effects are strain-specific, meaning that each type of bacterium, once it has become established, is likely to exert a specific influence as part of the intestinal flora. Strain identity is important to link a bacterium to a specific health effect, and to enable accurate surveillance of whether the microorganism remains in the colon.[12] When the strain can be demonstrated in feces in samples taken at intervals over a significant period of time, it can be assumed that the strain has colonized and is thriving in the bowel.

Because numerous studies have reported the ability of *Streptococcus themophilus* and *Lactobacillus delbrueckii* ssp. *bulgaricus* in yogurts to enhance lactose digestion in lactose-intolerant individuals, the identity of the individual strains is not considered to be highly critical. It is the final product—in this case, yogurt—that is important (see the discussion of yogurt that follows).

The World Health Organization[13] has recommended that each probiotic strain considered for therapeutic use in humans be investigated for its ability to

- Resist destruction by gastric acid

- Resist destruction by bile acid

- Adhere to the mucus and/or to human epithelial cells and cell lines

- Exert antimicrobial activity against potentially pathogenic bacteria

- Reduce the adhesion of pathogenic microorganisms to cell surfaces to prevent their establishment in the digestive tract

- Cause no harm to the human who consumes it

A thriving industry has developed to manufacture food products that contain live microorganisms able to sustain their growth within the food in the expectation of the organisms being delivered to the bowel to become established and thrive there. Probiotic bacteria may presently be delivered to the bowel via the oral route in yogurts (bioyogurts), fermented milks, fortified fruit juice, infant formula, powders, capsules, tablets, and sprays. Each country enforces its own regulation of probiotic foods, so some of these products may not be available worldwide.

Yogurt

Yogurt (also spelled "yogourt" or "yoghurt") is a semisolid fermented milk product that originated centuries ago in Bulgaria. It is now consumed in most of the world. Although the consistency, flavor, and aroma of yogurt may vary from one region to another, the basic ingredients and processes of manufacture are essentially the same worldwide. Although the milk of various animals has been used for yogurt production, cow's milk is used most frequently in large-scale manufacture. Whole milk, partially skimmed milk, skim milk, and cream may all be used to make yogurt.

Some manufactured yogurts contain a variety of ingredients in addition to milk, including:

- Other dairy products that increase the nonfat solids content, such as

  - Concentrated skim milk

  - Nonfat dry milk

  - Whey

  - Lactose

- Sweeteners, such as:

  - Glucose

  - Sucrose

  - Aspartame

- Stabilizers, such as

  - Gelatin

  - Carboxymethyl cellulose

  - Locust bean guar gum

  - Alginates

  - Carrageenans

  - Whey protein concentrate

- Flavors, which may be natural or artificial

- Fruit preparations, which may be natural or artificial (providing flavor and color)

Most yogurts produced in North America are based on a symbiotic blend of *Streptococcus salivarius* subsp. *thermophilus* (ST) and *Lactobacillus delbrueckii* subsp. *bulgaricus* (LB). These bacteria have been demonstrated to help lactose-intolerant people digest lactose.

The metabolic products of one strain stimulate the growth of the other. These microorganisms are ultimately responsible for the formation of typical yogurt flavor and texture. The yogurt mixture coagulates during fermentation as a result of the drop in pH. The streptococci are responsible for the yogurt mixture's drop in initial pH to approximately 5.0 (on a scale where 7.0 represents neutrality, with numbers lower than 7.0 representing increasing acidity, and numbers higher than 7.0 representing increasing alkalinity). The lactobacilli are responsible for a further decrease in pH to 4.0. The following fermentation products contribute to the flavor of yogurt:

- Lactic acid

- Acetaldehyde

- Acetic acid

- Diacetyl

How to Choose Yogurt for Its Probiotic Benefit

Only choose yogurt whose label includes the statement, "Contains live culture." The best is plain yogurt, which has only two ingredients: live cultures and milk (which may be whole milk, low-fat, or skim). These products should contain at least 100 million (10^8) colony-forming units (CFUs)[c] per gram at the time of manufacture.

In some highly sweetened yogurts, the consumer is getting more calories from the sweetener than from the yogurt. Be sure to read the protein and sugar values on the label's nutrition panel. The higher the protein content and the lower the sugar content, the more actual yogurt there is in the container.

Avoid yogurt whose label includes the statement, "Heat-treated after culturing." This statement means the yogurt was pasteurized after the microorganisms were added, which defeats yogurt's purpose as a probiotic. Pasteurization also deactivates the lactase that the microorganisms produced during the manufacturing process. Therefore, two health benefits of yogurt would be completely eliminated by heating. Heat-treating yogurt trades economic gain for nutritional loss. It may prolong shelf life, but it spoils the nutrition and health food value of yogurt. Lactose-intolerant persons who can tolerate yogurt that contains live bacteria will not be able to tolerate heat-treated yogurt.

A long line of products—including yogurt-covered candies, raisins, nuts, and pretzels; and yogurt-based salad dressings and dips—includes yogurt as an ingredient but contains no live culture. These products have no probiotic value. They should be eaten for their food content alone, and for whatever value exists in their additives.

As a general rule, commercially prepared yogurts can be grouped into Best Yogurts, OK Yogurts, and Don't-Even-Buy Yogurts. The Best Yogurt contains

---

[c] Colony-forming units (CFUs) are the number of living cells capable of multiplying to form a colony when cultured on laboratory media.

only live and active cultures and milk. This yogurt is often advertised as "organic yogurt." The "OK Yogurt" contains live and active cultures, milk, and a few filler ingredients. The "Don't-Even-Buy" yogurt has a label that reads "heat-treated," and it contains added sugar and stabilizers—and much more. This product might as well be pudding.

Probiotic Desserts and Other Treats for Children

Commercial fruit yogurts often contain sugar and a variety of unwanted additives. Don't buy such products for children. Instead, buy plain yogurt made with milk and live cultures only. For children under age 5, use whole-milk yogurt rather than yogurt made from skim or fat-reduced milk. Add fresh fruit, raisins, nuts, and other natural foods tolerated by your child. Take care to avoid adding to the plain yogurt any food to which your child is allergic, but otherwise make dessert fun by providing a new plain-yogurt-and-natural-fruit combination at each meal. Because yogurt can be frozen without destroying the bacteria, yogurt popsicles and other frozen yogurt treats make excellent probiotic desserts.

Make dips for vegetables by adding herbs, garlic, and other appropriate natural additions to plain yogurt.

Other Probiotic Foods

Probiotic foods are often marketed as "functional foods," indicating that they have an added health benefit over and above their intrinsic nutritional value. Most commercially promoted products with probiotic properties contain strains of the *Lactobacillus* or *Bifidobacterium* species of bacteria. These foods are often in the form of fermented milk products. Table 25-1 lists some of the more widely available fermented milk products. This list is not exhaustive, and does not endorse any particular product; it is meant to provide examples only.

Table 25-1 SOME FERMENTED MILK-BASED PROBIOTIC FOODS	
Product and Manufacturer	**Probiotic Strains**
Dannon Activia® (Available throughout U.S. and Canada)	*Lactobacillus bulgaricus* *Streptococcus thermophilus* *Bifidobacterium lactis*
Yakult: Milk-based, yogurt-like beverage (Available in more than 26 countries in the UK, Ireland, Asia, and Latin America; first developed in Japan)	*Lactobacillus casei* var. Shirota
Danone Actimel® (Available in UK) Dannon DanActive® (Available in U.S.)	*Lactobacillus casei* var. Immunitas
Yoplait® Everybody Developed in Ireland	*Lactobacillus rhamnosus* GG
Avonmore Milk Plus (by Glanbia Foods) Advertised as the only product on the Irish market that includes *Lactobacillus* GG (LGG)	*Lactobacillus rhamnosus* GG
Olympic Dairy Products' yogurts and sour creams (Available throughout Canada)	"All of our yogurts and sour creams contain combinations of the following active bacterial cultures: *Lactobacillus acidophilus* Bifidobacteria *Streptococcus thermophilus* *Lactobacillus paracasei* subsp. *casei* *Lactobacillus delbrueckii* subsp. *bulgaricus* *Lactobacillus delbrueckii* subsp. *lactis*

Table 25-1 (continued) SOME FERMENTED MILK-BASED PROBIOTIC FOODS	
Product and Manufacturer	**Probiotic Strains**
Olympic Dairy Products' yogurts and sour creams (Available throughout Canada) (cont'd)	Our certified organic yogurts combine all five of these beneficial bacteria, which make them a truly powerful and nourishing food."*

* Product statement furnished by Olympic Dairy Products.

PROBIOTICS FOR THE MILK-ALLERGIC CHILD

Most of the readily available probiotic products are based on bacterial cultures in milk. This is because probiotic microorganisms grow easily in the bacterial cultures in milk, and stay healthy and vigorous until their post-consumption delivery to the colon. However, for the many children who are allergic to milk, yogurts are unsuitable as a means of providing the live culture.

An alternative may be one of the variety of probiotics that are sold as supplements in capsule or powdered form. In addition to the probiotic supplements now on the market, there are a number of prebiotic supplements. These allow the establishment of beneficial organisms in the bowel, along with the nutrients to get the organisms started.

However, parents are advised to be cautious in selecting a probiotic for their milk-allergic child. Not all probiotics in capsule or tablets are entirely free from milk proteins. For example, one readily-available acidophilus powder is marketed with a product information enclosure that states that the product is free from the common allergens wheat; gluten; milk; soy; yeast; sugar; egg; maltodextrin; artificial sweeteners, colorings, and flavorings; stearates; preservatives; and salicylates, and that the product "*may contain a trace of casein.*" This final phrase should alert parents and caregivers of the milk-allergic child to be very careful with this product. A mere trace of casein may trigger a severe allergic reaction in a very sensitive child.[14]

A few vegetable- and cereal-based probiotic and prebiotic products are being developed that may be well suited for milk-allergic children, although much more research must be carried out to prove their efficacy in practice. The development of one of these probiotic food products was launched in Sweden in 1994. The product is a fermented oatmeal gruel that contains no milk constituents and is mixed into a fruit drink.[15] One liter of the gruel provides approximately 5×10^{10} colony-forming units of *L. plantarum* 299v. The strain *L. plantarum* 299v originated in the human intestinal mucosa and has been shown in rats to improve the immunologic status of the lining of the digestive tract and to reduce mucosal inflammation. Researchers familiar with the Swedish fermented oatmeal product and with *L. plantarum* 299v claim that it improves the bacterial flora of the intestine and may also regulate the host's immunologic defense.

THE PROBIOTICS, ALLERGY, AND FOOD INTOLERANCE: BOTTOM LINE

Yogurt with live cultures of *Streptococcus salivarius* subsp. *thermophilus* and *Lactobacillus delbrueckii* subsp. *bulgaricus* may help reduce the diarrhea and bloating experienced by children with lactose intolerance. (Please read the section Microorganisms and Lactose Intolerance in Chapter 8, Lactose Intolerance, for more information.)

At present, there is no indication that the practice of consuming *Lactobacillus rhamnosus* GG is viable as an eczema preventative. In research studies the probiotic *Lactobacillus rhamnosus* subsp. GG has seemed to help prevent eczema in the infant in families at high risk for allergy. This beneficial strain of bacteria was given to pregnant women and to their newborn infants in formula. It was also given to lactating mothers, and to their babies by spoon, to continue the beneficial effects after birth. This occurred in research settings, but subsequent studies have been unable to confirm the initial results.

Although some manufacturers voluntarily label their products with a list of the probiotic strains they contain, no laws require that labels identify the specific strains or amounts of probiotics in a product. Therefore, to purchase the best probiotic product, buy brands and types of yogurt whose labels list only milk and live culture. It is relatively simple to contact the manufacturer for information about the specific strains of live culture included in any commercial yogurt.

Milk-free probiotics, some in combination with prebiotics, are available in countries around the world and in such varied forms as powders, capsules, biscuits, fruit drinks, and meal supplements. If your child is allergic to some food that may be an ingredient in a probiotic product (for example, if your child is allergic to milk proteins) make sure the probiotic you choose is guaranteed to be free from that ingredient.

Large-scale, well-controlled trials must be conducted before it can be firmly determined whether and how probiotic products may be of benefit to children with food allergies. For now, the information discussed in this chapter is about the best available.

References

1. Thompson WG. Probiotics for irritable bowel syndrome: A light in the darkness? *European Journal of Gastroenterology and Hepatology* 2001;13(10):1135–1136.

2. Joint FAO/WHO Working Group Report on Drafting Guidelines for the Evaluation of Probiotics in Food. London, Ontario, April 30 and May 1, 2002.

3. FAO/WHO Working Group Report on Evaluation of Probiotics in Food; Shanahan F. Therapeutic manipulation of gut flora. *Science* 2000;289:1311–1312.

4. Rastall RA, Maitin V. Prebiotics and synbiotics: Toward the next generation. *Current Opinion in Biotechnology* 2002;13(5):490–496.

5. de Vrese M, Stegelmann A, Richter B, Fenselau S, Laue C, Schrezenmeir J. Probiotics–Compensation for lactase insufficiency. *American Journal of Clinical Nutrition* 2001;73 (suppl):421S–429S.

6. Bjorksten B, Sepp E, Judge K, et al. Allergy development and the intestinal microflora during the first year of life. *Journal of Allergy and Clinical Immunology* 2001;108:516–520.

7. Furrie E. Probiotics and allergy. *Proceedings of the Nutrition Society* 2005;64(4):465–469.

8. Murch SH. Probiotics as mainstream allergy therapy? *Archives of Disease in Childhood* 2005;90:881–882.

9. Kalliomaki M, Salminen S, Poussa T, et al. Probiotics and prevention of atopic disease: Four-year follow-up of a randomized placebo-controlled trial. *Lancet* 2003;361:1869–1871.

10. Brouwer ML, Wolt-Plompen SA, Dubois AE, van der Heide S, Jansen DF, Hoijer MA, Kauffman HF, Duiverman EJ. No effects of probiotics on atopic dermatitis in infants: A randomized controlled trial. *Clinical and Experimental Allergy* 2006;36(7):899–906.

11. Majamaa H, Isolauri E. Probiotics: A novel approach in the management of food allergy. *Journal of Allergy and Clinical Immunology* 1997;99(2):179–185.

12. FAO/WHO Working Group Report on Evaluation of Probiotics in Food. Shanahan F. Therapeutic manipulation of gut flora.

13. FAO/WHO Working Group Report on Evaluation of Probiotics in Food. Shanahan F. Therapeutic manipulation of gut flora.

14. Moneret-Vautrin DA, Morisset M, Cordebar V, Codreanu F, Kanny G. Probiotics may be unsafe in infants allergic to cow's milk. *Allergy* 2006;61(4):506–508.

15. Molin G. Probiotics in foods not containing milk or milk constituents, with special reference to *Lactobacillus plantarum* 299v. *American Journal of Clinical Nutrition.* 2001;73(2):380S–385S.

Dietary Considerations for the Expectant Mother

FOLLOWING THE PREGNANCY DIET

This section explains how to use the information in Table A-1, Pregnancy Diet Based on Three Major Food Categories.

The guidelines here differ in the categorization of the food groups according to the "Food Guides" published by the health departments of many countries, for example, the US "Pyramid"[1] and the Canadian "Rainbow"[2], but incorporate all of the directives of those publications. The goal here is the development of a diet that will provide you with complete balanced nutrition, taking into account any food allergy that you need to manage.

- Cross out any foods listed in the table that you are intolerant of or allergic to, and list in the appropriate columns any foods that you tolerate that were omitted from the table.

- Try to eat three meals a day, and one or two snacks between meals.

- Include in each meal **at least one food** from each of the **three major food categories** listed in column 1 of Table A-1:

  – Protein (**PRO**)

    – Grain (**GR**) or Starch (**ST**)

    – Fruit (**FR**) or Vegetable (**VEG**)

- Include in each snack one **protein** food, along with foods from the other two groups. (It would be ideal to include a food from all three groups in each snack, but this is not easy to do in practice. At minimum, always include a protein in your between-meal snacks.)

- Eat moderate-size portions of each of your selections, rather than a large portion of any one food. If you have an urge to eat a larger portion (e.g., more of a vegetable, or more cereal), choose a second food from the same column of Table A-1, rather than eating an extra-large portion of one food. Practicing this form of moderation will keep you from allergen overload. Some authorities believe allergen overloading may lead to allergic sensitization of the fetus in utero, although this consequence has not been proven by research.

- Distribute relative portion sizes among different meals as outlined below to boost energy early in the day, while promoting sleep at day's end—something every expectant mother wishes to do!

  - Consume a larger portion of protein at breakfast, with less grain and starch, and a smaller serving of fruit. (Protein provides long-sustaining energy and prevents the mid-morning craving for sweets that often follows a breakfast high in sugar and starch.)

  - Consume a midday meal consisting of equal portions from the three categories of protein, grain or starch, and fruit or vegetable foods.

  - Consume an evening meal with a larger portion of grain or starch foods and a sugar-containing fruit, to promote production of the sleep-inducing chemical serotonin.

- Take care to consume adequate amounts of all the micronutrients (vitamins and minerals) your body needs. The body's requirements for some micronutrients increase during pregnancy and lactation, for example:

  - Calcium and vitamin D requirements increase (see Tables A-2 and A-3). If you are allergic to milk, obtain the calcium you need through nondairy sources (shown in Table A-4) and through calcium supplementation (discussed in the paragraph following Table A-4).

– The requirement for folate increases during pregnancy and lactation. Adequate intake of folate (folacin) is critical for formation of the neural tube in the developing baby, from conception onward. All females, from puberty through menopause, should consume sufficient folate to avoid the risk of neural tube defect in their babies (see Tables A-5 and A-6).

Table A-1			
PREGNANCY DIET BASED ON THREE MAJOR FOOD CATEGORIES			
Food Category	**Food Subcategory**	**Examples of Specific Foods**	**Examples of Derived Foods**
Protein **(PRO)**	Meat	Beef	Veal
		Bison	
		Buffalo	
		Lamb	Mutton
		Pork	Bacon
			Ham
		Wild meats	Venison (deer)
			Moose
			Elk
			Bear
	Poultry	Chicken	
		Duck	
		Goose	
		Grouse	
		Ostrich	
		Partridge	
		Pheasant	
		Quail	
		Turkey	
	Fish	Bass	
		Catfish (basafish)	
		Cod	
		Halibut	
		Herring	
		Orange roughy	

	Table A-1 (continued) PREGNANCY DIET BASED ON THREE MAJOR FOOD CATEGORIES		
Food Category	Food Subcategory	Examples of Specific Foods	Examples of Derived Foods
Protein (PRO) (cont'd)	Fish (cont'd)	Perch	
		Pilchard	
		Plaice	
		Salmon	
		Sardine	
		Sole	
		Trout	
		Tuna	
		Whitebait	
		Whiting	
	Shellfish (crustaceans and mollusks)	Crab	
		Crayfish (crawfish, spiny lobster)	
		Lobster	
		Prawn	
		Scampi	
		Shrimp	
		Clams	
		Cockles	
		Mussels	
		Scallops	
		Whelks	
		Winkles	

Table A-1 (continued) PREGNANCY DIET BASED ON THREE MAJOR FOOD CATEGORIES			
Food Category	**Food Subcategory**	**Examples of Specific Foods**	**Examples of Derived Foods**
Protein **(PRO)**	Eggs	Chicken	
		Duck	
		Goose	
		Quail	
		Turkey	
	Nuts	Almond	Nut butters
		Brazil nut	
		Chestnut	Nut milks
		Coconut	
		Hazelnut (filbert)	
		Pecan	
		Pine nuts	
		Pistachio nut	
		Walnut	
	Seeds	Melon	Seed butters
		Poppy	
		Pumpkin	Seed milks
		Sesame	Tahini
		Sunflower	
	Legumes	Peanut	Peanut butter
		Soy	Tofu
	Milk*	Cow's milk	Homogenized Skim milk

Table A-1 (continued)			
PREGNANCY DIET BASED ON THREE MAJOR FOOD CATEGORIES			
Food Category	**Food Subcategory**	**Examples of Specific Foods**	**Examples of Derived Foods**
Protein **(PRO)**	Milk* (cont'd)	Cow's milk (cont'd)	2% Reduced fat milk 1% Reduced fat milk
		Fermented milks	Yogurt Kefir Buttermilk

		Cheese	Solid cheeses:
			  Brie
			  Camembert
			  Cheddar
			  Cheshire
			  Danish blue
			  Derbyshire
			  Double Gloucester
			  Farmer's cheese
			  Gorgonzola
			  Lancashire
			  Leicestershire
			  Monterey Jack
			  Others too numerous to list

		Goat's milk	Feta cheese
		Mare's milk	
		Sheep's milk	Romano cheese
Grains **(GR)** and starches **(ST)**	Cereal grains	Amaranth	Flours made from all cereal grains
		Barley	
		Buckwheat	
		Corn	Corn starch Corn flour

Table A-1 (continued) PREGNANCY DIET BASED ON THREE MAJOR FOOD CATEGORIES			
Food Category	**Food Subcategory**	**Examples of Specific Foods**	**Examples of Derived Foods**
Grains **(GR)** and starches **(ST)**	Cereal grains (cont'd)	Kamut	
		Millet	
		Oats	
		Quinoa	
		Rice	
		Rye	
		Spelt	
		Wheat	Whole wheat flour Cake and pastry flour All-purpose flour Semolina Durum Graham flour
	Starchy vegetables	Beets	
		Corn	
		Carrot	
		Cassava	
		Parsnip	
		Plantain	
		Potato	
		Rutabaga	
		Swede	
		Sweet potato	
		Taro	

Table A-1 (continued)			
PREGNANCY DIET BASED ON THREE MAJOR FOOD CATEGORIES			
Food Category	**Food Subcategory**	**Examples of Specific Foods**	**Examples of Derived Foods**
Grains **(GR)** and starches **(ST)**	Starchy vegetables (cont'd)	Turnip	
		Yam	
	Starchy fruit	Banana	
	Starchy legumes	Dried peas and beans (all types)	Black beans
			Black-eyed peas
			Brown beans
			Indian dals (all types)
			Kidney beans
			Lentils
			Navy beans
			Pinto beans
			Split peas
			White beans
		Green peas	
		Sugar peas	
		Romano beans	
		Fava beans	
		Broad beans	
Fruits **(FR)** and vegetables **(VEG)**[**]	Citrus fruit	Grapefruit	
		Kumquat	
		Lemon	
		Lime	
		Orange	
		Tangelo	
		Tangerine	

	Table A-1 (continued) PREGNANCY DIET BASED ON THREE MAJOR FOOD CATEGORIES		
Food Category	**Food Subcategory**	**Examples of Specific Foods**	**Examples of Derived Foods**
Fruits **(FR)** and vegetables **(VEG)****	Stone fruit	Apple	
		Applepear (Asian pear)	
		Apricot	
		Cherry	
		Damson	
		Dates	
		Nectarine	
		Peach	
		Pear	
		Plum	
		Prune	
		Quince	
	Seed fruits and berries**	Blueberry	
		Boysenberry	
		Cranberry	
		Fig	
		Gooseberry	
		Mulberry	
		Raspberry	
		Strawberry	
	Tropical fruits	Guava	
		Longan	

	Table A-1 (continued)		
PREGNANCY DIET BASED ON THREE MAJOR FOOD CATEGORIES			
Food Category	**Food Subcategory**	**Examples of Specific Foods**	**Examples of Derived Foods**
Fruits **(FR)** and vegetables **(VEG)****	Tropical fruits (cont'd)	Lychee	
		Mango	
		Papaya	
		Pineapple	
		Star fruit	
	Vine fruits	Grapes	
		Raisins	
	Melons	Cantaloupe	
		Honeydew	
		Melon	
		Watermelon	
		Others	
	Green leafy type	Beet greens	
		Celery	
		Lettuce (all types)	
		Parsley	
		Radicchio	
		Spinach	
		Swiss chard	
		Turnip greens	
	Onion	Chives	
		Garlic	

	Table A-1 (continued) PREGNANCY DIET BASED ON THREE MAJOR FOOD CATEGORIES		
Food Category	**Food Subcategory**	**Examples of Specific Foods**	**Examples of Derived Foods**
Fruits **(FR)** and vegetables **(VEG)****	Onion (cont'd)	Green onions	
		Leeks	
		Onions	
		Scallions	
		Shallots	
		Young onions	
	Cauliflower/ cabbage	Artichoke	
		Asparagus	
		Broccoflower	
		Broccoli	
		Brussels sprouts	
		Cabbage	
		Cauliflower	
		Collards	
		Cress	
		Kale	
		Kohlrabi	
		Radish	
		Watercress	
	Gourds	Winter squash	
		Summer squash	
		Cucumber	

Table A-1 (continued)			
PREGNANCY DIET BASED ON THREE MAJOR FOOD CATEGORIES			
Food Category	**Food Subcategory**	**Examples of Specific Foods**	**Examples of Derived Foods**
Fruits **(FR)** and vegetables **(VEG)****	Gourds (cont'd)	Gherkin	
		Pumpkin	
	Legumes	Green beans	
		Runner beans	
		French beans	
		Yellow wax beans	
	Vine vegetables	Tomato	
		Eggplant	
		Peppers (all types)	

* Milk is listed as a protein because protein is the major nutrient in milk. Other foods in this category will be substitute proteins when milk is excluded because of allergy. Milk also contains sugar (lactose) at a level of 4%, so for accuracy, when milk is included in a balanced meal, a small amount of "starch equivalent" (ST) is also present.
** Fruits and vegetables are categorized here for the convenience of identifying the foods, not to reflect botanical genera or species.

PREGNANCY DIET DAILY MEAL PLANS

The following pages provide sample plans for two days' meals and snacks based on the complete and balanced nutrition of the Pregnancy Diet.

Remember – this is only a sample menu: portion sizes and food selection should be adjusted for appropriate weight gain and other considerations for each mother individually. Check with your doctor about how much weight you should gain, and discuss any other dietary concerns, such as diabetes, you may need to address. The help of a registered dietitian in this process is strongly recommended.

Day 1

Breakfast

2 Eggs, cooked any way (**PRO**)

1 Slice of toast made with whole wheat or brown rice bread (**GR/ST**)

(spread with 2 teaspoons butter)

1 Cup unsweetened apple juice (**FR**)

Bottled water, still or sparkling, 1 cup

Mid-morning Snack

3 Rice crackers (**GR/ST**)

1 Tablespoon chunky peanut butter (**PRO**)

1 Mandarin orange (**FR**)

½ Cup skim milk (**PRO/ST**)

Lunch

Chicken, rice, mushroom soup (**PRO, GR/ST**) with additional vegetables such as:

2 Ounces chopped zucchini (**VEG**)

¼ Cup chopped green peppers (**FR/VEG**)

Bottled water, still or sparkling, 1 cup

Afternoon Snack

3 Graham crackers with cinnamon (**GR/ST**)

1 Tablespoon almond butter (**PRO**)

2 Teaspoons concord grape jelly (**FR/VEG**)

½ Cup milk (**PRO/ST**)

Evening Meal

3 Ounces baked halibut (**PRO**)

1½ Cups cauliflower (**VEG**)

1 Cup broccoli (**VEG**)

Baked potato (**GR/ST**) with:

1 Tablespoon sour cream

1 Tablespoon chopped fresh chives (**VEG**)

½ Cup peaches cooked in own juice (**FR/VEG**)

Bottled water, still or sparkling, 1 cup

24 Ounces additional water, any time throughout the day.

Day 2

Breakfast

3 Slices bacon (**PRO**)

2 Pork sausages (**PRO**)

Hashed brown potatoes (**ST**)

½ Cup orange juice (**FR**) diluted with ½ cup sparkling water

Mid-morning Snack: Ants on a Log

Celery, 2 medium-to-large sticks(**VEG**)

2 Tablespoons cashew butter (spread on celery) (**PRO**)

¼ Cup raisins (**FR**) (added along length of buttered celery)

Cut into 2-inch-long sections

½ Cup skim milk (**PRO/ST**)

Lunch: Tuna Salad Sandwich

2–3 Ounces canned tuna (**PRO**)

1 Tablespoon mayonnaise (**ST**)

Chopped or sliced tomato, ¼ cup (**FR/VEG**)

2 Slices whole wheat bread or lightly toasted brown rice bread
   (Tastes better when lightly toasted)

Dijon mustard, mild, ½ teaspoon

2 Lettuce leaves

6 Cucumber slices

Bottled water, still or sparkling

Mid-afternoon Snack

    1 cup small mixed fruit salad (**FR**) without added sugar

    ½ cup plain yogurt (**PRO**)

Dinner

    Steak, 3 ounces (**PRO**)

    1 cup cooked green beans (**VEG**)

    ½ cup cooked sliced beetroot (**ST**)

    Butter, 2 teaspoons

    1 cup rice with ¼ cup green peas (**ST**)

    Lettuce, 3 leaves

    Cucumber ¼ cup sliced

    Tomato ¼ cup sliced

Facts About Calcium

- The percentage of calcium in food that is actually absorbed, used, and retained by the body varies, depending on: (1) the individual's age; (2) the level of calcium intake; (3) the type of food eaten; and (4) what other nutrients are eaten at the same time.

- An average adult will absorb about 40% of the calcium consumed in his or her diet. The percentage absorbed increases during periods of growth, pregnancy, and lactation, and reduces over the span of the aging process.

- In general, the lower the dietary intake of calcium, the more the body retains (i.e., less calcium is excreted when dietary intake is low).

- An adequate level of vitamin D in the body is necessary for efficient absorption of calcium. Although foods such as milk, liver, and egg yolk

Table A-2
DIETARY REFERENCE INTAKE VALUES FOR CALCIUM AND VITAMIN D

Life Stage Group Male[a] and Female	Calcium Adequate Intake (mg/day)	Vitamin D Adequate Intake (mcg/day)
0–6 months	210	5
7–12 months	270	5
1–3 years	500	5
4–8 years	800	5
9–13 years	1300	5
14–18 years	1300	5
19–30 years	1000	5
31–50 years	1000	5
51–70 years	1200	10
>70 years	1200	15
Pregnancy:		
≤18 years	1300	5
19–50 years	1000	5
Lactation:		
≤18 years	1300	5
19–50 years	1000	5

Source: Data provided by the Food and Nutrition Board of the Institute of Medicine, National Academy of Sciences, 2002.

[a] Except for values associated with pregnancy and lactation, which do not apply to males.

provide some vitamin D, the best source of it is the action of sunlight (i.e., ultraviolet light) on the skin.

• A diet high in phosphorus and protein (i.e., the traditional high-protein American diet) tends to reduce the amount of calcium retained in the body.

Table A-3
CALCIUM CONTENT OF MILK AND MILK PRODUCTS

Food	Quantity	Milligrams of Calcium
Whole milk	1 cup	285
Skim milk	1 cup	296
Yogurt, low fat	1 cup	350
Swiss cheese	1 ounce	270
American cheese	1 ounce	170
Cream cheese (such as Philadelphia brand)	1 ounce	23
Ice cream	1 cup	180

Table A-4
NONDAIRY SOURCES OF CALCIUM
(FOR MILK-ALLERGIC INDIVIDUALS)

Foods in Table A-4 are listed according to their calcium (Ca) content. Foods with highest Ca content (300 mg Ca) are listed before foods with lower Ca content; foods with lowest Ca content (15 mg Ca) are listed last.

Note: **Do not eat any food that causes you to have an allergic reaction.**

Food	Portion	
	Metric Unit	U.S. Equivalent
More than 300 mg Ca		
Sardines, with bones, canned	85 g	3 oz
Rhubarb, frozen, cooked*	270 g	1 cup
Wheat flour, artificially enriched	125 g	1 cup
Collards, frozen, cooked*	170 g	1 cup
Arugula (Rocket kale)	170 g	1 cup
250–300 mg Ca		
Sockeye salmon, with bones, canned (213g/can) (7.5 oz can)	100 g	½ can
Rhubarb, cooked, fresh*	270 g	1 cup
Spinach, cooked*	190 g	1 cup
200–250 mg Ca		
Almonds	125 mL	½ cup
Pink salmon, with bones, canned (7.5-oz can) (213-oz can)	100 g	½ can

Table A-4 (continued)
NONDAIRY SOURCES OF CALCIUM
(FOR MILK-ALLERGIC INDIVIDUALS)

Food	Portion	
	Metric Unit	U.S. Equivalent
200–250 mg Ca (cont'd)		
Oysters, raw, meat only	250 g	1 cup
Sugar, brown, packed down	220 g	1 cup
Turnip greens, cooked*	165 g	1 cup
150–200 mg Ca		
Beet greens, leaves and stems, cooked*	145 g	1 cup
Kale, frozen, cooked	130 g	1 cup
Amaranth (cooked grain):	Uncooked weight = 100 g	Cooked = 1 cup
100–150 mg Ca		
Baked beans, canned	250 mL	1 cup
Brazil nuts	125 mL	½ cup
Scallops		7 medium
Sesame seeds	125 mL	½ cup
Soybeans, cooked	250 mL	1 cup
Tofu	1 Piece: 8 × 6 × 2 cms	3" × 2.5" × 1"
Shrimp, meat only	113 g	4 oz
Molasses, cane, blackstrap	20 g	1 tbsp

Food	Portion	
	Metric Unit	U.S. Equivalent
100–150 mg Ca (cont'd)		
Dandelion greens, cooked*	105 g	1 cup
Mustard greens*	140 g	1 cup
Okra pods, cooked	160 g	1 cup
Brussels sprouts*	156 g	1 cup
Broccoli, cooked	250 mL	1 cup
50–100 mg Ca		
Asparagus, fresh, cooked, drained	240 g	1½ cup
Lima beans, cooked	180 g	1 cup
Green beans, cooked	125 g	1 cup
Yellow beans (wax beans), cooked	125 g	1 cup
Cabbage, fresh, cooked*	217 g	1½ cup
Chinese cabbage (bok-choy)*	76 g	1 cup
Sauerkraut*	235 g	1 cup
Carrots, cooked	234 g	1½ cups
Parsnips, cooked	155 g	1 cup
50–100 mg Ca		
Onions, cooked	210 g	1 cup
Tomatoes, canned, solids and liquid	241 g	1 cup

Table A-4 (continued)
NONDAIRY SOURCES OF CALCIUM
(FOR MILK-ALLERGIC INDIVIDUALS)

Table A-4 (continued)
NONDAIRY SOURCES OF CALCIUM
(FOR MILK-ALLERGIC INDIVIDUALS)

Food	Portion	
	Metric Unit	U.S. Equivalent
50–100 mg Ca (cont'd)		
Chili con carne with beans	250 mL	1 cup
Red kidney beans, cooked	250 mL	1 cup
White beans, cooked	250 mL	1 cup
Beans, dry, cooked and drained	180 g	1 cup
Lentils, cooked	200 g	1 cup
Garbanzo beans (chickpeas), cooked	250 mL	1 cup
Wheat germ	113 g	1 tbsp
Oats, puffed	50 g	2 oz
Orange, raw		1 medium
Orange sections	180 g	1 cup
Hazelnuts, chopped	28 g	1 oz
Cereal, All-Bran	250 mL	1 cup
Cereal, 100% bran	250 mL	1 cup
Cereal, Branbuds	250 mL	1 cup
Cereal, granola	150 mL	⅔ cup
15–50 mg Ca		
Cereals:		
Bran flakes and raisins	250 mL	1 cup

Table A-4 (continued)
NONDAIRY SOURCES OF CALCIUM
(FOR MILK-ALLERGIC INDIVIDUALS)

Food	Portion	
	Metric Unit	U.S. Equivalent
15–50 mg Ca (cont'd)		
Cereals (cont'd):		
Corn bran	250 mL	1 cup
Cheerios	250 mL	1 cup
Oatmeal, cooked	250 mL	1 cup
Shredded wheat	(10 mg Ca @ biscuit)	2–5 pieces
Shreddies	250 mL	1 cup
Bread:		
Cracked wheat	(22 mg Ca @ slice)	1 slice
Mixed grain	(27 mg Ca @ slice)	1 slice
Rye, light	(19 mg Ca @ slice)	1 slice
White	(24 mg Ca @ slice)	1 slice
Whole wheat (100%)	(25 mg Ca @ slice)	1 slice
Whole wheat (60%)	(23 mg Ca @ slice)	1 slice
White bun, hamburger or hot dog	(37–44 mg Ca)	1
Pita, whole wheat, 16.5-cm diam.	(49 mg Ca)	1
Tortilla, corn	(42 mg Ca)	1
Vegetables:		
Cabbage, raw, shredded	250 mL	1 cup

Table A-4 (continued)
NONDAIRY SOURCES OF CALCIUM
(FOR MILK-ALLERGIC INDIVIDUALS)

Food	Portion	
	Metric Unit	**U.S. Equivalent**
15–50 mg Ca (cont'd)		
Vegetables (cont'd):		
Carrot, raw, medium		1
Cauliflower, raw, cooked	250 mL	1 cup
Celery, diced, raw	250 mL	1 cup
Turnip, cooked	250 mL	1 cup
Spinach, raw, chopped	125 mL	½ cup
Olives, black		5 large
Olives, green		5 medium
Parsley, raw, chopped	25 mL	2 Tbsp
Peas, boiled	250 mL	1 cup
15–50 mg Ca		
Fruit:		
Grapefruit, raw		1 medium
Kiwi		1 large
Fig, dried, uncooked		1 medium
Pear, raw		1 medium
Raisins	125 mL	½ cup

Table A-4 (continued)
NONDAIRY SOURCES OF CALCIUM
(FOR MILK-ALLERGIC INDIVIDUALS)

Food	Portion	
	Metric Unit	U.S. Equivalent
15–50 mg Ca (cont'd)		
Other foods:		
Chocolate	30 g	1 square
Egg, whole, cooked		1 large
Maple syrup	15 mL	1 Tbsp
Peanuts, roasted in oil	50 mL	¼ cup
Sunflower seeds, kernels	50 mL	4 Tbsp
Soymilk, liquid	250 mL	1 cup

* This food contains oxalic acid, which impairs calcium absorption. The calcium content of the food is as stated, but the oxalic acid acts to significantly reduce the amount of Ca that is absorbed by the body.

Calcium Supplementation

- One-half teaspoon (2.5 mL) calcium carbonate provides between 625 and 750 mg elemental calcium (Ca).

- Calcium citrate, malate, and calcium gluconate appear to be more effective supplements than calcium carbonate, and may interfere less than calcium carbonate in the absorption of iron.

- Some authorities find that chelated minerals are absorbed and utilized more efficiently than the unchanged mineral salts. Because magnesium intake tends to be reduced in diets rich in calcium, you may want to use a chelated calcium product with magnesium, which also ensures adequate magnesium intake. (Carefully read product labels and follow instructions for use.)

- A chelated calcium with magnesium product is available (read labels) that also ensures adequate magnesium intake (which tends to be reduced in diets rich in calcium).

Food Sources of Folate and Folic Acid

Western diets are often deficient in natural sources of folate. It is essential that the expectant mother consume adequate amounts of folate because of the risk of a condition in the baby such as neural tube defect, which can occur when the mother's diet is deficient in this nutrient. Females are strongly urged to consume adequate amounts of folate (400 mcg), from puberty through menopause. This is advised because the fetal neural tube is formed so soon after conception.

More than one-third of the folate in the American diet is provided by fruits and vegetables. Grain products contribute a little more than one-fifth and legumes, nuts, and seeds contributed a little less than one-fifth. Foods that contain small amounts of folate but are not considered good sources can contribute significant amounts of folate to an individual's diet if these foods are eaten often or in large amounts[3].

Table A-5 lists the amounts of folate recommended to be each day consumed at different life stages.

Table A-5
DIETARY REFERENCE INTAKE (DRI) VALUES FOR FOLATE

Life Stage Group Male[a] and Female	Folate Adequate Intake (mcg/day)[b]
0–6 months	65
7–12 months	80
1–3 years	150
4–8 years	200
9–13 years	300
14–18 years	400
19–30 years	400
31–50 years	400
51–70 years	400
>70 years	400
Pregnancy:	
≤18 years	600
19–50 years	600
Lactation:	
≤18 years	500
19–50 years	500

Source: Data provided by the Food and Nutrition Board of the Institute of Medicine, National Academy of Sciences, Washington, DC, 2002.

[a] Except for values associated with pregnancy and lactation, which do not apply to males.

[b] Dietary folate equivalent (DFE)

    1 DFE = 1 mcg food folate

        = 0.6 mcg folic acid from fortified food or as a supplement consumed with food

        = 0.5 mcg of a supplement taken on an empty stomach

Table A-6
FOOD SOURCES OF FOLATE[c]

Animal, Poultry, and Fish Sources

Liver	Eggs
Kidney	Fish of all types

Nuts and Legumes

Nuts (all types)	Chickpeas (garbanzo beans)
Beans	Soybeans (if tolerated)

Vegetables

Avocado	Cauliflower
Beans	Endive
Celery	Lettuce
Asparagus	Parsley
Broccoli	Spinach
Brussels sprouts	Turnip greens
Cabbage	

Fruit

Orange and orange juice

Other Food Sources of Folate

Nutritional yeast	Baker's yeast
Brewer's yeast	

[c] Data derived from multiple sources.

References

1. United States Department of Agriculture. My Pyramid Plan can be accessed at: http://www.mypyramid.gov/

2. Health Canada: Canada's Food Guide to Healthy Eating can be accessed at http://www.hc-sc.gc.ca/fn-an/food-guide-aliment/fg_rainbow-arc_en_ciel_ga_e.html

3. Ohio State University Extension Fact Sheet: Folate (Folacin, Folic Acid). Can be accessed at: http://ohioline.osu.edu/hyg-fact/5000/5553.html

Gluten- and Casein-free Diet

A TRIAL DIET TO REDUCE SYMPTOMS OF AUTISM

Each of the foods that this diet requires you to avoid are found in many products, and each of the restricted foods has many derivatives. It is therefore essential that you **carefully read all product labels on the foods you select** when planning meals to comply with this diet. Take care to use only the foods listed as "allowed" over the course of the diet. A trial of 1 to 3 months' duration should be long enough to assess whether the diet improves the symptoms of autism.

GUIDELINES TO ENSURE COMPLETE BALANCED NUTRITION

Compensate for Exclusion of Milk and Milk Products

- Although no milk products are allowed on this diet, the same proteins that are supplied in milk can be obtained from a good variety of meats and other alternative sources.

Table B-1
FOODS ALLOWED ON A GLUTEN- AND CASEIN-FREE DIET

Food Group	Foods Allowed
MILK AND MILK PRODUCTS *AVOID* Any food product containing • *Casein* • *Milk solids*	**Drink these as a beverage, or pour on cereal:** • Rice Dream® (made from brown rice and safflower oil) enriched with calcium (in the *white carton*) • Soy-based drinks with no milk component (such as SoGood®; SoNice®) • Non-dairy creamers such as Coffee Rich® • Darifree® (made from potato starch) • Whey powder (diluted with water per package directions) **In recipes, substitute these for milk:** • Whey powder (diluted with water per package directions) • Pure fruit juices • Pure vegetable juices • Homemade soup stock • Water from cooking vegetables, especially potatoes

Table B-1 (continued) **FOODS ALLOWED ON A GLUTEN- AND CASEIN-FREE DIET**	
Food Group	**Foods Allowed**

MILK AND MILK PRODUCTS (cont'd)	**Spreads**
	
	• Clarified light whipped butter (see recipe on page 431)
	
	• Margarines free from milk solids, such as:
	
	  – Fleischmann's® Unsalted Light Margarine
	
	  – Some diet spreads such as Parkay® Diet Spread
	
	  – Canoleo® 100% canola oil margarine
	
	Sauces
	
	• Use olive oil, vegetable oils, clarified butter, herbs, and dressings made with allowed ingredients

BREADS AND CEREALS *AVOID* Any food containing • *Wheat* • *Spelt* • *Kamut* • *Triticale* • *Semolina*	**Grains and Flours** Use grain, nut, seed, and legume flours such as: • Pea and bean flours • Rice and rice flour • Wild rice and wild rice flour • Arrowroot starch and flour • Chickpea or garbanzo flour (also known as besan flour)

Table B-1 (continued)
FOODS ALLOWED ON A GLUTEN- AND CASEIN-FREE DIET

Food Group	Foods Allowed
BREADS AND CEREALS (cont'd) ***AVOID (cont'd)*** • *Durum* • *Cous cous* • *Rye* • *Barley*	**Grains and Flours (cont'd)** Use grain, nut, seed, and legume flours such as: • Soy flour • Lentil or pea flour • Potato starch and potato flour • Tapioca, tapioca starch, and tapioca flour • Millet and millet flour (also known as bajri, or bajra, flour) • Sago flour • Amaranth and amaranth flour • Quinoa and quinoa flour • Buckwheat and buckwheat flour • Nut and seed flours • Corn, corn flour, corn starch • Oat and oat flour **Breads and Baked Goods** Baked goods and specialty baking mixes that contain allowed ingredients, including these: • Specialty breads such as Ener-G Rice®

Table B-1 (continued) FOODS ALLOWED ON A GLUTEN- AND CASEIN-FREE DIET	
Food Group	**Foods Allowed**
BREADS AND CEREALS (cont'd)	**Breads and Baked Goods (cont'd)** Baked goods and specialty baking mixes that contain allowed ingredients, including these: • Good 'n' Easy® bread and pastry mixes • Celimix® rice or flaxmeal bread mixes • Homemade baked goods made with allowed flours **Crackers and Snacks** • Rice crackers • Rice cakes • Cakes and muffins with no restricted ingredients • Potato chips, *unless a low-fat diet is being followed* • Popcorn without artificial flavours and colors • Oat cakes made from oats and oat flour – (Oat cakes cannot contain wheat flour or any other flour whose source is not identified.)

Table B-1 (continued)
FOODS ALLOWED ON A GLUTEN- AND CASEIN-FREE DIET

Food Group	Foods Allowed
BREADS AND CEREALS (cont'd)	**Cereals** • Cream of Rice® • Rice bran • Puffed rice • Puffed millet • Puffed amaranth • Corn flakes • Oat meal • Any allowed grain, cooked **Pasta** • Rice noodles and pasta • Brown rice pasta • Wild rice pasta • Mung bean pasta • Soy pasta • Buckwheat pasta • Corn pasta • Pasta made from any allowed grain (for example, the potato and quinoa pastas that are available in specialty stores)

Table B-1 (continued)
FOODS ALLOWED ON A GLUTEN- AND CASEIN-FREE DIET

Food Group	Foods Allowed
VEGETABLES	• **All tolerated vegetables** without prepared sauces • Pure vegetable juices

LEGUMES	**All tolerated legumes**, including:
	• Peanuts
	• Fresh peas and beans, including:
	  – Green peas
	  – Sugar peas
	  – Green beans
	  – Yellow wax beans
	
	All cooked dried peas and beans, including:
	• Lentils (brown, red, yellow, white)
	• Split peas (yellow, green)
	• Kidney beans
	• Navy beans
	• Pinto beans
	• Black-eyed peas
	• Soybeans

Table B-1 (continued) FOODS ALLOWED ON A GLUTEN- AND CASEIN-FREE DIET	
Food Group	**Foods Allowed**
LEGUMES (cont'd)	**Processed legumes**, including: • Pure smooth-style peanut butter without sweeteners • Plain tofu • Soybean flour • Chickpea flour • Black bean flour • Red bean flour
FRUIT	**All tolerated fruits** (fresh, frozen, or canned in fruit juice or water) **All tolerated fruit juices**, including these: • Freshly squeezed juices • Fruit juices in cans, bottles, or cartons • Pasteurized fruit juices **All tolerated preserved fruits**, including these: • Fruit conserves, jellies, and jams made with allowed fruits and sweeteners • Dried fruits

Table B-1 (continued) FOODS ALLOWED ON A GLUTEN- AND CASEIN-FREE DIET	
Food Group	**Foods Allowed**
MEAT, POULTRY, AND FISH	**All plain cooked meat, poultry, or fish** (fresh, frozen, or canned) • May be marinated in oil, herbs, lemon (cooked) • Fish canned in oil or water
EGGS	**All tolerated eggs**, provided egg dishes are prepared only with allowed ingredients
NUTS AND SEEDS	**All tolerated nuts and seeds**, including nut and seed flours, and nut and seed butters such as: • Almond butter • Cashew butter • Sesame tahini • Sunflower seed butter • Any nuts or seeds made into butters or milks in a blender

FATS AND OILS	• All pure vegetable oils, including canola, olive, sunflower, safflower, flaxseed, soy
	
	 • Milk-free margarines such as:
	
	   – Fleischmann's® Unsalted Light Margarine
	
	   – Parkay® Diet Spread

Table B-1 (continued) FOODS ALLOWED ON A GLUTEN- AND CASEIN-FREE DIET	
Food Group	**Foods Allowed**
FATS AND OILS (cont'd)	• Milk-free margarines (cont'd) such as: – Canoleo® 100% canola oil margarine • Meat drippings and poultry fat • Homemade gravy made with allowed thickeners • Lard
HERBS AND SPICES	All fresh or dried spices and herbs
SWEETENERS	• Sucrose (table sugar) • Glucose, dextrose • Fructose (fruit sugar), levulose • Honey (for children older than 1 year) • Lactose-free sugar substitutes (e.g., Sugar Twin®, Splenda®) (These are usually safe for children but are not recommended.)
BEVERAGES	• Plain water and mineral water • Coffee, tea, and herbal teas • Pure fruit and vegetable juices (may be diluted with water to reduce sugar concentration)

Table B-1 (continued) FOODS ALLOWED ON A GLUTEN- AND CASEIN-FREE DIET	
Food Group	**Foods Allowed**
OTHER	• Baking soda
	• Baking powder
	• Cream of tartar
	• Salt
	• Baker's yeast
	• Guar gum
	• Plain gelatin

• Soy-based beverages and Rice Dream® are good substitutes for milk to drink as a beverage, to use on cereal, or when milk is called for in a recipe. However, these substitutes do not contain the calcium and vitamin D that are provided in milk (unless the nutrients are added artificially).

• Because milk and milk products are the principal source of calcium in the Western diet, it is difficult to obtain adequate daily amounts of calcium from dietary sources alone when milk and milk products are eliminated.

• Vitamin D is required for uptake and utilization of dietary calcium. Adequate vitamin D is usually obtained from the action of sunlight on the skin (a half hour's exposure to the sun each day provides the daily vitamin D requirement for an individual). In situations where exposure to sunlight is limited, a supplementary source of vitamin D is recommended.

- The Institute of Medicine has compiled a dietary intake table (Table B-2) as a guide to the amount of daily calcium and vitamin D each individual should consume. During the period your child follows the gluten-and casein-free diet, you must take care to provide him or her adequate calcium and vitamin D from alternate sources. Please find details about your child's daily requirements for calcium and vitamin D in Appendix A.

For additional information on the requirements (by age) for calcium and vitamin D in the diet, please see Table A-2 in Appendix A. In addition, Appendix A also includes additional information on calcium supplementation and calcium absorption.

Calcium Dosage

- Calcium appears to be best absorbed when taken with food in three or four doses throughout the day, rather than in a single dose. For example, for a total daily requirement of 1000 mg, the calcium could be given as: (1) four 250-mg tablets (one at each meal and one with a snack before bed); (2) three 350-mg tablets (one with each meal); or (3) two 500-mg tablets, each broken in half and taken in four 250-mg doses.

- Liquid calcium (Ca) is usually available in 1-teaspoon doses of 100 mg Ca. If a child requires 500 mg liquid Ca per day, for example, it could be given in 2 teaspoons with breakfast, 1 teaspoon with lunch, and 2 teaspoons with supper to supply the total daily requirement.

GENERAL DIET GUIDELINES

Include in every meal or snack at least one food from each of these three categories: (1) protein; (2) grain or starch; and (3) fruits and vegetables.

Note: Because a number of basic foods are excluded from the gluten- and casein-free diet, in order to supply an adequate balance of nutrients, the categories outlined below may contain foods that would not traditionally be included in a particular food group.

Protein (PRO)

> Meat
>
> Poultry
>
> Fish
>
> Shellfish
>
> Egg
>
> Nut butters
>
> Seed butters
>
> Tofu

Grain (GRA) or Starch (ST)

> Any allowed whole grain
>
> Whole grain flour as allowed
>
> Lentils, split peas, and other legumes
>
> Lentil, pea, or bean flour
>
> Root vegetables, such as:
>
> > Potato
> >
> > Sweet potato and yam
> >
> > Carrot
> >
> > Parsnip
> >
> > Turnip
>
> Starchy fruit, such as banana

Fruits (FR) and Vegetables (VEG)

> All tolerated vegetables, including
>
> > Leafy vegetables, such as:

    Spinach

    Kale

    Chard

    Broccoli

    Lettuces of all types

    Cabbages

    Beet greens

    Brussels sprouts

    Asparagus

Cauliflower

Squashes of all types, including zucchini

Eggplant

Sweet peppers

Salad vegetables, such as:

    Cucumber

    Tomatoes

    Radishes

All fruits, including

Fresh, frozen, canned, and dried fruits

Fresh, frozen, and canned pure fruit juices

EXAMPLES OF BALANCED MEALS

Breakfast

Breakfast Cereals

PRO: Nuts or seeds and nut and seed butters (if tolerated)
Soy milk (if tolerated)

GRA/ST: Packaged cereal as allowed
Cooked cereal grain (see cooking directions below)

FR/VEG: Fruit (fresh, frozen, cooked, or canned in fruit juice)
OR 100% fruit jam sweetened with honey
OR fruit juice

Cooking Directions for Cereal Grains

- Cook amaranth, millet, quinoa (wash first), and buckwheat grain the same way you cook brown rice:

    Combine 1 cup of grain with 2¼ or 2½ cups of water.

    Bring to a boil, cover, lower heat, and simmer for 45–60 minutes.

- If cooked insufficiently, grain will taste slightly bitter and will irritate the digestive tract.

- The grains can be cooked in large batches (e.g., 4 cups of grain) to freeze in 1-cup quantities.

- Cooked grain can be reheated in a microwave oven to form the basis of an instant breakfast cereal.

Quick Blender Drink

PRO: Tofu; nuts; or seeds

GRA/ST: Rice bran

FR/VEG: Cooked fruit

- In a blender combine

  Medium or soft tofu (from produce section of grocery store)

  Any fruit

  2–4 tablespoons sesame tahini, seed, or nut butter

  1 tablespoon boiled lime juice

  1 tablespoon sugar or honey (or to taste)

  2 tablespoons rice bran

  Soy milk as desired (to thin mixture)

- Blend until well-combined.

Vegetable Omelette

PRO: Egg

GRA/ST: Potato

FR/VEG: Assorted vegetables; fruit juice

- Sauté these ingredients in an omelette pan in clarified butter (or in a combination of clarified butter and olive oil):

  - Zucchini, grated

  - Mushrooms, thinly sliced

  - Red and green peppers, chopped finely

  - Parsley, chopped

  - Carrots, grated

  - Garlic, pressed, to taste

- Whip together 2 or 3 eggs until foamy.

- Add whipped eggs to above cooked ingredients, with salt and herbs to taste.

- Cook until set on the bottom; slide onto a plate, cooked side down.

- Invert into the omelette pan, uncooked side down.

- Cook in omelette pan 1 or 2 minutes, until set on the bottom.

- Fold over into a half-circle; slide onto a heated plate.

- Garnish with parsley, serve with hashed brown potatoes and heated and cooled fruit juice.

Enriched Scrambled Eggs

> **PRO:**   Egg
>
> **GRA/ST:**   Potato; rice bread; rice or soy bread
>
> **FR/VEG:**   Green onions; black olives; fruit juice

- Sauté the following ingredients in clarified butter:

  - Green onions or chives, finely chopped

  - Black olives

  - Garlic, pressed, to taste

- Beat 2 or 3 eggs with a fork and add to above cooked ingredients.

- Cook, stirring until mixture is firm.

- Add salt to taste, and garnish with parsley.

- Serve with hashed brown potatoes, toasted rice, or rice or soy bread with fruit juice.

- If eggs are not tolerated, substitute firm tofu, broken with a fork.

Pancakes

½ cup	Rice flour	125 mL
½ cup	Soy flour	125 mL

1 tbsp	Allowed baking powder	15 mL
1 tbsp	Honey or fructose	15 mL
½ tsp	Salt	2.5 mL
¼ cup	Allowed oil	50 mL
2	Eggs	2
1 cup	Rice Dream® or soy milk	250 mL

- Sift dry ingredients three times and set aside.

- Beat eggs, oil, and milk together until well blended.

- Add egg mixture to flour and beat until batter is smooth.

- Heat a nonstick skillet. For each pancake pour 1–2 tablespoons of batter into skillet.

- When air bubbles appear on surface of pancake, flip to cook on other side.

These pancakes freeze well.

Pancakes as a Complete Meal (Breakfast Pancakes)

PRO: Nut or seed butter

GRA/ST: Flours used in pancake batter (see pancake recipe above)

FR/VEG: Fruit included in pancake batter
Fruit as topping
Fruit juice

- Make batter according to recipe (see above). Add frozen or fresh berries (blueberries, strawberries, raspberries) or any allowed fruit, chopped into small pieces.

- Cook individual pancakes on skillet (fruit will cook at the same time the batter does).

- Spread 2 teaspoons of any nut or seed butter on each pancake while still hot.

- Top with any cooked fruit, sweetened to taste, if desired.

- Serve with fruit juice.

Vegetable or Fruit Pancake Sandwiches

PRO: Nut or seed butter

GRA/ST: Flours used in pancake batter (see pancake recipe above)

FR/VEG: Grated vegetables (carrot; zucchini; red and green peppers)

OR: chopped fruit (apple; pear; peach; apricot; nectarine; pineapple)

OR: berries (blueberry; strawberry; raspberry)

- Make batter according to recipe. Add grated vegetables or chopped fruit or berries.

- Cook individual pancakes on griddle. Cool on a cake rack.

- For lunch box sandwiches, spread with nut or seed butters and honey, or 100% fruit jam without sugar (but add honey to taste if desired). Make square pancakes for variety.

- Include fruit juice and serving of cooked fruit (packed in small container for lunch box).

Lunch (Suitable for Lunch Box and Snacks)

1. Brown rice cakes spread with nut or seed butter (and honey to taste), 100% fruit jam
    (**PRO:** Nut or seed butter; **GRA/ST:** Brown rice; **FR/VEG:** Fruit jam)

2. Rice crackers spread with nut or seed butter and vegetable butter (recipes below)
    (**PRO:** Nut or seed butter; **GRA/ST:** Rice crackers; **FR/VEG:** Vegetable butter)

3. Rice cakes spread with meat butters (recipes below)
    (**PRO:** Meat, poultry, or fish; **GRA/ST:** Rice cakes; **FR/VEG:** Vegetables or fruits)

4. Rice cakes or crackers spread with nut or seed butter and fruit butter (see recipes at the end of this appendix)
   (**PRO**: Nut or seed butters; **GRA/ST**: Rice cakes or crackers; **FR/VEG**: Fruits)

Dinner or Supper

1. Stir-fried vegetables (**FR/VEG**) including bean sprouts, with chicken, tofu, fish, or shellfish (**PRO**) and served with rice (**GRA/ST**)

2. Rice pasta or any pasta made from allowed grains (**GRA/ST**), homemade meat (**PRO**) and tomato sauce with additional vegetables (**FR/VEG**)

3. Rice or pasta made from allowed grains (**GRA/ST**) with tuna (**PRO**) and black olive sauce (**FR/VEG**)

4. Bouillabaisse (fish and shellfish stew) (**PRO**) with a variety of vegetables (**FR/VEG**) served with toasted rice or allowed-grain breads (**GRA/ST**)

5. Roast meat or poultry (**PRO**) with a variety of vegetables (**FR/VEG**) and served with french fries or baked potato (**GRA/ST**)

6. Steamed, poached, or broiled fish (**PRO**) with a variety of vegetables (**FR/VEG**) and rice (**GRA/ST**)

7. Broiled steak (**PRO**), french fries (**GRA/ST**), and a variety of vegetables (**FR/VEG**)

8. Meat (**PRO**) and vegetable (**FR/VEG**) kebabs served with rice (**GRA/ST**)

A Few Useful Recipes

Cooking Directions for Cereal Grains

- Cook amaranth, millet, quinoa, and buckwheat grain the same way you cook brown rice:

– Combine 1 cup of grain with 2¼ or 2½ cups of water.

– Bring to a boil, cover, lower heat, and simmer for 45–60 minutes.

• If cooked insufficiently, grain will taste slightly bitter and will irritate the digestive tract.

• The grains can be cooked in large batches (e.g., 4 cups of grain) to freeze in 1-cup quantities.

• Cooked grain can be reheated in a microwave oven to form the basis of an instant breakfast cereal.

Clarified butter

• Heat regular butter gently until it melts.

• Milk solids will sink to the bottom, and also may rise to the top in a "foam".

• Skim off the top foam and discard.

• Allow the milk solids to fall to the bottom and pour off the clear oil.

• Discard the bottom solids.

• The **clear yellow oil** is clarified butter.

Light whipped butter

Clarified butter is very hard and difficult to spread once it has solidified. Making a light whipped butter, with the addition of a polyunsaturated vegetable oil such as canola oil makes the product softer, and also reduces the saturated:unsaturated fat ratio, which is beneficial in cholesterol-lowering diets.

• Add canola oil to the liquid clarified butter when it has cooled and just started to solidify, in the proportions:

– 1 cup clarified butter to ½-cup canola oil.

• Whip together in a blender, food processor, or by hand. The two oils blend together best when the butter oil cools and just starts to solidify.

• Pour into a plastic container and refrigerate.

Vegetable Spreads

- Combine clarified light whipped butter with one of the following vegetables

    - Pureed cooked carrot with honey

    - Cooked mashed yams with honey

    - Grated zucchini and chopped parsley or cilantro, cooked

    - Green peas and chopped mint, cooked

    - Mashed cooked mixed vegetables with herbs

    - Cooked mushrooms chopped finely with cooked green onion or chives

    - Cooked, mashed lentils with cilantro

- Whip with a fork, or in a food processor or blender until well mixed.

- Add salt, cooked pressed garlic, or herbs to taste.

Fruit spreads

- Combine the following in a food processor, blender, or mix by hand

    - Dates (remove pits) and nut or seed butter

    - Mashed cooked banana with nut or seed butter

    - Nut butters with raisins soaked in boiling water

    - Nut butters and pureed canned peaches or apricots

    - Apple sauce (apples cooked in a little water and mashed) with nut or seed butters

    - Pear sauce (pears cooked in a little water and mashed) with nut or seed butters

    - Cooked, mashed berries with nut or seed butters

Fish or meat spreads with fruit or vegetables

- Combine clarified light whipped butter with one of the following mixtures

  - Canned fish (tuna, sardine, salmon) with cooked lemon juice to taste

  - Chopped ham with canned pineapple

  - Finely chopped chicken or turkey with cooked cranberries

  - Chicken or turkey livers, pureed with chopped cooked onions or chives

- Whip with a fork, or in a food processor or blender until well mixed.

- Add salt, cooked pressed garlic and herbs to taste.

Humus as a dip or spread

  - 1 can chickpeas (garbanzo beans) in water. Drain and reserve *half* of the liquid.

  - 4 tablespoons sesame tahini

  - 1–3 cloves pressed garlic (to taste) cooked in 1 tablespoon lemon juice

- Put all ingredients with half of the liquid from the chickpeas into a blender.

- Blend on high until completely smooth.

APPENDIX C

Gluten-Free Diet for Management of Celiac Disease

This diet is designed to eliminate the gluten-containing grains associated with celiac disease, a chronic intestinal disorder that results in poor absorption of nutrients. The principal gluten-containing grains excluded from this diet include

- Wheat and grains related to or derived from wheat (such as triticale, kamut, and spelt)

- Rye

- Barley

- Oats[a]

---

[a] Research indicates that oats may be tolerated by many people with celiac disease. Your pediatrician can recommend whether you should exclude oats from your child's diet. As a compromise, consider avoiding oats and oat products initially; then reintroduce them after all symptoms have disappeared, to see whether eating oats causes recurrence of intestinal distress.

The gluten-free diet restricts consumption of the following

Wheat	Rye
Semolina	Oats
Spelt	Oatmeal
Triticale	Barley
Bulgur	Kamut
Couscous	Farina
Durum	

This diet restricts consumption of flours, breads, and crackers made from the above grains, including:

White bread	Rye bread
Whole wheat bread	Oat bread
Sourdough bread	Barley bread
All-purpose flour	Bread crumbs
Gluten flour	Cracker meal
Graham flour	Graham crackers
Phosphated flour	Matzos
Protein flour	Starch (unless identified as corn starch)
Cracked wheat flour	Cream of Wheat®
Durum flour	Wheat germ
Pastry flour	Bran
Self-rising flour	

***The following products are restricted because they
may contain gluten as a hidden ingredient:***

Frankfurters	Meatloaf
Sausages	Breaded meat or fish
Luncheon meats	Meat or fish in batter
Stuffing	Canned soups (some, read labels)
Spreads	Soups, gravies made with thickeners
Paté	Bouillon cubes
Pies	Ice cream cones
Pie fillings	Salad dressings (some, read labels)
Croquettes	Icing sugar
Patties	Cereal coffee substitutes (Postum®)
Root beer	Commercial baking powder
Mustard pickles	Soy sauces (some)
Any product containing bread or breadcrumbs	
Any product labeled "gluten-enriched"	
Malted milk	
Cheese spreads or "cheese foods" (some)	

***The following flours, starches, and grain products
are allowed on the gluten-free diet:***

Amaranth grain and flour	Potatoes and potato flour
Arrowroot starch or flour	Quinoa grain and flour

Buckwheat grain and flour

Cassava

Corn, corn flour, cornstarch

Lentil grains and flour

Millet grain and flour (bajri)

Nuts, nut meal, and
flour (any type)

Chickpeas and chickpea
flour (besan)

Rice (white and brown) grain and
flour

Sago flour

Seed grains, flours, and oils (any
type)

Soybeans and flour

Tapioca starch or flour

T'eff

Table C-1
FOODS ALLOWED AND RESTRICTED ON
THE GLUTEN-RESTRICTED DIET

Food Group	Foods Allowed	Foods Restricted
Breads, Cereals, and Substitutes	Breads, baked goods, cereals, pancakes, pasta, and snack foods made from any allowed grain, including: • Corn • Corn meal, corn-starch, corn flour • Rice flour and starch • Potato flour and starch • Millet flour • Buckwheat groats and flour • Kasha • Amaranth flour • Quinoa flour • Tapioca starch • Sago starch and flour • Soy flour • Lentil flour • Pea and bean flours • Chickpea flour • Arrowroot starch and flour • Nut meal and flour • Seed meal and flour	Breads, baked goods, cereals, pancakes, pasta, and snack foods made from any restricted grain, including: • Wheat • Kamut • Spelt • Triticale • Semolina • Durum • Bulgur • Farina • Couscous • Matzoh • Products labeled "gluten-enriched" • Malt • Rye • Oats • Barley

Table C-1 (continued)
FOODS ALLOWED AND RESTRICTED ON
THE GLUTEN-RESTRICTED DIET

Food Group	Foods Allowed	Foods Restricted
Milk and Milk Products	All milk and milk products made without restricted ingredients, including: • Milk • Yogurt • Buttermilk • Cheeses • Cream cheese • Cottage cheese • Butter • Ice cream (examine product label for inclusion of restricted ingredients)	Any milk product containing restricted ingredients, especially: • Cocoa powders • Chocolate mixes • Hot chocolate • Cheese sauces • Cheese spreads • Malted milk
Meat, Fish, and Poultry	All meat, fish, and poultry that is: • Plain, fresh, frozen, or canned without addition of any restricted ingredients • Battered with allowed grains, flours, or crumbs • A plain deli product made without any restricted ingredients	Meat products that might contain restricted ingredients (read labels carefully), including: • Luncheon meats • Frankfurters • Sausages • Patés • Spreads • Stuffing • Meat loaf

	Table C-1 (continued) FOODS ALLOWED AND RESTRICTED ON THE GLUTEN-RESTRICTED DIET	
Food Group	**Foods Allowed**	**Foods Restricted**

Meat, Fish, and Poultry (cont'd)		Meat products that might contain restricted ingredients (read labels carefully), including:
		
		• Croquettes
		
		• Battered meats
		
		• Breaded meats
		
		• Manufactured products containing:
		  – HVP
		  – HPP
		  – MSG

Eggs	All plain egg dishes prepared without any restricted ingredients	Egg dishes made with restricted ingredients, such as: • Quiche • Mousse • Pavlova • Soufflé
Nuts and Seeds	All plain (raw or roasted) uncoated nuts and all allowed seeds	Snack nuts and seeds coated with restricted ingredients and flavoring agents such as: • HPP • HVP • MSG

Table C-1 (continued)
FOODS ALLOWED AND RESTRICTED ON
THE GLUTEN-RESTRICTED DIET

Food Group	Foods Allowed	Foods Restricted
Vegetables	• All plain fresh, frozen, or canned vegetables • Vegetable dishes prepared with allowed ingredients • All allowed sprouted grains and seeds • All plain vegetable juices	Vegetable dishes prepared with restricted ingredients in the: • Coating • Breading • Marinade • Garnish • Sprouted form
Legumes	All plain peas, beans, and lentils prepared with allowed ingredients, including: • Dals prepared without any restricted flours and grains • Plain tofu • Soy products • Peanut butter	All legume dishes that contain restricted ingredients, such as: • Dals with added wheat • Tofu patties coated with wheat flour or bread crumbs
Fruits	All pure fruit (fresh, frozen, canned, or dried) and pure fruit juices	All fruit dishes that contain restricted ingredients, such as: • Pie fillings • Fruit sauces • Dessert fillings and toppings

Table C-1 (continued) FOODS ALLOWED AND RESTRICTED ON THE GLUTEN-RESTRICTED DIET		
Food Group	**Foods Allowed**	**Foods Restricted**

Fats and Oils	• Butter
	• Margarines made without restricted ingredients
	• All pure vegetable, nut, seed, and fish oils, including
	  – Olive
	  – Corn
	  – Sunflower
	  – Safflower
	  – Canola
	  – Avocado
	  – Grapeseed
	  – Soy
	  – Peanut
	  – Sesame
	  – Mustard
	  – Walnut
	• Lard
	• Meat drippings
		• Salad dressings made from restricted ingredients
		• Gravy thickened with any restricted flour or starch

Table C-1 (continued)
FOODS ALLOWED AND RESTRICTED ON
THE GLUTEN-RESTRICTED DIET

Food Group	Foods Allowed	Foods Restricted
Herbs and Spices	All plain herbs and spices	Seasoning mixes with restricted ingredients such as: • HPP • HVP • MSG
Sweeteners	• Sugar • Honey • Molasses • Maple syrup • Jams • Jellies • Preserves • Date sugar	Sweets containing restricted ingredients such as: • Icing sugar • Sorbitol • Marshmallows

Challenge Phase: Elimination and Challenge Protocols for Determining the Allergenic Foods

It cannot be stressed strongly enough that if you have any cause to suspect that your child has had a severe or anaphylactic reaction to a food, any challenge tests should be undertaken only under medical supervision in a suitably equipped facility.

Never challenge on your own a food that has caused a severe reaction in the past, or has elicited a strong reaction on a skin test, or your child has a high level of IgE to the food on a blood test!

Any food that has been avoided for a long period of time (6 months or more) because of a previous reaction to it should always be rechallenged under the supervision of a suitably qualified medical practitioner because reactions after long abstinence tend to be more severe than when the food has been eaten regularly.

Check with your child's doctor before proceeding with any food challenge.

In this section of the book, we provide you with a step-by-step procedure to carry out a food challenge test program for your child. All the steps in the program are important and they must be followed in the order presented to both protect the health of your child and identify the foods to which your child is sensitive.

THE SEQUENTIAL INCREMENTAL DOSE CHALLENGE OF INDIVIDUAL FOOD COMPONENTS

Always remember the early-warning test before you give a child any food for challenge after a period of avoidance. The early-warning test procedure is as follows:

- Rub the food on the child's cheek and wait for 20 minutes to see if a reddened area appears that indicates a reaction to the food.

- Then place a small amount of the food on the child's outer lip and wait 30 minutes and observe carefully for any reaction such as reddening, blistering, irritation (child rubs the area).

- If you want to be even more sure, place a tiny amount of the test food on the child's tongue and again observe for 30 minutes, this time looking for any reaction that the child has previously exhibited after eating a food.

If there are no signs of local reactions, then proceed to the challenge test as described below.

Two or Four Day Introduction

Once you have tested for local reactions, the next step is a two or four day introduction period. Continue all meals as consumed during the elimination phase. The test foods are introduced between meals. Because symptoms will have subsided during the elimination phase, any increase in symptoms, or reappearance of symptoms will be due to the new foods.

Day 1

Morning: Between breakfast and lunch

- The child eats a small quantity of the test food; quantities are given below.

- Monitor the child's response; be alert to any adverse reactions.

- If a reaction occurs, only the usual symptoms will be experienced, but they may be more severe than usual.

  Wait four hours before giving the test food again.

If <u>no</u> adverse reactions have been experienced, the reintroduction should proceed as follows:

Afternoon: Between lunch and dinner

- Double the quantity of the test food eaten in the morning.

- Monitor the child's response; be alert to any adverse reactions.

- If a reaction occurs, the usual symptoms will be experienced, but they may be more severe than usual.

  Wait four hours.

If no adverse reactions have occurred, proceed as follows:

Evening: After dinner

- Double the quantity of the test food eaten in the afternoon.

- Monitor the child's response; be alert to any adverse reactions.

- If a reaction occurs, only the usual symptoms will be experienced, but they may be more severe than usual.

IF AN ADVERSE REACTION OCCURS AT ANY TIME DURING THE CHALLENGE, DISCONTINUE THE TEST FOOD.

WAIT AT LEAST 48 HOURS AFTER AN ADVERSE REACTION HAS <u>SUBSIDED</u> BEFORE TESTING A NEW FOOD.

Day 2

Day two is the period during which you check for delayed reactions.

- Child does not eat any of the test food challenged on Day 1.

- He or she eats only the foods allowed on the elimination diet.

- Monitoring for any reactions should be carried out throughout the day.

- Any adverse response may be due to a delayed reaction to the food tested yesterday; if a reaction occurs, *discontinue testing that food component.*

- If there is no reaction, the food can be considered safe.

Day 3

If no adverse reactions have occurred, the next food on the list should be tested in the manner described for Day 1.

   If results of the Day 1 test are unclear:

   Test the same food as on Day 1 again on Day 3 as follows:

- At midmorning give the child a greater quantity of the test food than eaten at midmorning on Day 1.

- Continue to double the quantity every four hours and monitor all reactions as described for Day 1.

Day 4

Is another monitoring day, observing for delayed reactions as described for Day 2.

   If there is no evidence of an increased adverse reaction by the end of Day 4 the food can be considered safe.

   Continue in a similar fashion until all suspect foods have been tested.

Sequence of Testing Foods

The sequence for testing foods is an important consideration in a food challenge program. Here are the steps to follow to carefully sequence the foods you'll be testing.

- Choose the food **category** with which you would like to begin. This is usually one of the child's favorite foods. For example, he or she might miss ice cream: start with the milk category. Perhaps your child is particularly fond of muffins and cookies: choose the wheat category first. If he or she misses fruits, you can start with the fruit category, and so on.

- The **sequence** of testing in some of the categories is important because each test adds an extra ingredient to the previously tested food.

- When individual components of a food contain different allergens, each is tested separately so that only those to which your child reacts need to be avoided. For example, there are separate tests for casein and lactose in milk. This ensures that your child will be able to consume the maximum range of foods, and therefore nutrients, that he or she tolerates.

- The "test component" is highlighted as each is added in sequence in these cases.

- When the first food in a category is tested (for example, milk and milk products, grain, or vegetable), the foods in that category are tested in the sequence specified and should be continued until each has been tested and the limit of tolerance has been established.

- Do not switch between categories.

Quantity of the Test Food

Quantities given are for a child between 2 and 10 years. However, you can adjust these quantities according to your child's age, size, and appetite, as described below.

For an infant below the age of two, use smaller quantities of foods. Select the quantities as follows:

**Choosing the appropriate quantities for
testing if those given below are not suitable:**

- Determine an appropriate serving size of the food for your child.

- This will be the quantity that he or she eats for the **third test** (after the evening meal) on Day 1.

- A quarter of this quantity will be the child's first dose (after breakfast) on Day 1.

- Half of the serving size will be the second test dose between lunch and dinner on Day 1.

- The child will eat the full serving size for the third dose after the evening meal on Day 1.

If you need a second test day on Day 3 because the previous challenges were unclear, start with the half-size serving in the morning; give the full serving in the afternoon; and in the evening let the child eat as much as he or she can handle, over and above the full serving if possible.

Food Categories and Test Sequences

The food categories include milk and milk products, eggs, cereal grains, other grains and grain products (such as oils), fruits and vegetables, legumes (including peanuts), nuts, meat and poultry, (fin) fish, shellfish, and sugars (including honey).

Milk and Milk Products

Test 1: Test for **casein proteins**

> Test food: White hard cheese
>
> Suggested types: Mozzarella; Parmesan
>
> Use a block of about 2-3 ounces
>
> Cut into SEVEN equal cubes

Morning: one cube

Afternoon: two cubes

Evening: four cubes

Interpretation of results of Test 1

- If there is no reaction after Day 2 (monitoring day), **CASEIN PROTEINS** are tolerated.

- If there is an adverse reaction, casein proteins are not tolerated and Tests 2 and 3 should not be attempted, since all of these foods contain casein.

Test 2: Test for casein and **whey proteins**

Test food: Lactase treated milk

Suggested: Purchased Lactaid milk®; or Lacteeze milk®
(99% lactose free)

OR: Milk treated with Lactaid drops as follows:

- Add 15 drops to 1 litre of homogenized milk

- Leave treated milk in the refrigerator for 24 hours before the test to allow the enzyme (lactase) to break down the lactose.

Quantities:

Morning: ⅛ cup

Afternoon: ¼ cup

Evening: ½ cup

Interpretation of results of Test 2

- If there is <u>no</u> adverse reaction after Day 2 (monitoring day), **casein and whey proteins** are tolerated.

- If there <u>is</u> an adverse reaction to Test 2, but not to Test 1: casein proteins are tolerated, but whey proteins are not.

Test 3: Test for casein proteins, whey proteins and **lactose**

Test food: Regular Milk

Suggested: Skim; OR partially skimmed; OR 1%; OR 2%; OR homogenized milk.

Only use homogenized or whole milk for a child under 5 years of age.

Morning: ⅛ cup

Afternoon: ¼ cup

Evening: ½ cup

Interpretation of results of Test 3

- If there is <u>no</u> reaction after Day 2 (monitoring day), milk protein allergy and lactose intolerance have all been ruled out.

- When a lactose-intolerant person exceeds their limit of tolerance, gastrointestinal symptoms of gas, bloating, and sometimes abdominal pain and diarrhea will be experienced. If gastrointestinal symptoms occur after Test 3, but not after any of the previous tests for milk components, **lactose intolerance** is confirmed.

NOTE:

1 cup of homogenized (3.3% M.F.) milk contains 12.00 grams of lactose.

1 cup of 2% or 1% milk contains 11.2 grams of lactose.

1 cup of 1% milk contains 10.8 grams of lactose.

This means that you can estimate the amount of lactose that your child can tolerate. Here are some general guidelines:

- A child who tolerates ¼ cup of milk will be able to tolerate lactose in food and beverages to a total of about 3 grams.

- If ½ cup of milk is tolerated, lactose to a level of 6 grams in food and beverages will be safe.

- If 1 cup of milk is tolerated, lactose to a level of 12 grams in food and beverages will be tolerated.

The above challenge tests are usually quite sufficient in confirming milk allergy and lactose intolerance in children. For those people who would like a clearer idea of their reactivity to other components of milk (whey proteins and modified milk proteins) please refer to the directions in the companion book in this series.[1]

Most children love Test 4 and, since the child has usually not enjoyed the elimination part of the test, this is often used by parents as a "reward."

Test 4: Complete Milk Proteins and Lactose in a complex Product

Test Food: Ice Cream

Suggested: Pure cream ice cream, plain vanilla flavor:

Note on the Manufacture of Ice Cream:

In the manufacture of ice cream, vanilla is made first, then the lighter colored ice creams, usually ending with chocolate. If the vats are not cleaned adequately between different batches, residues from the previous batches may contaminate the later ones. Therefore, chocolate ice cream is likely to contain the greatest number of potential allergens and should be tested only after all other flavors have been shown to be tolerated. This is an important consideration if a child is allergic to nuts: the nut-flavored ice creams are usually made before the chocolate-flavored ones.

In cheaper brands of ice cream, a number of additives such as artificial and natural flavors, colors, preservatives, emulsifiers, and texture modifiers are used. If these are suspected to be triggers of adverse reactions, ice creams containing these additional ingredients should be tested only after ice cream made from pure cream has been tolerated.

Each flavor of ice cream may be challenged separately if vanilla ice cream is tolerated.

Quantities:

Morning:	⅛ cup
Afternoon:	¼ cup
Evening:	½ cup

Egg

Egg yolk and egg white are tested <u>separately</u> because each fraction contains different proteins. Eggs from different species of birds may be challenged in separate tests.

- Hard boil the egg.
- Separate the yolk from the white.

Test 1: Egg yolk

Morning:	½ teaspoon
Afternoon:	1 teaspoon
Evening:	2 teaspoons

Test 2: Egg white

Test exactly as described for egg yolk

Morning:	½ teaspoon
Afternoon:	1 teaspoon
Evening:	2 teaspoons

<u>Interpretation of Results of Egg Challenge</u>

- If egg yolk, but not egg white is tolerated (no adverse reaction to egg yolk), egg yolks *separated from the white* can be used in baking, making omelets, and providing other egg-containing dishes, but cannot be used in dishes that require egg white only.

- Egg Beaters® or other similar products that are made from egg white only (often advised in cholesterol-lowering diets) *cannot be used* if egg white is not tolerated.

- If the egg white (albumin) is tolerated, but egg yolk is not, egg whites, separated from the yolk, Egg Beaters,® and other products made from egg white only, can be used.

- Egg replacers made from vegetable oils and other nonegg ingredients can be used if egg yolk and egg white are not tolerated.

Cereal Grains

Challenges for cereal grains need to be taken in an organized, step-by-step approach.

- Each cereal grain is reintroduced as a single food before being challenged as an ingredient in baked goods such as crackers, breads, and so on.

- Most grains can be obtained as a "bulk food," so a small quantity suitable for the test can be purchased without incurring the expense of buying a large quantity of something that may not be eaten again.

Wheat

There are three tests for wheat.

Test 1: Wheat in its purest form

Test food: Pure wheat cereal, without additives

Suggested: Puffed wheat®

Or Shredded wheat® (without sugar coating or additives)

Or wheat flakes (cooked in water)

Or Cream of Wheat® (cooked in water)

Formula, fruit juice, Rice Dream® or soy beverage may be added *if allowed during the elimination phase of the program.*

Morning: ⅛ cup

Afternoon: ¼ cup

Evening: ½ cup

Test 2: Wheat flour with ingredients commonly included in baked products, but without yeast

Test food: Yeast-free wheat cracker

Suggested: Triscuit® crackers

Quantities:

Morning: 1 cracker

Afternoon: 2 crackers

Evening: 4 crackers

Test 3: Complete wheat product

Test food: Whole wheat flour, with yeast and the usual bakery ingredients

Suggested: Commercial whole wheat bread

Quantities:

Morning: ¼ slice

Afternoon: ½ slice

Evening: 1 slice

Other grains

Other grains, including oats, rye, barley, and corn, need to be tested individually.

- Test each grain in its purest form first.
- Follow with baked goods made from the flour (e.g. bread, crackers).
- Use the method and quantities as described above for wheat.

Oats   (1) Test food: Oatmeal

Suggested food: cooked natural oatmeal made into a breakfast porridge

(2) Test food: Oat cake

Suggested food: Scottish oat cake (wheat-free) made with oats and oat flour

Rye   (1) Test food: Rye grain

Suggested food: Rye flakes cooked in water, made into a breakfast porridge

(2)Test food: Rye cracker

Suggested food: Ryvita® rye cracker or Wasa® Light rye crispbread without wheat

(3) Test food: 100% rye flour

Suggested food: Commercial 100% rye bread (available in specialized bakeries)

Barley   (1) Test food: Barley grain

Suggested food: Pearl barley or barley flakes cooked in water or tolerated broth

(2) Test food: Barley flour

Suggested food: Barley bread made with wheat-free barley flour

Corn

Corn is widely used as a grain or a vegetable and appears in many derivatives. Because of its many forms, there are several steps in the challenge tests.

- Because corn is eaten in various ways such as the whole grain as a vegetable, or derivatives of corn are used as ingredients in the form of corn oil, corn syrup, corn starch, corn flour and corn meal, it may be necessary to challenge each separately.

- Not all components of corn have the same potential for triggering adverse reactions.

- Thus it is sometimes important that a child's tolerance of each should be assessed.

- If whole corn is not tolerated it is especially important to challenge corn derivatives because they are used in numerous manufactured foods.

- Eliminating corn from the diet is relatively simple and usually poses no nutritional risk; however, restricting all foods containing ingredients derived from corn can make life difficult, and may lead to nutritional deficiency if many convenience foods are included in the family's meals, because so many convenience foods contain ingredients derived from corn.

- If corn derivatives are proven to be safe, it will make dietary choices much easier.

<u>Test food:</u> Corn grain as a vegetable

Suggested: corn on the cob (cooked):

Quantities:

    Morning: ¼ cob

    Afternoon: ½ cob

    Evening: 1 cob

    OR:

Frozen or canned corn Niblets®, cooked and served without additional ingredients such as butter.

Quantities:

    Morning: 1 teaspoon

    Afternoon: 2 teaspoons

    Evening: 4 teaspoons

<u>Test food:</u>   Processed whole corn

Suggested food: Plain popcorn

<u>Test food:</u>   Corn meal

Suggested food: Corn meal bread

<u>Test food:</u>   Corn starch or corn flour

Suggested: Use as a thickener in gravy made from meat drippings where all the other ingredients are known and tolerated.

<u>Test food:</u>   Corn oil

Suggested: Add to pasta, or a salad with known and tolerated ingredients.

<u>Test food:</u> Corn syrup

Suggested: Pour over pancakes made from known and tolerated ingredients.

Soy

In our modern world, soy beans are components in hundreds of food products, many of which have names that do not sound like "soy." Thus, it is important to learn to recognize the various names for soy and soy products.

- Soy is consumed in a number of different forms, for example:

  – tofu (soy protein coagulated [not fermented] with calcium or magnesium sulfate)

  – soy beverage ("soy milk") made from (usually) uncooked ground soy beans diluted with water

  – soy sauce (fermented soy usually with wheat added)

  – tamari sauce (fermented soy without wheat)

- It is wise to challenge each one separately.

- The following schedule of challenge tests is designed to evaluate a child's reactivity to each of these.

Test 1: Test food: Tofu, cooked

Suggested: Extra-firm tofu cut into one-inch cubes, deep-fried in olive or canola oil and drained

Morning: 1 cube

Afternoon: 2 cubes

Evening: 4 cubes

Test 2: Soy beverage

Suggested: Commercial soy "milk"

Morning: ⅛ cup

Afternoon: ¼ cup

Evening: ½ cup

<u>Test 3:</u> Fermented soy derivative without wheat

> Suggested: Tamari sauce. May be added to any known tolerated food.

> Morning: ¼ teaspoon

> Afternoon: ½ teaspoon

> Evening: 1 teaspoon

Regular soy sauce (with wheat) can be used if wheat is tolerated.

FRUITS AND VEGETABLES

Fruits and vegetables need to be handled individually in challenge tests, so you should plan to take these foods one at a time.

- Heat can change the allergenicity of vegetables and fruits.

- The cooked form is usually less allergenic, and thus better tolerated than the raw.

- When challenging vegetables and fruits, test the cooked form first, and follow with the food in its raw state.

Fruits

There are some important points to remember in the fruit challenge process. These are:

- The heat generated in the canning process is usually sufficient to change the allergenicity of the food, so fruit canned in its own juice can be challenged as "cooked."

- Alternatively, fruits can be "poached" by boiling in a little water, or cooked into a purée, for example, cooking apples into "apple sauce", but without any added ingredient, such as sugar.

- Some varieties of fruits are more allergenic than others. Ideas for different species of a fruit have been provided; the ones considered lower in allergenicity are given first in the sequence.

Orange

<u>Test 1</u>: Test food: Cooked orange

> Suggested: Canned Mandarin orange

Quantities:

> Morning: 1 section
>
> Afternoon: 2 sections
>
> Evening: 4 sections

<u>Test 2</u>: Test food: Raw orange

> Suggested food: Fresh Mandarin orange

Quantities:

> Morning: 1 section
>
> Afternoon: 2 sections
>
> Evening: 4 sections

<u>Test 3</u>: Test food: Raw orange of a different variety

> Suggested: Fresh navel orange

Use the same quantities as given for raw Mandarin orange above.

Grapefruit:

> Test food: (1) Cooked or canned grapefruit
>
>   (2) Raw grapefruit

Challenge exactly as described for oranges above.

Grapes

There are several things to remember about testing grapes. These are:

- Wash fruit well before testing, preferably with a detergent made for washing foods, to remove surface molds. An example of a food detergent is Fit® Fruit and Vegetable Wash, manufactured by Proctor and Gamble.

- Sulfites used as a preservative will not be removed entirely by washing.

- People sensitive to sulphites should not eat grapes.

- Because grapes are not usually eaten cooked, they are challenged in the raw state only.

Quantities:

Morning: 2 grapes

Afternoon: 4 grapes

Evening: 8 grapes

Raisins

Raisin food challenges need to be handled carefully to identify whether an allergic reaction is caused by the raisin itself or by sulfite, a product often added to raisins as a preservative.

- Raisins are dried grapes. Raisins purchased in the grocery store or supermarket are raw.

- However, raisins are often eaten cooked in cakes, cookies, and other baked goods, whereas grapes are not.

- Occasionally a child will tolerate cooked raisins but will react adversely to raw raisins.

- It is wise to challenge cooked raisins before trying them raw.

- Most commercially produced raisins contain sulfite, which is added as a preservative.

- If sulfite sensitivity is suspected, nonsulfited raisins, available in health food stores, should be challenged before the sulfited kind.

- If nonsulfited raisins are tolerated, sulfited raisins should then be challenged.

- If sensitivity to raisins is suspected, raisins should be tested in the following sequence:

  1. nonsulfited cooked raisins

  2. nonsulfited raw raisins

  3. sulfited raw raisins

- This sequence of testing will determine whether the child is

  1. Sensitive to cooked raisins

  2. Sensitive to raw raisins

  3. Sensitive to sulfites

For each challenge, the following quantities of raisins are suitable:

Morning: ⅛ cup

Afternoon: ¼ cup

Evening: ½ cup

Apple

Test 1: Test food: Apple cooked in one of the ways suggested:

Boil

- Core and slice one large or two medium apples.

- Place in a saucepan with a little water and bring to the boil.

- Reduce heat and simmer until the apple is soft and mushy.

Microwave

- Alternatively, place cored, peeled, sliced apple into a covered dish.

- Microwave on high for five minutes.

Quantities for test:

Morning: ⅛ cup

Afternoon: ¼ cup

Evening: ½ cup

Test 2: Raw apple

- Peel and core apple.

- Cut one half of the apple into seven equal slices; use a whole apple for an older child, or a small apple for a younger child.

Morning: 1 slice

Afternoon   2 slices

Evening: 4 slices

Vegetables

There are many vegetables to which your child may be allergic. It is important to challenge each of these individually to identify which ones cause your child distress. There are several steps to follow to start a vegetable challenge test. Begin by offering cooked forms of the vegetable to be tested.

- Cook the vegetable until is soft and "limp." For most vegetables, choose one of the following methods of cooking:

  − 5-7 minutes at high in a microwave oven

  − 15-20 minutes boiled in water

  − Roast in an oven at 400°C for 20-30 minutes

- This is usually enough to change the structure of the molecules sufficiently for the food to be tolerated.

- Make sure that the food is cooked <u>all the way through</u>, otherwise the raw uncooked center might cause an adverse reaction.

- Adjust the times given above as needed to ensure thorough cooking.

A few representative examples of challenge tests for vegetables are provided below.

- Test each type of vegetable separately.
- Adjust cooking times and quantities, if necessary, depending on the characteristics of the vegetables being tested.

Tomato

Tomatoes should be eaten without dressing.

<u>Test 1</u>: Cooked or canned without additional ingredients

Morning:	⅛ tomato	or 1 slice cooked	or ⅛ cup
Afternoon:	¼ tomato	or 2 slices cooked	¼ cup
Evening:	½ tomato	or 4 slices cooked	½ cup

<u>Test 2</u>: Raw tomato

Morning:	⅛ tomato	or 1 slice cooked	⅛ cup
Afternoon:	¼ tomato	or 2 slices cooked	¼ cup
Evening:	½ tomato	or 4 slices cooked	½ cup

<u>Test 3</u>: Tomato ketchup

Commercial tomato ketchup contains additional ingredients to which your child may react. It is wise to test this separately if you suspect that ketchup may have caused a reaction in the past, but the child does tolerate tomatoes.

Test food: Commercial tomato ketchup

Carrier food: French fries (if tolerated)

- Ensure that the specified amount of ketchup is consumed.
- The number of French fries is unlimited (unless you want to limit them!)

  Morning   ½ tablespoon

  Afternoon   1 tablespoon

  Evening   2 tablespoons

Other fruits and vegetables

- Test each separately as described above.
- Adjust cooking times and quantities according to the characteristics of the food.

Juices

Both vegetable and fruit juices may be tested using the following steps:

- Test cooked juice first before the fresh, raw product.
- Fruit or vegetable juice can be heated in the microwave, or brought to a boil on the stove and cooled before drinking.
- Pasteurized juices will have been heated sufficiently to change the allergenicity of the fruit or vegetable antigens; pasteurized juices can be used in the challenge in place of ones you cook at home.

Lemon or lime

Squeeze juice from a fresh fruit into ½ cup of water.

  Add sugar or honey to taste.

  Morning: Juice from ⅛ fruit

  Afternoon: Juice from ¼ fruit

Evening: Juice from ½ fruit

Other fruit or vegetable juices (apple, orange, carrot, etc.)

Morning: ⅛ cup

Afternoon: ¼ cup

Evening: ½ cup

Legumes

Legumes include peanuts, peas, navy beans, mung beans, and soybeans. Peanuts are one of the most common allergens.

Peanut

Test 1: Cooked peanuts

- Roasted without added ingredients such as artificial barbecue flavor, and so on.

- Or: boiled peanuts

Quantities:

Morning: 2 peanuts

Afternoon: 4 peanuts

Evening: 8 peanuts

Raw peanuts are generally not available in North America. Those in the shell have been roasted. However, you are advised to read product labels carefully, especially for imported peanut products.

Peas, dried peas, and dried beans

Test 1: Cooked peas and beans of any type with skins such as:

Navy beans   Green peas

Pinto beans	Dried peas
Kidney beans	Black-eyed peas
Soybeans	Mung beans

Quantities:

Morning:	⅛ cup
Afternoon:	¼ cup
Evening:	½ cup

Test 2: Raw legumes

If legumes are sometimes eaten raw (for example, snow peas, green peas), challenge separately after testing them cooked.

Bean Sprouts

Many types of beans are used for sprouts, including soybeans, peanuts, mung, and more. Thus, you need to read labels carefully to determine the type of bean used to make the particular sprouts you are testing. Your child may—or may not—tolerate sprouts from several types of beans.

- Sprouting changes the composition of the bean.

- Bean sprouts are eaten cooked (as in stir-fries) or, more commonly, raw in salads and sandwiches.

- Both cooked and raw sprouts from any beans should be challenged separately.

- The following quantities are suitable for testing both cooked and raw sprouts:

Quantities:

Morning	⅛ cup
Afternoon	¼ cup
Evening	½ cup

- Challenge sprouts from grains (such as wheat) and seeds (such as alfalfa) in the same way.

Nuts

<u>Cooked nuts should be tested before raw nuts since roasting and other forms of heating can change the chemical composition of the nuts.</u>

<u>Test 1:</u> Cooked nuts

>   Suggested: Roasted nuts without additional ingredients such as artificial flavor, color, or preservatives

- Nuts are the reproductive parts of trees of many unrelated species.

- Allergy to one species of tree does not indicate that nuts from botanically unrelated trees will cause allergy.

- You may wish to challenge each type of nut individually, for example:

Almond	Cashew	Chestnut
Walnut	Pistachio	Hazelnut (Filbert)
Pecan	Macadamia	Pine nut (Pignoli)
Brazil nut	Coconut	

<u>Test 2:</u> Raw nuts from the shell

Quantities for cooked or raw nuts:

>   Morning: 1 teaspoon
>
>   Afternoon: 2 teaspoons
>
>   Evening: 4 teaspoons

Note: If a child is allergic to one nut, or even peanuts, it is wise to make sure that he or she avoids all nuts until they are old enough to distinguish one from another.

The danger of cross-contamination from one type of nut with another during processing and distribution is very high, and since nuts and peanuts are highly allergenic foods, total avoidance is advised in most cases.

The exception is when the child has only a mild reaction to one type of nut, and parents wish to feed the child pure nut and seed butters. This is particularly important for vegetarian, and even more so for vegan, families when nuts and seeds supply a significant proportion of the protein in their diets.

Seeds

Test food: Seeds, roasted, followed by raw if appropriate, without additional ingredients

Suggested:

Sesame seed	Sunflower seeds
Poppy seed	Flax seed
Pumpkin seed	Melon seed

Quantities:

Morning:	½ teaspoon
Afternoon:	1 teaspoon
Evening:	2 teaspoons

Meat and Poultry

Meats from any animal, including poultry, need to be tested one at a time since your child may be sensitive to meat from one animal but not meat from another.

- The easiest way to challenge meat of any animal and poultry is to start with pure ground meat, without additives such as preservatives, colors, or flavors. Ensure that no nitrates or nitrites have been added to preserve the color.

- Cook the meat well in a microwave, oven, or frying pan.

- Pour off excess fat and discard.

- The meat may then be consumed as a patty, or crumbled.

    Suitable quantities for challenge tests:

    Morning   ½ ounce (15 g)

    Afternoon   1 ounce (30 g)

    Evening   2 ounces (60 g)

Processed meats

Processed meats include any meat product that has been cooked, spiced, salted, or otherwise changed from its pure, raw state. Bacon, pepperoni, bologna, and sausage are just a few of the processed meats that are commonly available in grocery stores and food products.

Test 1: Sliced meats

   Suggested: Slices of any manufactured meats such as:

Pepperoni	Cured or smoked bacon
Salami	Cured or smoked ham
Bologna	Summer sausage

   Quantities:

   Morning   1 slice

   Afternoon   2 slices

   Evening   4 slices

Test 2: Sausages

   Suggested: Frankfurters, wieners, or other sausages.

   Quantities below are based on the small-size wiener that is usually used as a regular hot dog in North America.

Morning	¼ sausage
Afternoon	½ sausage
Evening	1 sausage

Fish

<u>Test 1</u>. Plain cooked fish without breading or batter, such as:

Cod	Perch	Halibut
Sole	Salmon	Mackerel
Red snapper	Tuna	Sea Bass
Whitefish	Pollock	Basa

<u>Test 2</u>. Fish canned in water or oil, but without spices or sauce, such as:

Tuna	Sardines
Salmon	Pilchards

Quantities:

Morning	½ ounce (15 g)
Afternoon	1 ounce (30 g)
Evening	2 ounces (60 g)

Shellfish

Note that clams, oysters, mussels, and other bivalve species are included in the category of shellfish.

- Test cooked fish before testing it raw.
- Canned shellfish is cooked, so it can be eaten from the can.

- Amounts depend on the type of shellfish being tested.
- The following quantities are meant as guidelines.

Test 1: Large shellfish such as:

Crab	Crayfish (crawfish)
Lobster	

Quantities:

Morning	½ ounce (15 g)
Afternoon	1 ounce (30 g)
Evening	2 ounces (60 g)

Test 2: Individual shellfish such as:

Shrimp	Mussel
Prawn	Clam
Oyster	Scallop

Quantities:

Morning	2 fish
Afternoon	4 fish
Evening	8 fish

Sugars

Sensitivity to specific sugars can be due to several causes. These include inborn errors of metabolism (for example, abnormal galactose transport and metabolism; abnormal fructose metabolism); conditions involving abnormal regulation of serum levels of glucose such as hypoglycemia, hyperglycemia, and diabetes; and to allergy.

- If a person is allergic to sugar, it is the plant from which the sugar is derived that is the source of the foreign protein allergen.

- In order to determine which sugar source causes the allergic symptoms, each is challenged separately.

- *The instructions below are designed strictly and exclusively for determining whether a person is allergic to a specific sugar. They are not for diagnosis of any other condition that leads to an adverse reaction to sugars.*

- The same quantity of sugar is taken in each case. If desired, the sugar can be added to half a cup of warm water.

Quantities;

Morning:	½ teaspoon
Afternoon:	1 teaspoon
Evening:	2 teaspoons

Suggested sugars to be challenged individually:

- Maple sugar or maple syrup

- Cane sugar

- Beet sugar

- Corn sugar or corn syrup

- Date sugar

- Fructose (Fruit sugar; sometimes called levulose)

- Honey (glucose and fructose)

Notes on allergy to honey

- *Do not feed honey to any child under the age of 1 year because of its association with* **Clostridium** **difficile** *bacterial infections in the intestines of infants.*

- *Pollen allergy*

  If a person is allergic to the pollen of the plant from which the honey is derived, eating the honey may cause symptoms, whereas honey from a different plant may be tolerated. For example, alfalfa honey may cause an allergic reaction when clover honey is tolerated. Thus, it is important to carefully read the labels of any honey product to determine the source of the pollen. If no source is specifically mentioned on the label and your child is sensitive to honey from specific plants, then you must assume the honey is from multiple plants and you should not provide it to your child.

- *Bee sting allergy*

  There is no evidence that allergy to bee sting is associated with allergy to honey. Bee venom is injected directly into the blood stream during a bee sting, whereas the honey is eaten and undergoes digestion before entering the circulation. In any case, it is extremely unlikely that honey would contain any bee venom.

References

1. Joneja JMV. *Dealing with Food Allergies: A practical guide to detecting culprit foods and eating a healthy, enjoyable diet.* Boulder Colorado; Bull Publishing Company, 2003.

APPENDIX E

Maintenance Diets

When the culprit food components and additives have been identified, a maintenance diet must be formulated which removes the reactive foods and supplies complete balanced nutrition from alternative sources. Because this diet will probably need to be followed for the long term, it is extremely important that it should supply every essential nutrient. At the same time, this diet must be appropriate for the child and for the mother, if the baby is being breast-fed. If a diet is difficult to follow because of its emphasis on foods that the child or mother finds unacceptable, and/or, if it requires the expenditure of excessive time, money, and effort on the part of the parents and care-givers, it will soon be abandoned. All of the effort and energy invested in identifying the culprit foods will have been for naught, and both the caregivers and the child will be left with the same degree of distress as before. Formulating the appropriate diet for the particular needs of the child and the family requires some time and effort. This process is best achieved with the help of trained professionals, preferably the child's doctor and a registered dietitian.

The maintenance diet should aim to meet several important goals. To accomplish the goals, the diet will have the following characteristics:

- Must *exclude* all foods and additives to which the child has reacted.

- Must be nutritionally *complete*, providing nutrients from nonreactive sources.

- Must be designed to take into account your family's lifestyle and financial status.

- Should include sufficient flexibility to accommodate "unusual" situations such as religious festivals, celebrations (such as birthdays and weddings), vacations, travel, and eating in situations where obtaining substitute foods might be a problem.

When parents are focusing on the foods that are making their child sick and following often complex restrictive elimination diets, it is easy to lose sight of the most fundamental principal of dietary practice: Good health can be achieved and maintained only by providing the body with all of the macro- and micronutrients essential for its optimal functioning. At each stage of the process of determining the foods that are responsible for a child's adverse reactions, complete balanced nutrition must be provided, preferably from foods, but if this is not entirely possible, by adding appropriate supplements.

- Good health can be achieved and maintained only by providing the body with all of the macro- and micronutrients essential for its optimal functioning.

ENSURING THAT ALL THE ESSENTIAL NUTRIENTS ARE PROVIDED

The process of devising the ideal diet in each particular case starts with the identification of the nutrients that may be deficient when specific foods are removed, and correcting the deficiency by substitution of different foods containing the same nutrients. The following guidelines will aid in this process. Tables E-1 to E-5 provide data that will aid in formulating a nutritionally complete diet while eliminating the allergenic foods.

Diet for Optimum Nutrition

The most important directive is: provide your child with a nutritionally balanced diet that supplies all the required macronutrients (protein, fat, carbohydrate) and micronutrients (vitamins and trace minerals) every day.

- To simplify the process, **each meal** should contain three components:

  1. Protein (PRO)

  2. Grain (GR) or Starch (ST)

  3. Fruit and/or Vegetable (FR/VEG)

In the tables provided below, cross out every food to which your child reacted adversely. Add others that he or she tolerated in the appropriate category, if they are missing. Then select at least one food from each category for every meal and, if possible, for every snack. The quantities of each food should be appropriate for the child's age, and the breast-feeding mother's nutritional requirements.

Table E-1

THE BALANCED DIET: EXAMPLES OF FOODS IN EACH IMPORTANT FOOD CATEGORY

Protein foods (PRO):

- Meat of all types
- Poultry
- Fish
- Shellfish
- Eggs
- Nuts
- Seeds

- Tofu
- Milk
- Milk products such as:
  - Cheese of all types
  - Yogurt
  - Buttermilk

Grains (GR):

Starches (ST):

Grains should be whole grains as often as possible.

- Wheat
- Rye
- Oats
- Barley
- Rice
- Corn
- Amaranth
- Quinoa
- Buckwheat
- Millet

- Flours and starches derived from grains listed under "Grains"
- Starchy vegetables and fruits, such as:
  - Potato
  - Sweet potato
  - Yam
  - High-starch root vegetables
  - Lentils
  - Dried beans
  - Dried peas
  - Garbanzo bean (chick pea)
  - Lima beans

Table E-1 (continued)
THE BALANCED DIET: EXAMPLES OF FOODS IN EACH
IMPORTANT FOOD CATEGORY

Grains (GR) (cont'd):	Starches (ST) (cont'd):

Grains should be whole grains as often as possible.
 	
• Varieties and derivatives of wheat, such as:
  – Spelt
  – Kamut
  – Bulgur
  – Triticale
  – Semolina
	• Starchy vegetables and fruits, such as: (cont'd)
	  – Broad beans (fava)
	  – Cassava
	  – Plantain
	  – Banana

Vegetables	**Fruits**

• Green leafy vegetables such as:
  – Lettuce
  – Chard
  – Spinach
  – Broccoli
• Beans:
  – Green
  – String
  – French
  – Runner
  – Yellow wax
	• Berries:
	  – Strawberry
	  – Raspberry
	  – Blueberry
	  – Cranberry
	  – Others
	• Stone fruits:
	  – Peaches
	  – Apricots
	  – Nectarines
	  – Cherries
	  – Plums

Table E-1 (continued)
THE BALANCED DIET: EXAMPLES OF FOODS IN EACH IMPORTANT FOOD CATEGORY

Vegetables (cont'd)	Fruits (cont'd)
• Peas	• Stone fruits (cont'd):
– Green peas	– Others
– Sugar peas	• Melons
• Green, red, yellow peppers	– Cantaloupe
• Squashes of all types	– Honeydew
• Onions	– Watermelon
• Garlic	– Others
• Tomatoes	• Citrus
• Carrots	– Orange
• Beets	– Grapefruit
• Radishes	– Lemon
• Cauliflower	– Lime
• Asparagus	• Tropical fruits such as:
• Eggplant	– Pineapple
• Others	– Mango
	– Papaya
	– Passion fruit
	– Lychee
	– Others
	• Apples
	• Pears
	• Rhubarb
	• Others

SUPPLEMENTS

When a food category supplying essential micronutrients (vitamins and minerals) needs to be restricted, supplemental sources of the nutrients should be provided. For example:

Multivitamin/mineral

- A multivitamin/mineral with iron once a day

- The supplement should be **free from**: artificial color, flavor, preservatives and additional ingredients such as wheat, yeast, corn, lactose, sugar, salt if they are restricted in the diet.

- If histamine intolerance is a problem the multivitamin should also be free from *niacin.* You will find multivitamins that replace niacin with *niacinamide.* This is acceptable.

    - Recommended brands include: Quest, Jamieson, Nulife, Nutricology, Natural Factors, Sisu

Note:
These manufacturers also make supplements which do not conform to these recommendations, and other companies not listed here market suitable products. *Please read all labels carefully* in order to find the right supplement for your child's needs.

Calcium

- When all milk and milk products are restricted: Calcium gluconate, or calcium citrate, or calcium carbonate with Kreb's cycle derivatives according to recommended levels (Please refer to Chapter 7, Milk Allergy, for calcium requirements in each age category)

Table E-2

IMPORTANT NUTRIENTS IN COMMON ALLERGENS

Equivalent nutrients must be provided from alternative sources when the following foods are eliminated from the diet.

Milk and milk products:

Calcium	*Smaller amounts:*
Phosphorus	Vitamin A*
Vitamin D*	Vitamin E
Vitamin B_{12}	
Pantothenic acid	
Riboflavin	
Potassium	

Alternative sources of these nutrients:
Fortified rice,* soy,* and oat beverages* can be a good source of calcium, vitamin D, and vitamin A. Calcium-fortified juices and cereal products are also available. Riboflavin, pantothenic acid, phosphorus, and vitamin E can be found in meats, legumes (such as peanuts, peas, beans, soybeans), nuts, and whole grains.

Egg:

Vitamin B_{12}	*Smaller amounts:*
Vitamin D	Vitamin A
Pantothenic acid	Vitamin E
Biotin	Vitamin B_6
Folacin	Zinc
Riboflavin	
Selenium	
Iron	

Table E-2 (continued)
IMPORTANT NUTRIENTS IN COMMON ALLERGENS

Alternative sources of these nutrients:
Meat, fish, and poultry products; legumes; whole grains; and vegetables

Soy:

Thiamin

Riboflavin

Vitamin B_6

Folacin

Calcium

Phosphorus

Magnesium

Iron

Zinc

Alternative sources of these nutrients:
Soy is typically used in commercial products in amounts that are too small to be considered a significant source for these nutrients. Therefore, elimination of soy from the diet does not compromise the nutritional quality of most diets.

Peanuts:

Niacin	*Smaller amounts:*
Vitamin E	Potassium
Manganese	Vitamin B_6
Chromium	Folacin
Pantothenic acid	Phosphorus
Magnesium	Copper
	Biotin

Table E-2 (continued)
IMPORTANT NUTRIENTS IN COMMON ALLERGENS

Alternative sources of these nutrients:
These nutrients may be replaced by including meat, whole grains, legumes, and vegetable oils in the diet.

Fish and shellfish:

Niacin	*Smaller amounts:*
Vitamin B_6	Potassium
Vitamin B_{12}	Magnesium
Vitamin E	Iron
Phosphorus	Zinc
Selenium	Vitamin A
Calcium (in shellfish and fish bones)	

Alternative sources of these nutrients:
These nutrients are also present in meats, grains, legumes, and oils.

Wheat:

Thiamin*	*Smaller amounts:*
Riboflavin*	Magnesium
Niacin*	Folacin
Iron*	Phosphorus
Selenium	Molybdenum
Chromium	

Alternative sources of these nutrients:
Alternative choices of foods to replace these include oats, rice, rye, barley, corn, buckwheat, amaranth, and quinoa, which are fortified with similar nutrients. Alternatives to wheat flour include flours and starches from rice, potato, rye, oats, barley, buckwheat, tapioca, millet, corn, quinoa, and amaranth.

Table E-2 (continued)
IMPORTANT NUTRIENTS IN COMMON ALLERGENS

Rice:

       Thiamin*

       Riboflavin*

       Niacin*

       Iron*

Corn:

       Thiamin*

       Riboflavin*

       Niacin*

       Iron*

       Chromium

* Indicates nutrient added to the food product. When such nutrients have been added, the product may be labeled "fortified" or "enriched."

Table E-3
SUMMARY: IMPORTANT NUTRIENTS IN COMMON ALLERGENS

Vitamins	Nutrient							
	MILK	EGG	PEANUT	SOY	FISH	WHEAT	RICE	CORN
A	+	+			+			
Biotin	+	+				+		
Folacin (Folate; Folic acid)	+	+	+		+			
B_1 (Thiamin)			+		+	+	+	
B_2 (Riboflavin)	+	+		+		+	+	+
B_3 (Niacin)		+		+	+	+	+	
B_5 (Pantothenic acid)	+	+	+					
B_6 (Pyridoxine)		+	+	+	+			
B_{12} (Coalmine)	+	+			+			
C								
D	+	+			+			

Table E-3 (continued)
SUMMARY: IMPORTANT NUTRIENTS IN COMMON ALLERGENS

	Nutrient							
	MILK	EGG	PEANUT	SOY	FISH	WHEAT	RICE	CORN
Vitamins (cont'd)								
E (alpha-tocopherol)	+	+	+		+			
K	+	+		+				
Minerals								
Calcium	+			+	+			
Phosphorus	+		+	+	+	+		
Iron		+		+	+	+	+	+
Zinc		+		+	+			
Magnesium				+	+	+		
Selenium		+			+	+		
Potassium	+		+		+			
Molybdenum						+		

Table E-3 (continued)
SUMMARY: IMPORTANT NUTRIENTS IN COMMON ALLERGENS

	Nutrient							
Minerals (cont'd)	MILK	EGG	PEANUT	SOY	FISH	WHEAT	RICE	CORN
Chromium			+			+		+
Copper		+						
Manganese			+					

Table E-4
ALTERNATIVE SOURCES OF NUTRIENTS

When Milk, Egg, Peanut, Soy, Fish, Wheat, Rice, and Corn are to be avoided

Vitamins

Vitamin A	Liver, fish liver oils, dark green and yellow vegetables, tomato, apricots, cantaloupe, mango, papaya
Vitamin D	Liver, fish liver oils, action of sunlight on skin
Vitamin E (alpha tocopherol)	Liver, legumes, green leafy vegetables, tomato whole grains, vegetable oils
Vitamin B_1 (thiamin)	Meats especially pork, dried and green peas, legumes, whole grains, nutritional yeast
Vitamin B_2 (riboflavin)	Organ meats, legumes, green vegetables, whole grains, nutritional yeast
Vitamin B_3 (niacin)	Organ meats, poultry, beef, legumes, whole grains, nutritional yeast
Vitamin B_6 (pyridoxine)	Meats especially organ meats, legumes, whole grains, green vegetables, carrots, potato, cauliflower, banana, prunes, avocado, sunflower seeds, nutritional yeast
Vitamin B_{12} (cobalamin)	Meats, especially organ meats; poultry
Vitamin B_7 (biotin)	Organ meats, nutritional yeast, mushrooms, banana, grapefruit, watermelon, strawberries

Table E-4 (continued)
ALTERNATIVE SOURCES OF NUTRIENTS

When Milk, Egg, Peanut, Soy, Fish, Wheat, Rice, and Corn are to be avoided

Vitamins (cont'd)

Vitamin B_5 (pantothenic acid)	Organ meats, chicken, beef, fresh vegetables, whole grains, nutritional yeast
Vitamin B_9 (Folic acid; Folate) (Folacin)	Organ meats, legumes, green leafy vegetables, asparagus, beets, broccoli, avocado, oranges, bananas, strawberries, whole grains, nutritional yeast

Minerals

Calcium	Amaranth, baked beans, rhubarb, green leafy vegetables, broccoli, dates, molasses
Phosphorus	Meats, poultry, legumes, whole grains, seeds, green peas, artichokes, potato, Brussels sprouts
Iron	Meats, liver, legumes, raisins, dried apricots, prunes, pumpkin, asparagus, broccoli, chard, green peas, spinach, molasses
Zinc	Meat, liver, green leafy vegetables, beets, green peas, oranges, strawberries, prunes, chocolate syrup
Magnesium	Legumes, whole grains, meat, poultry, dark green vegetables
Selenium	Whole grains, meat, broccoli, onions, tomato

Table E-4 (continued)
ALTERNATIVE SOURCES OF NUTRIENTS

When Milk, Egg, Peanut, Soy, Fish, Wheat, Rice, and Corn are to be avoided

Minerals (cont'd)

Potassium	Meats, oranges, banana, dried fruits, cantaloupe, honeydew melon, nectarines, papaya, tomato, avocado, dark greens, sweet potato, winter squash, potato, molasses
Molybdenum	Meat, legumes, whole grains, green vegetables (especially spinach), lettuce, Brussels sprouts, carrots, squash, tomatoes, apple juice
Chromium	Vegetable oils, meats, liver, nutritional yeast, whole grains
Copper	Liver, meat, whole grains, green leafy vegetables, broccoli, potato, pears, banana, apple juice
Manganese	Sunflower seeds, whole grains, legumes, nutritional yeast, green beans, broccoli, cranberry, grape, pineapple

APPENDIX F

A Useful Tool in the Dietary Management of Food Allergies

THE ALLERGEN SCALE

The so-called "Joneja Allergen Scale" has proved to be a useful tool for anyone trying to put together a diet in which specific foods are restricted.

It lists foods by their "relative allergenicity". The foods most frequently associated with allergy are at the top of the scale; those that infrequently trigger allergy are at the bottom.

This scale has evolved over many years, incorporating information from a wide variety of sources, and is revised each time more information about the allergenicity of foods appears.

It is most useful as a guide to what your child can and cannot eat. Cross out all of the foods to which you and your children are allergic. Then include all of the remaining foods in your family's diet.

This scale is based on the typical North American diet; diets of other ethnic groups will differ in the relative positions of the foods.

Table F-1
FOOD ALLERGEN SCALE

Foods are listed from the highest to the lowest allergenicity, based on reports from a variety of sources.
People vary in their reactivity to foods and show a different pattern of reactivity depending on their individual characteristics.
The scale is based on the typical North American diet. Persons following ethnic diets tend to show a different order of allergenicity.

GRAINS & FLOURS	VEGETABLES	FRUITS	NUTS & SEEDS	MEATS & ALTERNATES	MILK & MILK PRODUCTS
Wheat Triticale Semolina Bulgur Spelt Kamut	Tomato Spinach Celery (raw)	Strawberry Raspberry Orange Fig Mango Watermelon	Peanut Nuts: 　Hazelnut 　(Filbert)	Egg white Egg yolk	Ice cream Cow's milk: 　- Homogenized 　- Raw milk 　- 1%, 2% 　- Skim
Rye Corn	Carrot (raw) Green pea Lima bean Broad bean 　(fava bean) Cabbage (heart)	Apple (raw) Apricot (raw) Peach (raw) Date Cantaloupe Pineapple Raisin Apple (cooked)	Walnut Pecan Brazil nut Almond Sesame seed Cocoa bean Chocolate Coconut	Shellfish: 　- Crab 　- Lobster 　- Prawn/shrimp 　- Clam 　- Oyster 　- Scallop	Cheese: Fermented: 　- Cheddar 　- Camembert 　- Blue 　- Swiss 　- Edam 　- Mozzarella 　- Goat cheese
Oats Barley	Cauliflower Brussels sprouts Green bean Yellow wax bean	Kiwi Cherry Plum/prune Apricot (cooked)	Cashew Pistachio Macadamia	Fin fish: 　- Cod 　- Sole 　- Other white fish	- Cottage cheese - Cream cheese
White rice Brown rice Wild rice Millet	Avocado Cabbage 　(outer leaves) Onion Green onion Garlic	Loganberry Boysenberry Plantain Banana Grape	Legumes: 　Soy 　Dried peas 　Lentils Dried beans: 　- Navy 　- Pinto 　- Garbanzo Carob Sunflower seed Flax seed	- Tuna - Salmon Processed meats: 　- Pepperoni 　- Salami 　- Bologna 　- Wieners 　- Ham 　- Bacon	Cream Sour cream Canned milk (evaporated) Goat milk Sheep milk
Buckwheat (kasha)	Celery (cooked) Green/red 　peppers	Grapefruit Lemon Lime			
Amaranth	Potato Cucumber Lettuce	Currants (red/black)	Pumpkin seed	Pork	Processed cheese
Tapioca Cassava	Asparagus Broccoli Beets	Peach (cooked/ 　canned)	Bean sprouts	Chicken Beef Veal Turkey	Soft cheese (Philadelphia)
Sago Arrowroot Quinoa	Squashes (all types)	Cranberry Blackberry Blueberry	Poppy seed	Wild meats: 　- Deer 　- Elk 　- Moose 　- Bear 　- Buffalo	Yogurt Buttermilk Butter
	Carrot (cooked) Parsnip	Pear			
	Turnip Sweet potato Yam	Rhubarb		Rabbit Lamb	Clarified butter

SEQUENCE OF INTRODUCING SOLID FOODS FOR THE ALLERGIC BABY

Many parents of allergic babies find it very helpful to have a clearly defined schedule for the sequence of introducing solid foods. The following chart (Table F-2) is based on the Allergen Scale, so that the first foods introduced are those least likely to trigger allergy. The more highly allergenic foods are introduced later when the infant's immune system and digestive tract are more mature and allergic sensitization is less likely to occur.

How to use the chart:

• First cross out those foods to which you know that your baby is allergic, based on his or her previous reactions. These are the foods that mother should have been avoiding in her own diet during breast-feeding.

• Introduce all foods individually according to the protocols detailed in Chapter 3.

• Start at the top of each column.

• There is no particular order in which the different categories of foods should be introduced. However, if the baby has been exclusively breast-fed it is a good idea to introduce meats early since a food source of iron is important from 6 months of age onward.

• All foods should be in the purest form for baby's first exposure to them:

  – Grains should be introduced as the pure grain before baby cereals or pablum containing the grain. Some baby cereals contain ingredients in addition to the grain, such as soy lecithin or milk solids. If the cereal is a baby's first exposure to the grain, it is not possible to tell whether the baby is reacting to the grain or the additional ingredients when an allergic reaction occurs unless each has been introduced separately.

  – Some jarred baby foods contain additional ingredients; for example some baby lamb in jars has citric acid added as a preservative.

  – Do not give combined foods such as baby apple/apricot until all of the foods in the mixture have been introduced separately and tolerated.

- If a food is not tolerated, avoid that food for at least 3 months. Babies mature quite quickly, and a food that caused a mild reaction at the age of 7 months, may well be tolerated at 10 months or later. However, if the food caused a strong reaction, wait until the baby is at least 18 months of age before trying it again.

- If the food that caused a reaction is one of the "Top Six Allergens" (cow's milk, egg; peanut, tree nuts, fish, shellfish), many authorities recommend reintroduction at a later time under medical supervision to avoid the risk of anaphylaxis.

Table F-2
SEQUENCE OF ADDING SOLID FOODS FOR THE ALLERGIC BABY

Time of Introduction	Grains and Cereals	Vegetables	Fruits	Meat and Alternates	Milk and Dairy	Nuts, Seeds, Other
6 to 9 months	Rice Millet	All cooked Yam Sweet potato Squash (all types) Carrot Beets Broccoli Potato Green beans Cabbage	All cooked Pear Peach Banana Apricot Nectarine Blueberry	Lamb Turkey	Breast milk If absolutely necessary, casein hydrolysate formula	None
9 to 12 months	Barley Rye Oats	Asparagus Avocado Cauliflower Brussels sprouts	Plum Prune Pineapple Grape Apple Cranberry Raisins	Chicken Veal Beef	Breast milk or casein hydrolysate formula	None except vegetable oils in formula
12 to 24 months	Corn Wheat Other grains	Green pea Spinach Tomato Celery Cucumber Lettuce Onion Garlic Lima beans Broad beans Other legumes; soy Raw vegetables	Citrus fruits (orange, lemon, lime, grapefruit) Strawberry Raspberry Other berries Melons Mango Fig Date Cherry Any raw fruits	Ham Pork Egg[a]	Yoghurt (plain) Whole milk White cheese Cottage cheese	Sesame seed Flax seed Seed oils: Canola Safflower Sunflower
After two years	All	All	All	Fish[b] Shellfish[b]	All others including ice cream	Peanut[b] Nuts[b] Chocolate Seeds

[a] Some authorities recommend waiting until 24 months to introduce egg.
[b] Some authorities recommend waiting until after 3 years of age to introduce peanut, tree nuts, fish, and shellfish.

APPENDIX G

Vitamin B$_{12}$

Vitamin B$_{12}$ is necessary for the synthesis of red blood cells, the maintenance of the nervous system, and growth and development in children. Deficiency can cause pernicious anemia. Degeneration of nerve fibers and irreversible neurological damage can also occur.

Some people have difficulty in absorption of vitamin B$_{12}$. The process of absorption involves a glycol-protein which is made by cells (called parietal cells) in the stomach. This glycol-protein is called intrinsic factor. People lacking this factor are in danger of vitamin B$_{12}$ deficiency.

Efficient absorption of vitamin B$_{12}$ also depends on the acid that occurs naturally in the stomach. The vitamin is tightly bound to proteins in meat, eggs, fish, and dairy products and requires high acidity to cut it loose. Sometimes the stomach contents are not acidic enough to do this. Aging, the use of antacids, and other conditions that affect the release of gastric acid may reduce the acidity of the stomach, and ultimately lead to a vitamin B$_{12}$ deficiency.

People who are unable to efficiently absorb vitamin B$_{12}$ for any of these reasons require injections of the vitamin, which delivers it directly to the blood stream.

FOOD SOURCES OF VITAMIN B$_{12}$

The vitamin is made by bacteria, and deposited in the tissues of the organism in which it is synthesized. The most important food sources are meats (especially organ meats like liver), poultry (especially the liver), milk and milk products, eggs, fish, and shellfish.

There are some plant sources of vitamin B$_{12}$; however, humans are virtually unable to absorb the vitamin from these sources. Vegans who consume no animal sources of food therefore require supplemental B$_{12}$ in order to avoid a deficiency.

A list of food sources of vitamin B$_{12}$ can be found at: Nutrition Data: Nutrition Facts, Level of Vitamin B$_{12}$ in a list of 999 foods. The list can be accessed at:

http://www.nutritiondata.com/foods-00011600000000000000.html

In addition to naturally-occurring B$_{12}$, supplements such as multivitamin tablets, and vitamin B complex tablets, will provide the vitamin in an absorbable form. Read labels to ensure that vitamin B$_{12}$ is included in the supplement you choose.

Some breakfast cereals are fortified with the vitamin, which is sprayed on rather than incorporated into the plant food material, and thus is more like a supplement than a food source.

APPENDIX H

Sulfite Sensitivity

Sensitivity to sulfites is most common in people with asthma. Of these people, individuals who are steroid dependent are considered most at risk for sulfite-sensitivity. Although the incidence of adverse reactions to sulfites is estimated to be as high as 1 percent of the U.S. population, sulfite sensitivity in people without asthma is considered rare. Reported symptoms have occurred in most organ systems, including the lungs, gastrointestinal tract, and skin and mucous membranes. Reports of life-threatening anaphylactic reactions in persons with asthma may occur, but are very rare.

SYMPTOMS OF SULFITE SENSITIVITY

Symptoms that have been reported in sulfite sensitivity include:

- Asthma in asthmatics

- Severe respiratory reactions, including bronchospasm, wheezing, and a feeling of tightness in the chest

- Flushing, feeling of temperature change

- Onset of hypotension (low blood pressure)

503

- Gastrointestinal symptoms (abdominal pain, diarrhea, nausea, vomiting)

- Swallowing difficulty

- Dizziness, loss of consciousness

- Urticaria (hives), angioedema (swelling, especially of the mouth and face)

- Contact dermatitis

- Anaphylaxis (in persons with asthma

There is no evidence that avoiding all dietary sources of sulfites improves asthma.

For people who are not sensitive to sulfites, exposure to sulfiting agents poses very little risk. Toxicity studies in volunteers showed that ingestion of 400 mg of sulfites daily for 25 days produced no adverse effects.

SULFITES IN FOODS AND MEDICATIONS

Sulfites are used as preservatives in beverages, fruits, vegetables, prepared and pre-sliced foods, and packaged snack foods. The active component is sulfur dioxide, which has been used as a preservative since Roman times, especially for wine. Today it is the most versatile food additive in use.

Sulfites are also used as preservatives in some medications, including inhalable and injectable drugs, where they act as antioxidants and prevent browning. Some forms of epinephrine (adrenalin) contain sulfite as a preservative. However, the action of epinephrine appears to overcome any adverse effects of sulfite, and administration of epinephrine in anaphylactic emergencies is the recommended treatment.

Cooking foods does not cause sulfites to lose their effect. In addition, because sulfites bind to several substances in foods, such as protein, starch, and sugars, washing foods, even if a detergent is used, will not remove all traces of sulfites.

Sulfates in foods do not cause the same adverse reactions as sulfites, and need not be avoided by persons who are sensitive to sulfites.

Many countries have requirements that sulfites be listed on ingredient labels because of the increasing numbers of people (predominantly asthmatics) who are sensitive to sulfite.

U.S. government regulations state that if any food contains 10 parts per million or more, the sulfite must be identified in the ingredient list on the label.

Canadian government regulations require that if sulfites are used, they must be listed on the label.

SULFITES IN MANUFACTURED FOODS

Sulfites are permitted for use in the form of:

- Sodium metabisulfite

- Potassium metabisulfite

- Sodium bisulfite

- Potassium bisulfite

- Sodium sulfite

- Sodium dithionite

- Sulfurous acid

- Sulfur dioxide

These terms may appear on food labels. The term "sufiting agents" can refer to any of these.

In the European labeling system, sulfites have the designations: E 220, E 221, E 222, E 223, E 224, E 225, E 226, E 227, E 228.

SULFITES IN NATURAL FOODS

The use of sulfites on fresh fruit and vegetables, except sliced potatoes and raw grapes, has been banned in the United States by FDA regulation since 1986, and in Canada since 1987. However, a specified level of sulfites (calculated in parts per million) may be added to the following foods and beverages because no suitable alternatives are currently available:

(Note: As in all food lists in this book, this list may not be complete and ingredients may change. Also, food imported from other countries may not be produced by the same food manufacturing processes as in the United States and Canada, and may not comply with the same labeling standards.)

Fruits and Vegetables

- Dried fruits and vegetables such as apples, apricots, coconut, mincemeat, papaya, peaches, pears, pineapple, raisins, and sun-dried tomatoes

- Fruit and vegetable juices (except frozen concentrated orange juice)

- Frozen sliced apples

- Frozen sliced mushrooms

- Grapes

- Sliced potatoes (e.g., frozen French fries, dehydrated, mashed, peeled, or pre-cut)

- Glazed/glacéed fruits (e.g., apples, grapes, and maraschino cherries)

- Soy products

- Starches (e.g., corn, potato, noodles, and rice mixes)

Beverages

- Alcoholic

- De-alcoholized wines and beers

Sweeteners

- Glucose solids and syrup

- Dextrose (used in making confectionery)
- Molasses

Fish

- Crustaceans (shellfish)

Others

- Jams, jellies, marmalades (sulfite is in the pectin)
- Mincemeat
- Pickles and relishes
- Tomato paste, pulp, ketchup, purée
- Gelatin
- Pectin
- Snack foods
- Candies and confectioneries
- Frozen pizza dough
- Frozen pastry shells

Not all manufacturers of these products use sulfites.

Some Foods Do Not Require Labels

The presence of sulfites in the following may not be listed:

- Some bulk foods
- Individually sold candies
- Individually portioned foods such as those sold in vending machines, mobile canteens, and delis

- As a secondary ingredient in a manufactured food. For example, if one of the ingredients in a prepared cake is jam that contains sulfites, the jam must be listed, but not the sulfite contained in it. This is because the final level of sulfite in the finished product is below the amount required by law to be disclosed.

- Restaurant food. When eating in restaurants, *ask* whether sulfiting agents are present in the foods.

Alcoholic Beverages

In the United States, if sulfite levels are 10 parts per million (or more in wine, distilled spirits, and malt beverages), sulfites must be listed on the labels. In Canada at present, ingredients of alcoholic beverages, including sulfites, *need not* be listed on the label.

Medications

Sulfites are used in a wide range of medications and pharmaceuticals. The Compendium of Pharmaceuticals and Specialties (CPS) provides a list of sulfite-containing products. Consult your pharmacist about the sulfite content of any medications you require.

Other Sources of Sulfites

Food processing equipment, and food packaging materials (e.g. plastic bags) may be sanitized with sulfites. These sources of sulfites will not be listed on any labels.

Sulfite-sensitive individuals should avoid opening any packages likely to contain sulfites, especially sealed plastic bags containing dried fruits.

Note:

Some food manufacturers publish quite extensive lists of their products in which they specify ingredients to which food and food-additive sensitive consumers might react. Persons with sulfite sensitivity are advised to obtain these publications if they wish to purchase manufactured foods such as cookies, breakfast cereals, boxed entrees, and so on.

Additional information about foods that are likely to contain sulfites can be found on the Web site of the Canadian Food Inspection Agency department of Health Canada at:

http://www.inspection.gc.ca/english/fssa/labeti/allerg/sulphe.shtml.

GLOSSARY

When you don't know the meaning of a word used in this book, look it up in the following list. Used as a dictionary, this will increase your knowledge of the text of the book, especially the scientific sections, and help you to understand a great deal of additional material on allergies, immunology, and food science that you will find in other sources.

acetylcholine—One of the chemical substances known as neurotransmitters that relay nerve impulses across the spaces between nerves and muscles. Neurotransmitters are released at the synapses of the parasympathetic nerves and at neuromuscular junctions.

acidosis—The accumulation of acid or depletion of alkali (bicarbonate) in the blood and body tissues.

adrenaline—See **epinephrine**.

aerosol—A suspension of solid or liquid particles in a gas.

albumin—A type of protein classified on the basis of its solubility. Albumins are soluble in water at pH 6.6 (see also globulins; prolamins; glutelins). Albumins occur in different forms according to their function. For example, serum albumins occur in animals and humans; ovalbumin in eggs; parvalbumin in fish; lactalbumin in milk.

allergen—An antigen or hapten that causes a hypersensitivity reaction (allergy) in a sensitized individual.

allergen overload—A term used by allergists to indicate an excessive amount of antigen that, in theory, may result in a large volume of antigen entering circulation and triggering an immunological response when a lower quantity of antigen may be tolerated.

allergy—Hypersensitivity to an environmental, drug, or food antigen (allergen) caused by an altered or unusual immune system reaction to the antigen.

511

amino acid—An organic compound containing amino (nitrogen-hydrogen) and carboxyl (carbon-oxygen) chemical groups. Amino acids are the building blocks of all proteins.

anamnestic response—The rapid production of antibody in response to an antigen following a first exposure. Examples of anamnestic response include a natural reinfection or a booster shot of vaccine. An anamnestic response requires the presence of memory B and T cells remaining in the body from the first exposure.

anaphylactic reaction (anaphylaxis)—An immediate, severe reaction, characterized by breathing difficulty (dyspnea); swelling, especially of the face (angioedema); and a drop in blood pressure (hypotension). It is the result of the release of inflammatory mediators from mast cells and basophils . Food, insect venom, and drugs are the most common antigens that cause this extreme IgE-mediated reaction.

anaphylactic shock—An acute generalized allergic response (anaphylaxis) to an allergen in which edema; constriction of smooth muscles in the lungs, stomach, and blood vessels; a fall in blood pressure; circulatory collapse; and heart failure can lead to death.

anaphylactoid reaction—A bodily reaction with anaphylactic symptoms that is not induced by an antigen-antibody complex.

anaphylatoxin—A substance produced during a complement cascade (specifically complement components C3a and C5a) that causes the release of histamine and other vasoactive chemicals from mast cells and basophils. Vasoactive chemicals have an effect on the blood vessels causing changes in their size or actions.

anaphylaxis—See **anaphylactic shock**.

angioedema—A localized swelling (edema) in tissues below the surface of the skin or mucous membrane. It is caused by increased permeability of the capillaries from which fluid moves into the tissues to cause the swelling.

antibiotic—A substance that can kill or inhibit the growth of microorganisms by interfering with their metabolism. Antibiotics are often used as medications (drugs) to control infections.

antibody—A protein of the gamma-globulin type (immunoglobulin). Antibodies are produced by lymphocytes in the blood in response to a foreign antigen. Humans produce 5 types of antibodies called IgA, IgD, IgE, IgG, and IgM.

antiendomysial antibody—An sIgA antibody detected in celiac disease. The presence of the antiendomysial antibody in a test indicates active celiac disease. The antigen involved in eliciting the antibody has been identified as tissue transglutaminase.

antigen—A foreign substance that induces the production of a specific matching (homologous) antibody by the immune system of the host it enters.

antigen determinant site—A part of an antigen's molecular structure. These sites induce the production of antibodies. Each cell has several different antigen determinant sites.

antigen processing—The engulfment and degradation of the antigen into its constituent parts by antigen processing cells such as macrophages, and the display of the antigenic molecules on the surface of the macrophage (antigen presentation); a preconditioning for recognition and response by T cells.

antihistamine—A drug (for example, chlorpheniramine, diphenhydramine, mepyramine) that inhibits the action of histamine. Antihistamines are widely used to treat hypersensitivity reactions in which histamine is the main cause of symptoms. These reactions include hay fever, hives (urticaria), and itching (pruritus).

antiserum—The fluid portion (serum) of blood containing antibodies to specific known antigens. Antiserum is used in diagnostic blood tests (serology) to identify unknown antigens and in passive immunization to transfer temporary immunity against a disease-causing (pathogenic) microorganism.

antitoxin—An antiserum containing antibodies against a toxin or toxoid.

arachidonic acid—A polyunsaturated essential fatty acid that is a component of membrane phospholipids. Tissue disruption by any cause, especially immunological mechanisms, allows enzymes to separate the arachidonic acid from the phospholipid, and the arachidonic acid to be metabolized into a large number of chemicals known as eicosanoids. Among the eicosanoids are prostaglandins and leukotrienes that contribute to an inflammatory response.

atopy, atopic allergy —An IgE-dependent hypersensitivity reaction with rapid onset of symptoms.

atopic dermatitis—A chronic inflammatory skin disorder seen in individuals with allergy (atopy). Also called allergic dermatitis, allergic eczema, or atopic eczema.

autoantigen—An antigen that is part of the body's own cells and induces the production of autoantibodies. The presence of autoantigens often leads to autoimmune disease.

autoimmunity—The production of antibodies against antigens of the body's own tissues. Autoimmunity often leads to autoimmune disease and tissue damage.

avirulent—A word used to describe a strain of microorganism that cannot cause disease.

azo-—A prefix denoting a nitrogen-containing (nitrogenous) compound. One example is the yellow azo dye, tartrazine.

B cell—A cell of the type called lymphocytes that produce antibodies in response to a specific antigen. B cells may be found in blood, lymph, and lymphoid tissues.

basophil—A white blood cell containing granules that stain with basic (alkaline) dyes. When the granules break down (a process called degranulation) in hypersensitivity reactions, the cells release mediators of the allergic response.

bifurcated—Having two branches; forked.

biogenic amines—Biologically active derivatives of amino acids that play a role in the functions of the nervous system. The most well-known biogenic amines include histamine, tyramine, serotonin, dopamine, and acetylcholine.

biopsy—The removal of living tissue from a body site and the examination of that tissue sample, usually under a microscope, to establish a precise diagnosis of a condition or disease.

blister—A localized raised portion of the skin containing a liquid. Causes include the body's reaction to abrasion or an immune response to an allergen.

bradykinin—One of several chemicals known as vasoactive peptides. Bradykinin is released during a hypersensitivity reaction. The release of bradykinin causes pain, dilation of blood vessels, edema, and smooth muscle contraction.

bronchitis—An inflammation of lung passages (bronchi) caused by infection with a microorganism or by other agents that damage the lining of the lung passages.

bronchoconstriction—A narrowing of the lung passages (bronchi) by contraction of their smooth muscle sheath.

bronchodilation—An opening of the lung passages (bronchi) by relaxation of their smooth muscle sheath.

bronchospasm—A narrowing of the lung passages (bronchi) due to spasmodic contraction of their smooth muscle sheath. The spasmodic contraction is caused by some stimulus. The spasmodic contraction usually allows air to be inhaled but requires great effort to expel air effectively. Bronchospasms occur in such conditions as asthma and bronchitis.

bronchus (pl. bronchi)—Air passages in the lungs that branch off from the windpipe (trachea). They are lined with mucus-secreting cells and sheathed with smooth muscle.

brush border cells—These cells are found in the epithelium lining the digestive tract. The name is derived from the appearance of the cells. There are numerous appendages, called villi (sing. villus), projecting from the cell surfaces, giving the impression of a brush. The villi increase the surface area available for the absorption of nutrients.

carbohydrates—Compounds containing carbon, hydrogen, and oxygen with the general formula $C_x(H_2O)_y$. They are one of the three main constituents of food (protein and fat are the others). Both sugars and starches are carbohydrates. Carbohydrates are an important source of energy in cellular metabolism. These compounds constitute three-quarters of the biological world and about 80% of the caloric intake of humans. The most abundant carbohydrate is cellulose, the principal constituent of trees and other plants. The major food carbohydrate is starch.

celiac disease—A chronic intestinal disorder characterized by the malabsorption of nutrients. It is caused by an immunologically-mediated sensitivity to gluten. Celiac disease is also known as gluten-sensitive enteropathy.

celiac sprue—Another term for celiac disease. This term is no longer widely used.

chelated calcium—A form of calcium in which the calcium element is bound as part of a ring.

chelated mineral—A form of a mineral in which the mineral is bound inside a ring (sequestered). Chelated forms of minerals are stable. This allows them to be excreted without further interaction with a living body.

chemotaxin—A chemical that promotes movement of a cell or microorganism toward a target in the process of chemotaxis.

chemotaxis—Movement of a cell or microorganism toward a target in response to a concentration gradient of a chemical known as a chemotaxin.

chitin—One type of carbohydrate. It is a white, insoluble, horny polysaccharide. Next to cellulose, it is the most abundant natural polysaccharide. It is a major component of the exoskeletons of many insects, spiders, and shellfish.

chitinase—An enzyme that decomposes (hydrolyses) chitin to produce a linear homopolymer acetyl glucosamine.

cholinergic—Describes nerve fibers that release the neurotransmitter acetylcholine.

colostrum—The first secretion from the breast after childbirth. Colostrum contains serum, protein nutrients, antibodies, lymphocytes, and macrophages.

complement—A group of over twenty enzymatic proteins in the blood that act together in response to antigens and antibodies to destroy foreign cells by breaking through the membrane and outer structure of the foreign cell and allowing the foreign cell contents to escape. This type of cell destruction is called lysis.

complement cascade—The sequential activation of complement proteins resulting in the destruction (lysis) of a target cell. The cascade releases various chemical by-products that act as opsonins, chemotaxins, and anaphylatoxins to help destroy a threat to the body.

complement system—A system within the body that consists of over 20 serum proteins, related cellular receptors, and other regulatory proteins.

conjunctiva (pl. conjunctivae)—The membrane covering the front of the eye and lining the eyelids.

conjunctivitis—Inflammation of the conjunctivae, causing redness, swelling, and a watery discharge.

control test—A test conducted in parallel with a test for a specific disease, reaction, or condition. Control tests are used to determine the response of normal or typical individuals to the test procedure(s). The results of control tests help determine the value of the treatment, medication, or procedure being tested.

cross-reacting allergens—A rather loose term that indicates that a person sensitized to one allergen will react to another allergen related to the first, because it is structurally very similar.

cyto-—A prefix denoting cell. For example, a cytocide is an agent that kills cells.

cytokines—Collective name for lymphokines and monokines (for example, the interleukins and interferons). These are peptides produced by immune system cells such as lymphocytes and macrophages. Cytokines are involved in sending signals between cells.

cytolysis—The destruction (lysis) of a cell, usually by disruption of its membrane and other outer structures.

dalton—A unit of measure used for the weight of molecules. It is an atomic mass unit, equal to 1.6605×10^{-27} kg, $\frac{1}{12}$ the mass of an atom of carbon 12. A kilodalton (kd or kD) is one thousand daltons.

DBPCFC—See **double-blind placebo-controlled food challenge**.

degranulation—A step in the process of inflammation involving the release of chemicals from the intracellular granules of leukocytes.

dermatitis—Inflammation of the skin.

dermatographism—A skin reaction in response to moderately firm stroking or scratching with a dull instrument. The reaction appears as a pale raised welt or wheal, with a red flare on each side.

double-blind placebo-controlled food challenge (DBPCFC)—A provocation test in which the identity of the food to be challenged is unknown to both the patient and the supervisor of the test. A placebo is similarly concealed and the response to the food is compared to the response to the placebo. A positive test is the appearance of symptoms after consumption of the food, with no symptoms in response to the placebo.

eczema—An inflammatory condition of the skin (dermatitis) caused by a variety of agents that is characterized by reddening, itching, oozing, crusting, and scaling. Also known as atopic dermatitis.

eicosanoids—The collective name for chemicals (such as leukotrienes, prostaglandins, and thromboxanes) derived from arachidonic acid (sometimes called eicosanoic acid), a fatty acid with a 20-carbon chain.

ELISA—See **enzyme-linked immunosorbent assay**.

endo-—Prefix denoting inside. For example, endogenous means originating from inside an organism or body.

endocrine system—A system of ductless glands and other structures that are critical in the life of a living mammal. The endocrine system includes the pituitary, thyroid, parathyroid, and adrenal glands, the ovaries, testes, placenta, and part of the pancreas, and the hormones these organs secrete internally and release into the bloodstream.

endorphins—Chemicals in the brain derived from beta-lipotropin and produced by the pituitary gland. Endorphins appear to influence the activities of the endocrine glands and have pain-relieving properties similar to those of the opiates.

endotoxin—Lipopolysaccharide (lipid [fat] linked to a carbohydrate) that is part of the cell wall of gram-negative bacteria and liberated only when the bacteria disintegrate. Endotoxins are responsible for the fever, gastrointestinal disorder, and shock of infections caused by pathogenic enterobacteria such as salmonella and shigella.

enteritis—Inflammation of the small intestine.

enterocolitis—Inflammation involving both the small intestine and the colon.

enteropathy—A general term that refers to any disease of the intestine.

enzyme—Protein produced by a living organism that catalyses (potentiates) a biological reaction without itself being affected. Enzymes are essential for the normal functioning of the body.

enzyme-linked immunosorbent assay (ELISA)—Immunological test for identification of antigen-specific antibody in blood serum. This laboratory test is usually used to identify IgE or IgG antibodies to allergens. The "indicator system" for positive reactions is antibody linked to an enzyme; the enzyme acts on the enzyme substrate to form a product that is usually indicated by a change in color.

eosinophil—A white blood cell that helps defend the body against parasites and contributes to allergic reactions. These cells contain granules that stain with acidic dyes such as eosin. When activated, the granules release bioactive chemicals (inflammatory mediators) that act on the surrounding tissues and cause symptoms.

eosiniphilic esophagitis—An inflammation of the esophagus characterized by the presence of eosinophils. Eosinophils are not normally found in the esophagus.

eosinophilic gastroenteritis—A form of intestinal inflammation in which eosinophils are present in the lining of the small intestine. The lining of the stomach may also be involved. The symptoms may include pain in the abdomen, diarrhea, general swelling (edema), fever, nausea, and malabsorption of food depending on the exact location of the inflammation.

epinephrine (adrenaline)—A hormone secreted by the adrenal gland that prepares the body for "fight or flight." It plays an important role in the control of blood circulation, muscle action, and sugar metabolism.

epitope—A molecule in the antigen (antigenic determinant) that triggers a response of the immune system, resulting in production of antibody. Functionally it is the portion of an antigen that combines with the antibody at a site called the paratope.

erythema—Abnormal reddening of the skin caused by dilation (enlargement) of small blood vessels.

erythrocyte—A red blood cell. Its color comes from hemoglobin which transports oxygen around the body.

esophagitis—Inflammation of the esophagus, the muscular tube that connects the mouth to the stomach.

estrogens—Steroid hormones, such as estrone and estradiol, that are produced mainly in the ovaries and control female sexual development.

etiology—The study of the cause of disease. An etiologic agent is the specific cause of a disease.

exo-—A prefix denoting outside. For example, exogenous means originating outside the organism or body.

exotoxins—Soluble toxic proteins, secreted by bacteria, that cause a variety of life-threatening diseases including botulism, gas gangrene, tetanus, and diphtheria. Exotoxins are among the most poisonous substances known.

expression—In the medical area, this term refers to the appearance of symptoms of a particular condition or disease.

FAST—See **fluorescence allergosorbent test**.

fat—A chemical composed of one or more fatty acids. Fat is the principal form in which energy is stored in the body.

fluorescence allergosorbent test (FAST)—A laboratory test of the type called an immunoassay, that is used to identify allergens. In the FAST the indicator reagent is a derivative of fluorescein, a chemical that emits polarized light.

folate—A form of folic acid, an important B vitamin.

folic acid (folacin)—A vitamin of the B complex and an essential component in many major metabolic reactions in the body.

food allergy—An inappropriate response by the immune system to foods that have been consumed. The immune system is activated when the body reacts as if the food were "foreign and unsafe."

food intolerance—A reaction to food involving a defect in the processing of food, either during digestion or after the food parts or components have been absorbed into the body. The immune system is not involved in a food intolerance reaction.

food protein enteropathies—Any of several diseases of the intestinal tract that are associated with proteins in foods. These diseases include celiac disease, inflammatory bowel disease, milk protein enteropathy, soy protein enteropathy, and others.

food tolerance—A normal reaction to the consumption of a food. The food is processed and absorbed normally and there is no immune or adverse response.

fructo-oligosaccharide (FOS)—A form of sugar that is sometimes called "oligofructose" or "oligofructan." Oligosaccharide is a short chain of sugar molecules (oligo = few; saccharide = sugar). In the case of FOS, the sugar molecules are fructose molecules. FOS is not digestible by human enzymes and passes unchanged into the large bowel where it acts as a substrate for microbial activities.

fructose intolerance—An inability to normally digest the sugar fructose. This intolerance may be either inherited or brought on by conditions or diseases. If the condition is not inherited (genetic), then the condition will pass once the condition or disease causing the intolerance is controlled or cured.

galactosemia—Refers to three types of genetic (inherited) metabolic disorders. The disorders are the result of a recessive trait that causes a deficiency of the enzyme needed to convert the sugar galactose to glucose. The result is a build up of galactose in the blood. Classic galactosemia is often fatal for newborns while galactokinse deficiency may cause cataracts in infants and children. Galactose epimerase deficiency is usually harmless.

galactose—A hexose sugar consisting of a chain of 6 carbon atoms combined with oxygen and hydrogen in a structure indicated by the formula $CH_2OH(CHOH)_4CHO$. The major source of galactose is milk, where it is found combined with glucose in a 1:1 ratio to form lactose. Other food sources of galactose include sugar beets, several gums, seaweeds, and flax seed mucilage.

GALT—See **gut-associated lymphoid tissue.**

gamma globulins—Blood proteins, rich in antibodies, that move in the "gamma" region in electrophoreses. Includes the five classes of immunoglobulin found in humans (IgA; IgG; IgM; IgD; IgE).

gliadin—An alcohol-soluble protein component of wheat and other gluten-containing grains. Several forms of gliadin occur in wheat; alpha-gliadin is the fraction most frequently associated with celiac disease.

globulin—Type of protein classified according to its solubility. Some globulins (for example, β-lactoglobulin in milk) are soluble in dilute salt solutions at pH 7.

glucan—A chemical compound (polymer) of glucose, often formed by the breakdown of sucrose by streptococci, especially *Streptococcus mutans*, in the mouth.

gluco-oligosaccahride (GOS)—A short chain of glucose molecules (gluco = glucose; saccharide = sugar). Also known as oligoglucan. GOS is not broken down by human digestive enzymes and passes into the colon unchanged. In the colon, it acts as a substrate (food source) for microbial activities and growth.

gluten—A protein which is found in some cereal grains, especially wheat, rye, and barley, combined with starch. It is composed of gliadins and glutenins. Gluten makes up to 80% of the proteins in wheat. It is responsible for the elasticity of kneaded dough, which allows leavening (rising) with yeast, and gives the "chewy" texture to baked products such as bagels.

glutenin—A protein classified on the basis of its solubility in acids (pH 2) or alkalis (pH 12). Glutenins are insoluble in water or ethanol. They are major proteins in wheat and other cereal grains.

glyco-—A prefix denoting the combination of a sugar molecule (often glucose or galactose) with another type of chemical. For example, glycoprotein means sugar combined with a protein; glycolipid is a sugar combined with a lipid (fat) molecule.

glycogen—The main form of carbohydrate storage material in animals. It is a long chain of glucose molecules which is formed in and mainly stored in the liver. To a lesser extent, glycogen is found in muscles.

glycogen storage disease—Any of several genetic (inherited) conditions which prevent the normal storage of glycogen in the body. There are eight major recognized types of glycogen storage diseases. They are categorized based on the absence of specific enzymes or transporters involved in the processing and storing of glycogen. These are recessive traits and most are rare.

granulocyte—A white blood cell with a lobed nucleus, characterized by numerous granules within its cytoplasm (see polymorphonuclear granulocyte).

growth hormone—(somatotropin)—A hormone secreted by the pituitary gland that controls growth of the long bones and promotes protein synthesis.

gut-associated lymphoid tissue (GALT)—Tissues where lymphocytes take part in immune responses.These tissues include the tonsils, Peyer's patches, the lamina propria of the intestine, and the appendix.

hapten—A molecule too small to be an antigen by itself, but that induces the production of antibody when combined with an antigen or a body protein.

heme iron—A chelate of iron (the iron is sequestered, or bound, within a ring) that forms part of the hemoglobin molecule. This is the form of iron that is found in animal tissues.

heparin—Anticoagulant chemical that inhibits the enzyme thrombin in the final stage of blood coagulation. Heparin is produced by various cells, including white blood cells. It is found predominantly in the liver and lungs.

histamine—A chemical derivative of the amino acid histidine. It is produced in all body tissues, especially by mast cells. An important mediator of inflammation, it causes contraction of smooth muscle and increases the permeability of small blood vessels. It is the principal mediator of the wheal-and-flare skin reaction.

HLA—See **human leukocyte antigens**.

homologous—The same. Homologous describes the relationship between an antigen and the specific antibody whose production it induces.

hormone—A chemical produced by the body (for example, by the endocrine glands) that circulates in the bloodstream and has a specific regulatory effect on certain cells or organs.

human leukocyte antigens (HLAs)—Antigens on the surface of body cells that are coded for the major histocompatibility complex (MHC) and unique to the individual. They allow the immune system to recognize self and non-self.

hydrolase—A class of enzymes that catalyze the addition of the elements of water to a substance thereby breaking it into two products.

hydrolysis—The process by which a molecule is broken apart with the addition of water. The process occurs under the influence of enzymes known as hydrolases.

hyper-—A prefix indicating excessive, more, or above normal. Examples include hyperactivity, hypersensitivity, hyper-responsive, and hypertension (high blood pressure).

hypo-—A prefix indicating deficiency, less, or below normal. For example, in hyposensitive, hyporeactive, and hypotension (low blood pressure).

hypolipoproteinemia—A disease characterized by abnormally low levels of lipoproteins in blood serum.

IBS—See **irritable bowel syndrome**.

idiopathic—Describes a disease of unknown cause.

immunity—Resistance to a disease.

immunoglobulin (Ig)—A glycoprotein that functions as an antibody. The five classes of immunoglobulins (IgA, IgD, IgE, IgG, and IgM) differ in the structure of their polypeptide heavy chains. Immunoglobulins make up gamma globulin; all antibodies are immunoglobulins.

immunosorbent assay—See **enzyme-linked immunosorbent assay**.

inter- —A prefix meaning between. For example, the word intercellular means between cells.

interferons—Cytokines typically produced by cells infected with viruses. The known interferons (alpha, beta, and gamma) play a variety of roles in immunity, particularly the inhibition of viral multiplication. Usually written as INF- followed by the identifying Greek letter of the specific cytokine (e.g. INF-α; INF-γ, etc)

interleukins—Cytokines, produced principally by macrophages and T cells, act as signals in controlling various stages of the immune response. Usually written as IL-followed by the number that identifies the specific cytokine (for example, IL-1; IL-2. IL-4 and so on)

International Unit (IU)—A unit used in pharmacology to measure the amount of a substance in a sample. The unit is based on its measured biological activity (or effect). This measure is used for vitamins, hormones, some drugs, vaccines, blood products, antibodies, and similar biologically active substances. The precise definition of one IU differs from substance to substance and is established by international agreement. The Committee on Biological Standardization of the World Health Organization (WHO) provides a reference preparation of the substance, determines the number of IUs contained in that preparation, and specifies a biological procedure to compare other preparations to the reference preparation. Thus, different preparations with the same biological effect will contain the same number of IUs.

intolerance—A word used to describe the inability of a body to normally process foods. The immune system and immune system responses are not involved in intolerance.

intra- —A prefix indicating inside, or within, for example, in intracellular (inside a cell), intracytoplasmic (within the cytoplasm).

in utero—A phrase meaning in the uterus or womb.

inulin—A group of oligosaccharides (a short chain of sugars) that are typically found in roots or rhizomes where they are a means of storing energy (instead of the usual starch). They belong to the class of carbohydrates known as fructans, which are classified as soluble fiber.

in vitro—A phrase meaning in glass. This phrase describes biological activity made to occur outside a living body, usually under experimental conditions in a laboratory.

in vivo—In life. This phrase describes biological activity within a living body.

irritable bowel syndrome (IBS)—A chronic non-inflammatory disease characterized by abdominal pain, altered bowel habits (diarrhea, or constipation, or both) with no detectable pathology. Also called spastic bowel, or spastic colon.

Kd—Kilodalton. One thousand Daltons. See **dalton**.

ketone or **ketone bodies**—A class of organic compounds with a specific structure (the carbon atom of a carbonyl group [C=O] is attached to two other carbon atoms) that forms as a result of unusual metabolic events in the body. Their presence of ketone or ketone bodies is often indicative of a pathological condition.

Kilodalton—One thousand daltons. See **dalton**.

lactoferrin—An iron-containing compound, present in secretions such as milk, that has a slight antimicrobial action due to its ability to bind the iron required by the microorganism.

lactose (milk sugar)—A carbohydrate (disaccharide) present in milk that is metabolized by the body into glucose and galactose.

leaky gut—A descriptive term used to indicate a situation in which fluids and solids move more readily through the lining of the digestive tract than normally. Usually results from inflammation caused by infection, allergy, or other insults to the epithelium. Synonymous with hyperpermeable digestive tract membrane.

leukocytes—White blood cells that defend the body against disease. There are three major types of leukocytes: granulocytes, monocytes, and lymphocytes.

leukotrienes—Hormone like chemicals derived from precursor fatty acids (such as arachidonic acid) via the lipoxygenase pathway. Leukotrienes contribute to inflammatory and allergic reactions. They are powerful chemotaxins and some cause constriction of smooth muscles.

lipids—These organic substances include fats, steroids, phospholipids, and glyco-lipids. They are important as cell constituents and a source of energy, certain vita-mins, and essential fatty acids.

lipo-—A prefix denoting fat or lipid.

lipopolysaccharide—A molecule composed of a fatty acid (lipo-) and a sugar (-poly-saccharide). One lipopolysaccharide is a major component in the endotoxin in the cell walls of gram-negative bacteria that cause the symptoms of many intestinal infections.

lymph—The transparent fluid in the lymphatic system that bathes body tissues. Lymph is similar in composition to blood plasma but with less protein and some lym-phocytes.

lymphatic system—The network of vessels that convey lymph from body tissues to the bloodstream. The lymphatic system is a pathway for exchange of electrolytes, water, proteins, and other chemicals between the bloodstream and body tissues.

lymphocytes—White blood cells that mature within the lymphatic system. They are classified as B cells and T cells; both are essential in immunity.

lymphokines—Chemicals produced by lymphocytes that act as control signals between cells of the immune system. Lymphokines are commonly grouped under the general heading of cytokines.

lymph nodes—These glands are small swellings, distributed in groups over the lym-phatic system, that filter lymph and prevent foreign particles from entering the bloodstream. The most noticeable lymph nodes are in the groin, armpit, and behind the ear.

lymphoid tissue—A lattice-work of reticular (resembling a network) tissue, the interstices of which contain lymphocytes. Lymphoid tissue may be loosely organized or densely gathered into lymph nodes and nodules.

lysis—The destruction of a cell by disruption of its membrane and outer structures allowing cell contents to escape.

macrophage—A type of phagocytic cell that surrounds and consumes foreign material. Large phagocytes, closely related to monocytes, are present in many organ systems such as connective tissue, bone marrow, the spleen, lymph nodes, liver, and the central nervous system. Fixed macrophages (histiocytes) are stationary; wandering macrophages move freely and accumulate at the site of infection or trauma where they remove foreign microorganisms and damaged tissue by phagocytosis. Macrophages could be described as the vacuum cleaners of the body since they remove foreign, dangerous, and dead materials.

MHC—See **major histocompatibility complex**.

major histocompatibility complex (MHC)—Genes located on chromosome 6 and encoded for the human leukocyte antigens (HLAs). HLAs are present on all body cells and are the identifying factors that distinguish self from non-self. Their products are primarily responsible for the rapid rejection of grafts between individuals. The function of the products of the MHC is signaling between lymphocytes and cells expressing antigens.

MALT (mucosa-associated lymphoid tissue)—Term for lymphoid tissue associated with any mucous membrane lined organs such as the intestinal tract, bronchial tree, etc.

mast cell—A large blood cell that is fixed within body tissue and characterized by numerous granules within its cytoplasm. The granules contain chemicals (inflammatory mediators) such as histamine, heparin, and enzymes released during an inflammatory or allergic reaction.

metabolic pathway—Series of reactions whereby enzymes transform organic molecules into forms that the body can use or store.

metabolism—The sum of the chemical and physical processes by which nutrients are converted into body tissue and energy. Metabolism includes both catabolism (destruction) and anabolism (construction).

microbiota—Very small forms of life. These forms of life are so small that it requires a microscope or other powerful magnifier to see them. Usually refers to the collection of micro-organisms inhabiting a specific area. For example, intestinal microbiota refers to all of the micro-organisms resident within the intestines (mainly the large bowel). Sometimes used as a synonym of microflora.

microflora—A term used to collectively describe the entire population of microscopic life residing in a specified location or area or typically present in a specified location or area.

monocytes—Single-nucleus, granulocytic white blood cells that surround and consume (phagocytose) foreign particles such as bacteria, viruses, and dead body cells. They function somewhat like vacuum cleaners for the body. See also **macrophage**.

mucus—A viscous fluid, composed largely of glycoproteins, secreted by the mucous membranes lining many body organs (such as the respiratory, gastrointestinal, and urogenital tracts).

natural killer (NK) **cell**—A specialized lymphocyte that destroys foreign cells, particularly aberrant cancer cells, apparently by releasing digestive enzymes that perforate the cells' membranes and cause cell contents to leak out.

neuropeptide—A peptide with significant effects on the nervous system but not, strictly speaking, a neurotransmitter. Neuropeptides include the encephalins, endorphins, somatostatin, substance P, thyrotropin-releasing hormone (TRH), and luteinizing hormone-releasing hormone (LHRH).

neurotoxin—Any chemical or substance that acts as a nerve poison.

neurotransmitter—A complex chemical substance (for example, acetylcholine, norepinephrine, dopamine, and serotonin) that transmits signals across the synapses between nerve cells and across the minute gaps between nerves and the muscles or glands they control.

neutrophil—A granulocytic white blood cell containing a lobed nucleus and numerous granules within its cytoplasm that stain with neutral dyes. Neutrophils are powerful phagocytes that remove microorganisms and other foreign particles by phagocytosis.

norepinephrine—A hormone produced by the adrenal gland and also released as a neurotransmitter from nerve fibers of the sympathetic nervous system. Its actions include constriction and relaxation of smooth muscles (especially in blood vessels and intestinal walls), and regulation of heart rate. Norepinephrine also has an influence on the rate and depth of breathing.

OAS—See **oral allergy syndrome**.

oligo-—A prefix meaning a few; little or scanty; deficient; or less than normal.

oligoantigenic diet—A diet consisting of only a few antigenic foods; also called a "few foods diet".

opsonins—Components of the immune system that facilitate attachment of antigen to the surface of phagocytes. Opsonins are antibodies and the C3b component of complement.

opsonization—A process by which opsonins aid the attachment of antigen to the surface of a phagocyte.

oral allergy syndrome (OAS)—A complex of clinical symptoms (for example, itching, swelling of lips and tongue, or blistering) in the mucosa of the mouth and throat that result from direct contact with food allergens in a sensitized individual who also exhibits respiratory allergy to inhaled allergens. OAS is usually caused by tree, grass, or weed pollens (pollinosis) and is triggered by raw foods that contain antigens with the same molecular structure as the pollen.

ovalbumin—A major protein in eggs. This protein is classified as an albumin on the basis of its solubility in water at pH 6.6.

parasite—An organism that lives in or on another living thing (the host), receiving food and shelter but contributing nothing to its host's welfare. Parasites may harm their hosts. Human parasites include bacteria, viruses, fungi, protozoa, and worms.

pathogen—A microorganism that causes disease.

pathogenesis-related proteins (PRs)—Proteins that are induced by pathogens, wounding, or certain environmental stresses in plants. PRs are presently classified into 14 distinct families of proteins, and include chitinases, antifungal proteins, lipid transfer proteins, inhibitors of alpha-amylases and trypsin, profilins, and proteases, among others.

parvalbumin—A major protein in fish. This protein is classified as an albumin on the basis of its solubility in water at pH 6.6.

peak flow meter—A measuring device, usually held in the hand, that measures the amount of air expelled from the lungs in a forced exhalation.

peptide—A chemical that forms proteins. A peptide consists of a chain of two or more amino acids linked together by peptide bonds between the end amino group of one amino acid and the beginning carboxyl group of the next.

phagocyte—A white blood cell that is able to engulf and digest microorganisms, cells, cell debris, and other small particles. Macrophages and monocytes are phagocytes.

phagocytosis—The process of engulfment and digestion of microorganisms and other small foreign particles by phagocytes.

phenylketonuria—A genetic (inherited) disease resulting from deficiency in the enzyme phenylalanine hydroxylase. This enzyme is required to metabolize phenylalanine, an amino acid in many proteins. Management of phenylketonuria requires following a diet very low in phenylalanine. The diet prevents the neurological damage that can occur if the condition remains untreated.

plasma—The fluid portion of blood in which blood cells are suspended.

plasma cell—A cell, derived from a B cell, that produces antibody.

platelet (thrombocyte)—A disc-shaped blood cell principally involved in coagulation.

platelet activating factor (PAF)—A phospholipid produced by leukocytes that causes aggregation of platelets and other effects (such as an increase in vascular permeability and bronchoconstriction). It also acts on various other cells. The active form is known as PAF-acether.

polymorphonuclear granulocyte (polymorph, granulocyte)—A white blood cell distinguished by a lobed nucleus and fine granules within its cytoplasm. These cells are classified according to the type of stain absorbed by the granules, which causes them to assume a specific color.

polysaccharide—A carbohydrate composed of monosaccharides (sugar molecules) joined together in chains.

prebiotic—The nutritional substrate (foundation) on which probiotic micro-organisms will grow and produce the by-products that give the food its health benefit. The substrate usually consists of non-digestible fiber such as an oligosaccharide.

probiotic—A culture of living micro-organisms within a food designed to provide health benefits beyond the food's inherent nutritional value.

profilins—These are actin-regulatory proteins. Profilins are ubiquitous in plants and are usually associated with reproductive processes.

prolactin—A hormone secreted by the pituitary gland that stimulates milk production after childbirth and the production of progesterone in the ovaries.

prostacyclin—A hormone-like chemical related to the prostaglandins.

prostaglandins—A group of hormone-like chemicals derived from precursor fatty acids (such as arachidonic acid) by the cyclo-oxygenase pathway. They have many important controlling functions in the body, including smooth muscle contraction and relaxation.

prolamins—These proteins are usually found in plants. They are classified on the basis of their solubility in 70% ethanol. Zein and gliadin are examples of major plant proteins of the prolamin class.

proteins—Organic substances, composed of chains of amino acids linked by peptide bonds. They are essential as structural components of body cells and as regulators of function. Both enzymes and hormones are proteins. They are one of the three main components of food.

pruritus—Itching.

pyogenic—Pus forming. For example, a pyogenic microorganism causes pus to form in a body.

pyrogen—A substance that produces fever.

radioallergosorbent test (RAST)—A technique (laboratory test) for measuring allergen-specific antibody in serum using radio-labeled reagents. This laboratory test is often used to measure allergen-specific IgE or IgG.

RAST—See **radioallergosorbent test**.

receptor—A molecule on the surface of a cell that provides a selective attachment site for a particular substance, usually a protein.

reticulin—A protein derived from the fibers of reticular (= net-like) connective tissue.

reticuloendothelial system (RES)—Aggregates of phagocytes (monocytes and macrophages) spread throughout body tissues that take up particles and remove them from cirulation.

rhinitis—An inflammation of the mucous membrane lining the nose.

rhino-—A prefix meaning nose.

rhinorrhea—Runny nose with watery discharge. Rhinorrhea is characteristic of the common cold.

scarifier—An instrument with sharp points used to scratch or puncture the skin (hence, scarify; scarification) usually for introduction of a vaccine or skin test reagent.

secretory—Describes chemicals that are produced by tissues or organs in a body or conditions that relate to the process of secreting fluids.

secretory IgA (sIgA)—A specific type of human antibody that is found in mucous secretions. It differs from serum IgA (written simply as IgA) in having an additional secretory piece that protects the antibody from acid and digestive enzymes. Thus, sIgA remains active and protective as it moves along the length of the alimentary canal.

sensitization—Alteration of a body's responsiveness to a foreign substance, usually an allergen. The immune system produces antibody to the allergen without symptoms on first exposure; this is the sensitizing event. Subsequent exposure releases more of the antibody and induces an allergic reaction.

serum (pl. sera)—The fluid portion of blood remaining after separation from clotted blood or clotted blood plasma. Serum is similar to plasma but lacks fibrinogen and other coagulatory components.

serology—The study of serum, especially of its constituents (such as antibodies and complement) involved in the body's defense against disease.

serological tests—Immunological techniques used in a laboratory to identify antigen-specific antibodies in serum.

serologic reactions—1. The response of sera to laboratory tests. 2. The use of reactions to locate antigens to either infectious diseases or allergens in a serum sample.

serologically related—Applied to antigens, the term indicates that antigens have been demonstrated to be related because they react with the same antibody

somatostatin—A hormone that inhibits the secretion of growth hormone by the pituitary gland.

spirometer—An instrument used for measuring the amount of air taken into and expelled from the lungs.

sprue—A term once used for celiac disease.

synapse—The gap between nerve fibers across which neurotransmitters carry impulses from one nerve cell to the next.

symbiotic—A process in which two dissimilar organisms live together. The two organisms may both benefit from this association, only one may benefit from the relationship, or one may benefit and one be harmed.

synbiotic—The combination of probiotic micro-organisms with their specifically designed prebiotic nutrient source.

synergism—A cooperative interaction between two systems that produces a greater effect than the sum of two systems acting alone.

T-cells—Specialized lymphocytes that produce cytokines and participate in all functions of the immune system.

thrombocyte—See **platelet**.

thymus—An organ at the base of the neck. The principal function of the thymus appears to be the maturation of lymphocytes into T cells.

titer—A measure of the amount of antibodies in serum.

tolerance—The ability of a body to recognize that a substance (such as food) is "foreign but safe." Once a body has developed tolerance to a foreign substance, it will not mount a defensive immune reaction to that substance.

tolerize—The process of "educating" the body to recognize a substance (such as food) as "foreign but safe" and not to mount a defensive immune reaction to that substance.

transglutaminase—One of a family of enzymes that catalyze the formation of a bond between proteins; the bond occurs between a free amino acid, for example, lysine on one molecule and a glutamine on the other. The enzyme is important in celiac disease because IgA antibodies formed against it are characteristic of the disease, and detection of these antibodies in a laboratory test is a sign of active celiac disease.

urticaria—An itchy rash, commonly called hives, characterized by round red wheals ranging in size from small spots to large patches several inches in diameter.

vascular—Relating to blood vessels.

vascular system—The network of blood vessels that circulates blood throughout the body.

vaso-—A prefix meaning vessel, especially relating to blood vessels.

vasoactive amine—A chemical (an amine) that acts on smooth muscle, especially those surrounding blood vessels, either increasing or decreasing their diameter.

vasoconstriction—A decrease in he diameter of blood vessels due to contraction of the muscles in their walls. Vasoconstriction causes an increase in blood pressure.

vasodilation (also vasodilatation)—An increase in the diameter of blood vessels due to relaxation of the muscles in their walls.

villus (pl. villi)—A small projection from a cell that is part of a membrane. Intestinal villi are threadlike projections that cover the surface of the mucous membrane of the small intestine and absorb fluids and nutrients.

virulence—A measure of the disease-producing ability of a microorganism. The measure includes factors such as the organism's ability to invade the host, to evade the host's immune defenses, and to cause damage to the host's tissues.

wheal—A smooth, slightly elevated area on the skin, paler or redder than the surrounding area. Wheals are caused by the release of histamine and its action on the local tissues. The area is often itchy, and the wheal may change in size and shape. Wheals usually disappear within a few hours.

wheal and flare—A positive response to a skin test. The wheal is a central "blister" which is surrounded by a flat reddened area (the flare). The reaction is caused by the release of histamine and other inflammatory mediators from mast cells in the skin in response to the application of the matching (homologous) antigen (allergen) applied in the test reagent.

INDEX